POCKET GUIDE TO

Intravenous Therapy

POCKET GUIDE TO

Intravenous Therapy

Shirley E. Otto, MSN, CRNI, AOCN

Clinical Nurse Specialist
Via Christi Regional Medical Center
Wichita, Kansas

Fourth Edition

with 122 *illustrations*

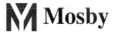 Mosby

An Affiliate of Elsevier Science

St. Louis   London   Philadelphia   Sydney   Toronto

Mosby

An Affiliate of Elsevier Science

Vice President; Nursing Editorial Director: Sally Schrefer
Executive Editor: N. Darlene Como
Developmental Editor: Barbara Watts
Project Manager: Deborah L. Vogel
Book Design Manager: Bill Drone
Cover Image: Arrow International

FOURTH EDITION

NOTICE

Pharmacology is an ever-changing field. Standard safety precautions must be followed, but as new research and clinical experience broaden our knowledge, changes in treatment and drug therapy may become necessary or appropriate. Readers are advised to check the most current product information provided by the manufacturer of each drug to be administered to verify the recommended dose, the method and duration of administration, and contraindications. It is the responsibility of the licensed prescriber, relying on experience and knowledge of the patient, to determine dosages and the best treatment for each individual patient. Neither the publisher nor the author assumes any liability for any injury and/or damages to persons or property arising from this publication.

Mosby, Inc.
An Affiliate of Elsevier Science
11830 Westline Industrial Drive
St. Louis, Missouri 63146

Printed in the United States of America

ISBN 0-323-01179-9

02   03   04   GW/RDC   9   8   7   6   5   4   3

*To staff nurses everywhere who have generously
shared their hints along the way*

Contributors

Conrad Boettger, BSN, RN
Manager Center for Technology and Innovation
Via Christi Research, Inc.
Wichita, Kansas
Professional Issues

Karon I. Giles, MSN, ARNP, CCRN
Critical Care Clinical Nurse Specialist
Via Christi Regional Medical Center
Wichita, Kansas
*Parenteral Nutrition, Vascular Access
   in Adult Critical Care*

Kimberly A. McAlpine, BSN, RN
Bone Marrow Transplant Coordinator
Oncology Patient Services
Karmanos Cancer Center
Detroit, Michigan
Pediatric Intravenous Therapy

Leslie Metivier, MSN, RN, AOCN
Manager Home Care and Hospice
Karmanos Cancer Institute
Detroit, Michigan
Home Care Infusion Therapy

Preface

All health care professionals are practicing in a rapidly changing, highly complicated environment in which IV therapy is a major treatment modality. Tremendous technological and reimbursement changes have necessitated proficiency not only in clinical skills but also in documentation, patient teaching, demonstrated continuous performance improvement, and risk management. Implantable ports, peripherally inserted central venous catheters, infusion pumps, state-of-the-art pain management, and complex home or ambulatory care IV medication and infusion regimens have challenged the nurse's practice climate. Increasingly, greater numbers of patients with serious illness—for example, bone marrow or stem cell transplantation, solid organ transplantation, cancer, and chronic organ failure—require astute, long-term IV medication management. *Pocket Guide to Intravenous Therapy* has been designed to give nurses working in diverse patient care settings and with varying clinical preparation an easily accessible, accurate, and concise reference based on recognized national standards of practice. This book is an ideal study guide for those entering IV therapy practice and/or reviewing for the Intravenous Nurses Society certification examination.

The advent and increased use of multiple and diverse IV products and equipment in all settings have added a new dimension of complexity to the demands on the busy nurse. Now more than ever, advanced IV skills are sought by all nurses. For the nurse entering practice, returning to practice, or changing areas, learning these skills can be intimidating. This book features practical strategies and tools for patient teaching, sample physician orders for heparin nomogram, heparinization of venous access devices, and parenteral nutrition, as well as *nursing clinical competencies for each chapter* that can be readily adapted to all settings to enhance the nurse's knowledge and clinical skills.

Each chapter discusses a major aspect of IV therapy. All chapters contain pertinent information, clinical alerts to clarify topics, tables for convenient reference, documentation recommendations, nursing diagnoses, patient/family teaching for self-management, home care considerations, and geriatric considerations. The content of this book has been organized in the manner in which nurses think and perform while providing care.

Chapter 1, Infusion Therapy, presents an overview of IV therapy principles and guidelines.

Chapter 2, Venipuncture, examines skills, product selection, and infection control issues.

Chapter 3, Central Venous Catheters, contrasts and compares all of the central venous catheters and provides step-by-step procedures for each device.

Chapter 4, Peripherally Inserted Central Catheters, provides guidelines on catheter placement, indications, contraindications, products, maintenance procedures, troubleshooting tips, and potential complications.

Chapter 5, IV Fluids, reviews the assessments and interventions required for the basic electrolytes. A table of replacement fluids is included.

Chapter 6, IV Medication Administration, describes all modalities of IV medication administration. Information on all the most commonly administered IV medications is included: analgesics, antiemetics, antimicrobials, antifungals, antivirals, biotherapy, cardiotonics, vasopressors, and immunosuppressants. Brief content information is presented about the drug category, drug administration guidelines, and patient monitoring practices.

Chapter 7, Blood and Blood Component Administration, presents all blood and blood product components and transfusion reactions in readily available tables.

Chapter 8, Chemotherapy Administration, explains theoretical information and nursing management for preparation, delivery, and disposal of cytotoxic drugs in the hospital or outpatient setting.

Chapter 9, Parenteral Nutrition, explains assessment parameters and nursing interventions and emphasizes teaching needs for self-management; examples of physician orders and parenteral nutrition calculation are also included in this chapter.

Chapter 10, Vascular Access in Adult Critical Care, discusses aspects of IV therapy for the patient receiving varied multimodality infusion therapy; specifics on drug/infusion dose calculations, compatibilities, and therapeutic monitoring guidelines are provided.

Chapter 11, Pediatric Intravenous Therapy, provides multiple IV topics: fluid and electrolyte balance, IV site access, central venous catheters, and intraosseous infusion, as well as administration of IV medications, blood products, chemotherapy, and parenteral nutrition for the pediatric patient.

Chapter 12, Home Care Infusion Therapy, provides multiple nursing assessment and intervention strategies for venous access devices, infusion pumps, and the varied infusates administered in the home care setting.

Chapter 13, Calculations for IV Infusions, illustrates the use of all formulas required for accurate administration of IV therapy.

Chapter 14, Professional Resources, includes education topics such as core curriculum for IV therapy and adult learning principles; pharmaceutical and device research and development; risk management; device, product, and infusion pump manufacture listings; and professional organizations and government agencies listings pertinent to IV therapy.

The Bibliography contains suggested readings for each chapter for those who desire more information.

Pocket Guide to Intravenous Therapy continues to be an excellent clinical resource for many nurses in all practice settings. This edition contains separate chapters on Home Care Infusion Therapy and Professional Resources to address core curriculum education for IV therapy; pharmaceutical and device research and development; risk management; and manufacture listings for products, devices, and infusion pumps. In addition, listings of the professional organizations and government agencies pertinent to IV therapy are provided. Each clinical chapter has 10 multiple choice study questions with answers. The editor and contributors continue to strive for excellence in all aspects of IV therapy.

The editor and contributors are indebted to the following persons: our families for consistent encouragement and support, representatives of the manufacturers of IV supplies and equipment for information and assistance, and Mosby for guidance.

Contents

Intravenous Therapy

Infusion Therapy

1

Objectives

1. Describe the sequential steps for administration of intravenous (IV) infusion solutions.

2. Discuss the safety recommendations that reduce exposure to needlestick injuries and exposure to patient body fluids during IV therapy.

3. List the factors that interfere with the delivery of accurate IV flow rates by gravity infusion and the interventions that promote accurate infusion delivery.

4. Verbalize the nursing strategies that prevent IV therapy–related problems.

5. Identify requirements for documentation of IV infusions.

The use of IV therapy continues to increase because of improved catheter and pump technology, resulting in multiple therapies administered to increasing numbers of patients. Inpatient hospital stays continue to shorten, and therefore patients are receiving complex multimodality IV therapy in outpatient and home care settings. These changes have required nurses in all settings to enhance their IV therapy skills. Astute clinical management and specialized IV therapy skills have become the norm in acute, ambulatory, home, clinic, and extended care settings.

This chapter focuses on observations and interventions required when administering IV infusions and on supplies and equipment commonly required for delivering IV infusion therapy.

Accurate Flow Rates

Achieving accurate flow rates is always an important concern in IV therapy because accuracy decreases the incidence of complications. Complications may include infiltration, phlebitis, loss of patency, metabolic alterations, and circulatory overload. When gravity is the force for fluid delivery, a combination of factors causes fluctuations in flow rates. Time-taping fluid containers (Fig. 1-1), using flow control regulators and volumetric chambers, and selecting tubing with the appropriate drop size all aid in establishing accurate fluid delivery by gravity. IV pumps provide the greatest accuracy of fluid delivery.

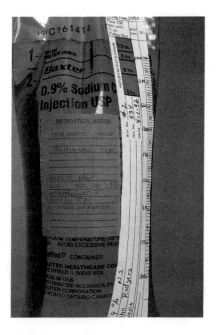

Fig. 1-1
Infusion bag with time strip.
(From Perry AG, Potter PA: *Clinical nursing skills and techniques,* ed 4, St Louis, 1998, Mosby.)

Observations

Nursing observations required to maintain an accurate flow rate include determining any mechanical factors that interfere with fluid delivery, evaluating patient factors that can alter the flow rate, and observing the patient for complications at the venipuncture site. The following mechanical factors may interfere with gravity flow rate:

1. Positioning the fluid container less than 36 inches above the IV site does not allow gravity to overcome vascular pressure and thus prevents the infusion of IV fluids.
2. Kinks in either the IV tubing or catheter tubing prevent or minimize effective fluid flow.
3. Taping at the catheter site can obstruct the catheter lumen, particularly if a piece of tape is tightly placed directly over the bevel of the IV catheter.
4. Small-gauge IV catheters can impede fluid delivery and may require the use of a positive-pressure infusion device or may have to be replaced with a larger-gauge IV catheter.
5. IV catheters placed near joints may occlude when the patient moves.

Additional factors such as tortuous veins and venous spasms may alter the IV flow rates. Pain or infection may cause increased patient restlessness, resulting in increased movement at or near the IV site. Infiltration, phlebitis, and/or loss of patency may all occur at the IV site and terminate the infusion.

Infusion System Evaluation

The following clinical elements should be confirmed during periodic evaluations of the entire infusion system:

1. The correct infusate is being used.
2. The IV infusion is flowing at the prescribed rate.
3. All tubing and IV catheter connections are intact.
4. The IV tubing is placed correctly—not hooked on other equipment or kinked.
5. The drop chamber contains the correct fluid level.
6. The IV catheter is securely taped.
7. The tubing and infusate are verified and replacements are considered.

CLINICAL ALERT: IV tubing and solutions need to be changed according to the manufacturers' recommendations and in the following situations that reflect guidelines of the Centers for Disease Control and Prevention and the Intravenous Nurses Society:

1. On a scheduled frequency, usually every 72 to 96 hours and when the IV catheter is changed
2. If the tubing tip and/or injection port becomes contaminated from touch
3. If blood backs up in the tubing and is not immediately flushed out
4. After piggyback administration of blood or lipid products
5. When the flow stops in tubing equipped with an in-line filter and no other cause can be found

Problems during IV Therapy

Most patients are able to assist with problems encountered during IV therapy if provided with the necessary information (see Patient Education, p. 20). Infiltration is the most common problem. Infiltration occurs when fluid infuses into tissue surrounding the venipuncture site because one of the following occurs:

- The IV catheter passes through the wall of the vessel.
- The catheter slips out of the vein.
- The tip of the catheter remains in the vein, and the vessel wall allows some fluid to infuse into the vein and some to infiltrate the tissue.

When the catheter passes through the vein wall or slips completely out of the vein, a blood return does not occur. It is possible to obtain a blood return if the catheter tip remains in the vein. Swelling is caused by fluid leakage into the tissue and is most likely to occur proximal to the insertion site. Puncturing the vein wall at the time of IV catheter insertion may cause leakage from the insertion site. A narrowing of the vessel wall may also cause a buildup of pressure in the vein, forcing the IV fluid out at the venipuncture site.

Common measures to assess for infiltration include the following:

- Asking patients about their level of discomfort
- Observing the site for swelling
- Palpating for coolness of the tissues surrounding the IV site
- Checking for a blood return

If the patient experiences *pain,* the IV infusion should be restarted *regardless* of whether other symptoms are absent.

Early identification and intervention for the problems reduces the severity of most adverse outcomes. Refer to Table 1-1 for troubleshooting tips and preventive measures for common IV therapy infusion problems.

Systemic Complications of IV Infusions

Although most IV therapy–related problems are localized to the infusion system or the catheter site, systemic complications can occur, including circulatory overload, air embolism, foreign body embolism, and septicemia (Table 1-2).

Common Infusion-Related Supplies and Equipment

Supplies and equipment commonly required for IV therapy include IV poles, infusion pumps, disposable infusion systems, labels for the infusion container and IV tubing, tape, IV boards, administration sets, filters, and flow regulation devices. Each IV admixture needs a label listing the following information: patient's name and identification number; additives, concentrations, and volumes; primary solution and total volume; flow rate; preparation and expiration dates; storage requirements (when applicable); and identification of the person preparing and hanging the infusion. All IV tubing(s) should also be labeled with information on the date and time with the initials of the person initiating and/or changing the tubing.

Priming Volumes (Dead Space)

Products for IV infusion include injection caps, extension tubings, IV connectors, and IV tubings.

These devices are available from various manufacturers, but all of them have similar essential information regarding packaging, sterility, expiration date, Luer-Lok connection, single and/or dual lumen, and *priming volume requirements specificities.* In clinical practice, priming volumes are sometimes referred to as *dead space* in the specific device (Fig. 1-2). Read and follow all product equipment instructions regarding priming volume requirements. *If the device is not filled with the required priming volume* of a sterile infusate (e.g., normal saline), the dead space becomes a portal entry of air into the vascular system. Depending on the device, gauge, size, and extension tubing and/or IV tubing length, the priming volume can vary from 0.1 ml to 20 to 30 ml per device or tubing.

Text continued on p. 12

Table 1-1   Troubleshooting tips—infusion therapy

Nursing Assessment	Nursing Interventions
Infiltration Infusion slows or stops Infusion device sounds occlusion alarm Tissue induration or swelling with cool tissue	Relocate IV site to other arm or above area of infiltration; if infiltration is severe, apply warm compresses and elevate the arm. *Prevention:* Observe site hourly during continuous infusions, especially if using a positive-pressure pump.
Phlebitis Two or more of the following present: pain, redness, swelling, induration, cord	Relocate catheter to other arm or above area of phlebitis; if infiltration is severe, apply warm compress. *Prevention:* Filter solutions; rotate sites on a planned basis every 48 to 72 hours; secure catheter to prevent motion in vein; flush catheter after each medication.
Runaway IV Dry IV or greater amount infused than scheduled	Notify physician and observe patient for signs of fluid overload and effects of IV additives. *Prevention:* Recheck flow rate after tubing changes; time-tape all infusions; use electronic pumps, controllers, or volumetric chambers for patients at greatest risk of developing complications.
Sluggish IV Amount to be infused behind	Observe entire system for mechanical schedule or patient factors, such as kinked tubing or patient lying on IV tubing; reposition or relocate IV device. *Prevention:* Verify that gauge of catheter is appropriate for type of infusion.

Tubing disconnection
Dampness from leaking fluid

Replace tubing if contamination occurs.
Prevention: Tape all connections or use locking devices for piggyback connections; use Luer-Lok connections for central venous catheters and other high-risk situations, such as for a human immunodeficiency virus (HIV) seropositive patient.

Blood backup in tubing

Flush tubing with normal saline if blood backed up only briefly; change tubing if backup time is unknown.
Prevention: Place arm restraints below a venipuncture site; avoid dry IVs; keep fluid container 36 inches above site; teach patient not to raise arm above heart.

IV line obstruction
Resistance met when flushing attempted

Remove catheter or needles; do not force flush; relocate IV.
Prevention: Flush IV locks at least twice daily; in active children flush every 4 hours; change IV container before infusion runs dry.

Table 1-2 Potential complications (systems)—infusion therapy

System	Clinical Features	Contributing Causes	Nursing Interventions	Complications
Circulatory overload	Dyspnea, cough, and pitting edema in dependent areas; puffy eyelids; weight increase especially during the past 24 hours	Patient has a history of compromised cardiac or renal condition, liver disease, or cerebral damage; an IV solution was inadvertently infused at a rapid rate; or the patient has received saline solution in excessive amounts, especially at night when renal function is normally reduced.	Decrease IV rate, elevate head of bed at least 30 degrees, dangle the patient's feet if possible, obtain frequent vital signs, auscultate breath sounds for presence of moist crackles, and notify the physician regarding clinical changes from baseline status.	Congestive heart failure and pulmonary edema

| Air embolism | Chest pain, shoulder pain, shortness of breath, cyanosis, air hunger, low back pain, hypotension, weak pulse, loss of consciousness | Air inadvertently enters into the venous system, a greater problem with central venous access placement than peripheral IV access; use Luer-Lok connections for all central venous access devices or catheters. | Immediately place the patient on left side in Trendelenburg position and notify the physician; remain with the patient, obtain vital signs and respiratory oxygen saturation status, maintain IV site patency, and consider medication(s) and/or oxygen administration. | Shock and death |

Continued

Table 1-2 Potential complications (systems)—infusion therapy—cont'd

System	Clinical Features	Contributing Causes	Nursing Interventions	Complications
Foreign body embolism	Similar to those with an air embolism; foreign body embolism rare complication	Portion of the IV catheter was severed or another foreign body such as a needle fragment inadvertently entered the IV catheter.	Immediately place the patient on left side in Trendelenburg position and notify the physician; obtain vital signs; apply a tourniquet to the extremity above the venipuncture site to confine embolus to the affected extremity; remain with the patient.	Occlusion of blood flow to a body part; shock and death

| Septicemia | Sudden or gradual rise in temperature, chills and shaking; increased pulse and respiratory rate, headache, nausea and vomiting, diarrhea | IV products were contaminated or a break in aseptic technique occurred, especially in immunocompromised patients. | Symptomatic as prescribed by the physician; save IV catheter, tubing, and solution for possible culture; if IV supply is suspect, follow steps for alerting manufacturer of need for a product recall; establish another IV site for administration of drugs. | Septic shock and death |

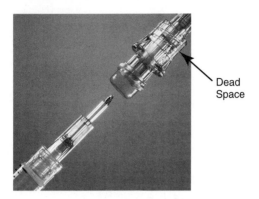

Dead
Space

Fig. 1-2
Dead space. Interlink System, BD Blunt Plastic Cannula.
(Courtesy Becton, Dickinson and Company.)

Any dead space or priming volume deficit can result in potential harm to the patient.

Selecting an Administration Set

Because many options are available for IV tubings, the choice of IV set depends on the solution container (glass, plastic bag, or syringe), allergy of the patient to latex, infusate (requirement for nonpolyvinylchloride), desired flow rate, gravity flow, and infusion pump. Some important considerations follow.

Drop size

Drop chambers deliver either microdrops (60 drops/ml) or macrodrops (10 to 15 drops/ml). A macrodrop system should be selected when large quantities of solution or rapid infusion rates are required. Microdrop systems are used most often for children younger than 16 years of age, elderly adults, or patients requiring limitations on volume or infusion rate.

Vents

Vents permit air to enter the vacuum in the bottle and to displace the solution as it flows out. Unlike rigid glass containers, flexible IV containers do not require vents. The tubing that is appropriate for either the flexible or the rigid IV container should be selected.

IV ports

Ports are required to administer secondary infusions and medications. Continuous-flow sets are designed with a back-check valve that allows a piggyback infusion to run and the solution to begin infusing again after the piggyback infusion is completed. The type, frequency, and number of secondary and/or bolus infusates the patient requires must be considered.

Volumetric chamber

Volumetric chamber IV sets are used to deliver small doses of medication or fluid over an extended period. They are commonly used for children and elderly adults and in acute care settings to reduce the risk of infusing large amounts of fluids too rapidly.

IV Filter Considerations

Infusion-related phlebitis is common and may result from particulates and microbes in the IV system or irritation caused by the IV catheter. IV filters are designed to remove particulates and microbes from IV infusions. However, filters are designed to complement IV therapy and not to replace aseptic technique.

Filtering may be done in a pharmacy area before delivery to the patient care area or with a filter attached to the IV tubing. Filter sizes range from 5 to 0.22 μm. The 0.45-μm filter may have an air-eliminating capacity, but like the 0.5- to 5-μm filters, it retains particulate matter. However, the 0.22-μm filter removes all particulate matter, fungi, and bacteria and is also air eliminating. The benefits of in-line filters and add-on filters have not been universally supported. However, no studies have contraindicated filter use, and many strongly encourage it. Problems associated with filters include clogging, which may slow or stop the flow rate when debris accumulates on the filter surface; drug binding to the surface of the filter, which may occur with some drugs, such as insulin and amphotericin B; and unnecessary cost increases for basic IV systems when filters may not be indicated for short-term infusions.

Flow Control Devices

Flow rates can be regulated with clamps, accessory devices, or IV pumps and controllers.

Clamps

Every IV administration set has one or more clamps to regulate flow. Roller clamps adjust tubing diameter and restrict or increase the flow rate. A slide clamp either stops or starts IV flow and should not be used in conjunction with a roller clamp.

Accessory devices

Small accessory flow regulation devices may be added to administration sets to control the drop rate more precisely than a roller clamp. Most of these devices depress a larger area of tubing than do roller clamps, although they are less precise than electronic pumps and controllers.

Elastomeric balloon device

A transparent outer shell houses a balloonlike reservoir that can be inflated to a predetermined volume—from approximately 25 to 375 ml. When the fluid or drug is poured into the reservoir through the opening at the top, positive pressure forms inside. Releasing the slide clamp starts the infusion. A preset restriction device in the tubing controls the flow. Rates range from approximately 2 to 200 ml/hr.

IV pumps and controllers

Electronic devices deliver fluids with the highest degree of accuracy. Their ability to sound an alarm when an occlusion occurs may assist with early identification of flow problems. These electronic devices may be stationary (attached to an IV pole), ambulatory (battery-operated; varied volume infusion, placed in case that is attached to patient's clothing), or implantable (preprogrammed pump that is implanted into a pocket of subcutaneous tissues in the abdomen or subclavian fossa). A pump has the ability to add pressure to an infusion under conditions of restricted flow. Controllers do not add pressure to the line to overcome resistance. (Pumps and controllers are discussed more completely in Chapter 6.)

Infection Control Practices
Patient Protection

Patients may be exposed to IV therapy–related infections in a variety of ways. Nosocomial infections are best prevented by ensuring that nurses wash their hands before making contact with

Table 1-3   Potential sources of IV-related patient infection

Source of Contamination	Protective Measures
Manufacture or storage	Verify integrity of all packaging before use (Fig. 1-3, *A*); discard a cracked bottle; assess IV solutions against a light and a dark background for particulate matter; verify expiration dates on packaging.
Break in aseptic technique during therapy	Avoid touch contamination when spiking bags (Fig. 1-3, *B*), priming tubing, or adding medications; change tubings if touch contamination occurs; do not reconnect disconnected or contaminated equipment. All admixture solutions should be prepared under laminar flow hoods by personnel adhering to strict aseptic technique.
Blood in tubing	Flush IV catheter immediately when blood backs up or change tubing if the time since backed up unknown; teach patients not to raise arm with IV line above heart; do not use IV access for routine blood drawing.
Injection ports	The injection port must be cleaned with an accepted antiseptic (e.g., 70% isopropyl alcohol, povidone-iodine solution) before injection of any infusate and/or connection to needleless devices allowing secondary infusion solutions.

any part of IV therapy systems. Product and equipment contamination can occur during manufacture, storage, or therapy. If a break occurs in aseptic technique during the course of therapy, tubing or containers should be changed immediately because the patient is at risk of developing a systemic infection. Potential sources of patient infection are summarized in Table 1-3.

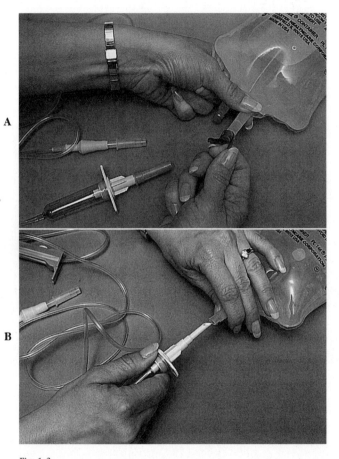

Fig. 1-3
A, Removing protective covering on the IV bag. **B,** Inserting spike into the IV bag.
(From Perry AG, Potter PA: *Clinical nursing skills and techniques,* ed 4, St Louis, 1998, Mosby.)

Nurse Protection from IV Therapy–Related Infection

Needlestick injuries are a compelling issue for all nurses and are a special concern for nurses working with IV therapy. Despite an increased awareness of the dangers involved with handling sharps and the incorporation of universal blood and body precautions into practice, injuries involving needlesticks remain unacceptably frequent occurrences in health care settings. Needlesticks can occur any time a needle is used, particularly if a patient moves unexpectedly or if a caregiver recaps a needle.

Of the high-risk percutaneous injuries (injuries from blood-filled needles), approximately 75% relate to blood drawing and 25% to IV line placement. Current research reports that 80% of needlestick injuries can be prevented with improved product safety design. Ideally, devices should eliminate hazards without sacrificing efficiency or requiring special training. Many products that eliminate exposure to sharps are available. The use of needleless devices or blunt-tipped needles or the substitution of plastic cannulas for needles can reduce needlestick injuries. Some shielded or recessed needles are designed for use with IV piggyback medications.

Needleless systems eliminate the needle by using one of four choices: prepierced septum, blunt cannula, a valved connector, and/or a capped Luer-Lok connector with a manual clamp to prevent fluid flow. Other optional devices include recessed needles that have a fixed shield in place (Fig. 1-4); joined by a secondary set to the Y-site of the IV tubing; disposable protective syringes; or safety syringes that protect against injury by shielding the needle after use. *Agency and OSHA guidelines must be followed in using all products for IV therapy.* Besides using these new products, everyone working in patient care has a responsibility to reduce sharps use whenever possible. Nonneedle alternatives should be sought for an IV procedure; for example, the practitioner can connect the IV tubing directly to the venous access device.

Other important needlestick prevention strategies include awareness and avoidance of unsafe practices such as recapping needles (responsible for about 25% of all needlestick injuries) and disposing of needles in containers that are not puncture resistant. In the event that a procedure is interrupted and a needle must be recapped, the practitioner should cover the needle using a scoop

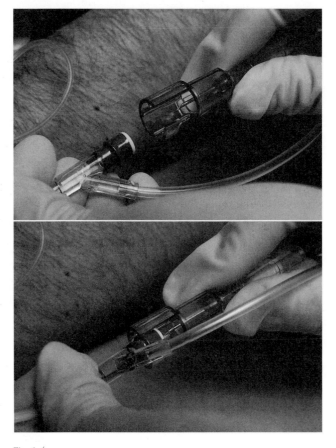

Fig. 1-4
Example of needleless device.
(From Perry AG, Potter PA: *Clinical nursing skills and techniques,*
ed 4, St Louis, 1998, Mosby.)

technique. This involves positioning the cap on its side on a table
and scooping up the cap with the tip of the needle. When a rigid
container is not available at the bedside, needles should be placed
in a plastic cup or other small container for transporting to the rigid
container. Finally, the practitioner should clean up after a procedure

methodically. All sharps that were assembled and/or used for the procedure should be accounted for.

Documentation Recommendations
Medical Records

Medical records are maintained to provide an accurate and easily retrievable account of patient care and treatment. Complete records are a principal means of communication among health care team members. Increasingly, records are used by insurers to justify supply and equipment costs, by review organizations to evaluate quality of care, and by courts for malpractice claims. Therefore IV therapy must be documented accurately and completely. Efficient chart forms can facilitate complete, concise documentation. IV therapy easily lends itself to flow sheet documentation.

Documentation Elements of Infusion Therapy

- Date and time of tubing changes; list of all accessory tubings
- Date, time, and contents of IV fluids
- IV flow rate, including subsequent rate changes
- Electronic and/or accessory equipment used to regulate the flow
- Regular site assessments
- Presence of any complications and action taken to correct the problem
- Time/date IV therapy was discontinued and whether the catheter was intact when removed
- Completion of patient teaching and demonstration of understanding through patient's repetition of action or information

Labeling IV Containers

In addition to documentation in the patient record, specific information needs to be placed on labels attached to the IV container. All IV containers should be labeled with the patient's name and identification number, the name of the IV solution, a list of additives (including dosage), the date and time initiated or changed, initials of the person hanging the infusion, and the expiration date or time of the infusion.

Nursing Diagnoses

- Infection, potential for, related to invasive procedure
- Injury, potential for, related to obstruction of catheter
- Skin integrity, impaired: actual

- Fluid volume excess: actual or potential
- Fluid volume deficit: actual or potential

Patient/Family Teaching for Self-Management

Patients need to know the purpose of their therapy, the approximate duration of the treatment, and any activity or movement restrictions to observe during the course of the infusion. In addition, patients should be taught to recognize and report the early signs and symptoms of infiltration or phlebitis. With electronic infusion devices, the patient should be instructed to call the nurse when an alarm sounds. Teaching activities to encourage patient cooperation and participation in care include the following measures:

- Discuss the signs and symptoms of possible infiltration or phlebitis, such as swelling, pain, burning, soreness, redness, or a cool feeling at the insertion site.
- Teach the importance of promptly reporting symptoms to the nurse.
- Discuss the importance of not readjusting the flow rate or bending or lying on the tubing.
- Show the patient how to avoid placing pressure on the venipuncture site when attempting to sit up in bed, pushing the IV pole, and positioning the arm with the IV catheter.
- Demonstrate how to wash the arm and hand in the area of the IV to ensure that the IV site remains clean and dry.

Geriatric Considerations

Many elderly people have compromised cardiovascular and renal systems. It is important to closely regulate and monitor infusions so that a rapid infusion does not cause fluid overload and become a precipitating factor for congestive heart failure or pulmonary edema. Frequent and scheduled observations may be necessary to minimize potential complications. Neuromotor and sensory deficits (e.g., memory, vision, and mobility) may interfere with educational strategies and prompt reporting of IV therapy–associated problems.

Resources
Patient Education—IV Therapy

The following information is designed to assist in answering patients' commonly asked questions about IV therapy.

What Is IV Therapy?

IV stands for *intravenous,* meaning inside the vein. For IV therapy, a catheter (a soft plastic tube about the size of a needle) or needle is inserted into a vein, usually in the hand or arm. The catheter or needle is attached to tubing and a fluid container that provides a way to give you medications and fluids.

How Long Will the IV Line Stay in?

Your IV therapy may last only a few hours or up to several days. Your physician decides the duration of IV therapy.

Is IV Therapy Painful?

When the IV infusion is initiated, you will feel the insertion of the needle placing the catheter into your vein. As the IV solution enters your vein, it may sting for a few minutes, but the discomfort should stop in a short time.

If you feel any discomfort after the initial insertion, ask your nurse to check your IV site. Once the IV system is in place and secured, it should cause you minimal, if any, discomfort.

Is It Possible to Walk Around?

If you have permission to get out of bed, you may do so even while receiving IV therapy. If a pump or controller is regulating your IV infusion, ask for assistance to unplug the instrument before you get up. It will be plugged in again when you return to bed.

While you are up and walking, push the pole slowly with your free arm while holding your arm with the catheter lower than the level of your heart. Keeping your IV arm lower than your heart prevents blood from backing up into the tubing and keeps the IV fluid flowing at the correct rate. Never take the IV bag off the pole.

Is Bathing or Showering Allowed?

Depending on the type and location of your IV therapy, you may be allowed to shower or take a tub bath. Check with your nurse for permission or instructions regarding bathing or showering.

What Is Intermittent IV Therapy?

When continuous IV fluids are not needed, your IV catheter is disconnected from the IV tubing, and an IV lock is attached to it. The IV lock is a device that allows IV medications to be given as needed.

What Happens after the IV Catheter Is Removed?

Immediately after your IV catheter is removed, pressure will be applied to the spot to seal the vein. After that, you may use your arm as you normally would.

If you have further questions about your IV therapy, ask your nurse or physician.

HELPFUL HINTS

Observing the following precautions will help your IV procedure go smoothly:

- Promptly report to your nurse problems such as unusual swelling, redness, tenderness, or burning at the catheter site.
- Do not touch any of the clamps or controls on the IV tubing. Ask the nurse to make all adjustments.
- Do not remove the fluid container from the IV pole.
- Be careful not to pull on the IV tubing.
- Minimize your arm movements, particularly at the joints closest to the catheter site.
- Do not raise your arm too high; the catheter site must be below the IV fluid container for it to flow properly.
- Do not lie on your arm or any part of your body receiving the IV infusion.
- Avoid lying on the tubing or letting it get tangled in the bed.
- Ask for help. Many tasks can be difficult with an IV in place.

Clinical Competency—Infusion Therapy

	Yes	No	NA
Infusion Administration			
1. Correctly selects type and volume of infusion solution.			
2. Validates IV access patency and flushes IV access according to procedure.			
3. Hangs a new bag of IV solution after verifying physician order.			
4. Uses aseptic technique to set up the IV pump, prime the IV device, extension tubing, or IV tubing; adjusts rate and/or applies pump sensor.			

Clinical Competency—Infusion Therapy—cont'd

	Yes	No	NA
Infusion Administration—cont'd			
5. Verifies correct IV pump for rate and volume of infusion.			
6. Troubleshoots IV pump alarms.			
7. Changes IV tubing and/or solution according to agency policy and procedure.			
8. Documents IV therapy on designated form: solution, rate, IV site status, any tubing change, pump.			
Documentation in the Medical Record			
1. All IV solutions are sequentially recorded.			
2. IV rates including rate changes are documented.			
3. IV controller or pump use is documented at least every 24 hours according to agency policy.			
4. All nurses document a venipuncture site and infusion assessment.			
5. Flushes are documented in conjunction with IV medication administration.			
6. IV tubing changes are documented at least every 72 to 96 hours.			
Patient and Infusion Solution Assessment			
1. IV solution hanging corresponds to the physician's order, and information in the medical record.			
2. IV bag has a time strip marked in hourly increments (includes bags regulated by controllers or pumps).			
3. The nurse hanging the bag initials the time strip.			

Continued

Clinical Competency—Infusion Therapy—cont'd

	Yes	No	NA
Patient and Infusion Solution Assessment—cont'd			
4. The solution is being infused on time, within 30 minutes of schedule.			
5. The IV tubing is labeled with date and time of last tubing change.			
6. The patient has been instructed not to adjust flow rate of the IV infusion. "Did the nurses tell you not to make any adjustments to your IV?"			
7. Controller/pump: "What have you been told to do if the alarm sounds?"			
8. The patient has been informed to report complications of IV therapy to the nurse. "What have you been told to report to your nurse?"			

Study Questions

1. Appropriate selection of IV administration sets include:
   a. Drop size, IV port, IV catheter, IV access site
   b. Drop chamber, drop size, IV catheter, IV port
   c. Drop size, IV port, vent, volumetric chamber
   d. Drop chamber, vent, IV port, IV catheter

2. IV tubing changes are recommended under the following conditions:
   a. Kink in IV tubing
   b. Intermittent medication infusion
   c. Tubing tip contamination
   d. Routinely every 24 hours

3. Select the intervention that will assist in improving IV flow rate via gravity flow:
   a. Position the IV solution at least 36 inches above the patient's heart

b. Restart the IV access with a larger-gauge IV catheter

c. Retape the venipuncture site using sterile technique

d. All the above

4. Which of the following statements *best* describe an infiltrated IV?

a. The area around the IV catheter is inflamed and warm to touch.

b. The IV fluid is flowing sluggishly.

c. There is tissue swelling and the surrounding tissue is cool to touch.

d. There is a palpable cord along the vein.

5. Which of the following is a nursing intervention that is *not recommended* for an IV solution not infusing?

a. Remove the IV catheter and relocate the IV access site.

b. Flush the IV tubing and IV access with normal saline in a tuberculin syringe.

c. Raise the height of the IV solution container.

d. Place the IV solution on an infusion device.

6. Phlebitis is identified as the presence of two or more of the following clinical features:

a. Tenderness, pitting edema, dyspnea, cough

b. Chest pain, cyanosis, hypotension, weak pulse

c. Headache, nausea, diarrhea, chills

d. Pain, erythema, induration, swelling

7. Nursing interventions for IV therapy–related septicemia include all of the following *except*:

a. Elevate the head of the bed at least 30 degrees.

b. Establish another IV access site for drug and solution administration.

c. Follow steps to alert the manufacturer for potential product recall.

d. Save the IV catheter, tubing, and solution for culture procedure.

8. IV therapy circulatory overload may be related to:

a. Contamination of IV solution

b. Infusion solution infused at a rapid rate

c. Inadvertent entry of air into the venous system

d. Use of Luer-Lok connections

9. *After* an infiltration the IV should be restarted _____.
    a. Above the area of infiltration
    b. Below the area of infiltration
    c. Lateral to the area of infiltration
    d. Do not restart for 24 hours

10. Patient instructions for reporting problems include:
    a. IV tubing changes
    b. IV rate changes
    c. IV pump setting changes
    d. IV therapy–related clinical features

Answers   1. c   2. c   3. d   4. c   5. b   6. d
7. a   8. b   9. a   10. d

Venipuncture

2

Objectives

1. Discuss important aspects of patient preparation for insertion of an IV cannula.

2. Compare and contrast the characteristics between veins and arteries.

3. Identify advantages and disadvantages of selecting each hand or arm vein for IV therapy.

4. Contrast characteristics and uses of the various venipuncture devices.

5. Describe the clinical sequences for a successful IV cannulation technique.

Venipuncture is a skill that is basic to IV therapy and can be learned and developed through frequent practice. Thorough understanding of both vein location and the venipuncture procedure increases confidence. Important elements of the procedure include patient preparation; assessment of the patient's diagnosis, vein condition, and type and duration of therapy; vein selection; device selection; accurate insertion technique; knowledge of troubleshooting; and patient instruction.

Patient Preparation

Reviewing the patient's record for allergies and verifying the physician's order with available laboratory results should be completed before approaching the patient. Supplies should be selected according to the type, purpose, and duration of therapy along with the patient's age and physical condition.

Patients who are unfamiliar with IV therapy may be anxious. When the patient is tense, the veins can constrict, making the venipuncture more painful and the vein difficult to cannulate. Instructing the patient to inhale and exhale slowly, to avoid looking at the IV site, and to focus on a pleasant image can lessen extreme anxiety. The following steps can encourage patient cooperation:

1. Ensure patient privacy; for example, ask visitors to leave the room during the procedure.
2. Assume a confident attitude.
3. Greet the patient by name.
4. Introduce yourself.
5. Validate the patient's identification.
6. Explain the procedure in a way easily understood by the patient.
7. Ask for the patient's cooperation in holding his or her extremity as still as possible.

Vein Selection

In general, distal veins of the hands and arms should be used initially, and subsequent venipunctures should be proximal to previous sites. Arm veins are preferred for patients who do not have compromised vasculature. Veins commonly used for IV therapy include the basilic, cephalic, and metacarpal (Fig. 2-1). The extremity should be observed and palpated before a vein is chosen. Resiliency and location should be assessed. An ideal vein is unused and relatively straight. The vessel should be verified as a vein and not an artery. The differences between veins and arteries include the following qualities:

Veins	Arteries
Dark-red blood	Bright-red blood
Slow blood return	Rapid, pulsating blood return
Valves at point of branching	No valves
Blood flow toward heart	Blood flow away from heart
Superficial location	Deep location surrounded by muscle
Multiple veins supply an area	Single artery supplies an area

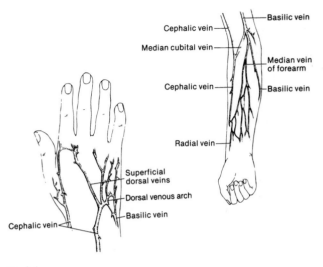

Fig. 2-1
Venous anatomy.
(From Perry AG, Potter PA: *Clinical nursing skills and techniques,*
ed 4, St Louis, 1998, Mosby.)

Careful vein selection and assessment are crucial to a successful
venipuncture procedure and the sequential medication or solution
infusion. The practitioner should observe the guidelines for vein
selection presented in Box 2-1.

Advantages and Disadvantages of Hand and Arm Veins

Digital veins flow along the lateral aspect of the fingers and are
joined to the dorsal veins by communicating branches.

> *Advantages:* They may be the only veins available and are
> usually secured with an IV splint device.
>
> *Disadvantages:* They may require small-gauge catheters, infil-
> trate easily, and are unsuitable for long-term therapy or
> infusion of irritating fluids and medications.

Superficial dorsal/metacarpal (hand) veins arise from the union
of the digital veins.

> *Advantages:* They permit arm movement and are easy to see and
> palpate; the IV access lies flat between the joints and the
> metacarpal bones of the hand, providing a natural splint.

Box 2-1   Guidelines for Vein Selection

1. Use distal veins first.
2. Use the patient's nondominant arm if possible.
3. Choose a vein above areas of flexion.
4. Select a vein that is large enough to allow adequate blood flow around the catheter.
5. Palpate the vein to determine its condition, e.g., soft, full, unobstructed veins.
6. Ensure that the site selected will not interfere with the patient's activities of daily living.
7. Select a site that will not interfere with planned surgery or procedures.

The following types of veins should be avoided if possible:

1. Veins previously or recently used
2. Veins injured by infiltration or phlebitis
3. Veins that are bruised, red, swollen, sclerotic, and/or hard
4. Veins of a surgically compromised limb (e.g., mastectomy or a dialysis access placement)
5. Veins near inflamed or infectious area
6. Veins used for laboratory blood sampling
7. Veins of an affected extremity after a cerebral vascular accident or neurologic trauma
8. Veins near areas of flexion, including the antecubital fossa
9. Leg veins, because circulation is sluggish and complications are more frequent (e.g., phlebitis)
10. Small, thin-walled branches of main arm veins

Disadvantages: Active patients may dislodge the catheter or get the dressing wet with handwashing; elderly patients may have inadequate tissue and thin skin in this area.

Cephalic veins are located in the lower arm on the radial (thumb) side of the arm. They ascend along the outer region of the forearm into the antecubital region. Cephalic veins are smaller and usually curve more than basilic veins.

Advantages: The clinician may use a large-gauge catheter for rapid infusions and/or administration of blood products. These veins are splinted by arm bones and are a good choice for infusion of irritating solutions.

Disadvantage: Cephalic veins curve more on the ascent up the arm than do the basilic veins; this is usually a disadvantage only when long-line catheters are inserted.

Basilic veins are located on the ulnar side of the forearm, ascend up the posterior—or back—of the arm, and then curve toward the anterior surface or antecubital region. They extend straight up the arm and enter the deep tissues.

Advantages: Advantages are the same as those for cephalic veins; however, basilic veins are usually straighter than cephalic veins. When other veins have been exhausted, the basilic vein may still be available. Request the patient to flex the elbow and bend the arm up to bring the basilic vein into view.

Disadvantages: Basilic veins may be prone to rolling movement; awkward positioning of the patient's extremity may be required during venipuncture.

Median/antecubital veins arise from the veins of the forearm and commonly divide into two vessels: one that joins the *basilic,* and one that joins the *cephalic.* They are commonly used for blood sampling.

Advantages: They are easily accessed, accommodate a large catheter, and have less tendency to roll.

Disadvantages: They may restrict patient arm movement and are often required for blood sampling.

The median cephalic vein crosses in front of the brachial artery, allowing the potential for puncturing the artery during the venipuncture procedure.

Venipuncture Device Selection

Choosing the correct IV catheter is important to the outcome of therapy. Catheters are made of many materials (e.g., silicone, steel needle). Steel-winged infusion devices (butterfly needles) are used in limited, short-term situations. They are easy to insert but infiltrate easily. Improved product design has resulted in many choices in short, peripheral, inside-the-needle and over-the-needle catheters (Fig. 2-2).

Differences among the various catheters include the following:

▪ Thickness of the catheter wall	*Effect:* Rate of flow
▪ Sharpness of the insertion needle	*Effect:* Slight alteration in insertion technique

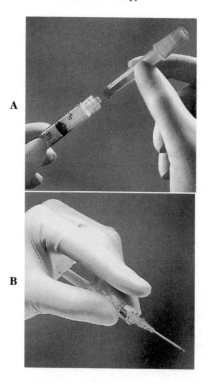

Fig. 2-2
A, BD TwinPak™. **B,** BD Insyte™ AutoGuard™ Shielded IV
catheter.
(Courtesy Becton, Dickinson and Company.)

- Softening properties of
  the catheter (Teflon does
  not soften; Vialon softens by a factor of 4;
  Aquavene softens by
  a factor of 50.)

  Effect: Catheter dwell time

- Safety design for pre-
  vention of needlestick
  injuries and blood
  contact

  Effect: Occupational safety
  (Fig. 2-3)

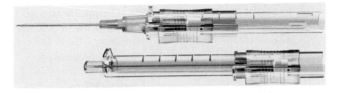

Catheter Safety System. The safety system covers the needle as the catheter is advanced.

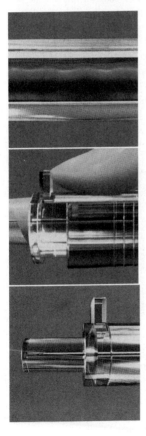

Optically clear yet radiopaque OCORLIN polyurethane is shown to reduce the occurrence of infusion-related phlebitis.

Push-off tab facilitates one-handed threading and helps keep both hands behind the needle until it is safely locked within the needle guard.

A built-in needle guard securely encases the entire needle to help prevent needlestick injuries. A "click" confirms the needle is safely locked within the needle guard.

Fig. 2-3
PROTECTIV® PLUS I.V. Catheter Safety System
(Courtesy Johnson & Johnson Medical, Division of Ethicon, Inc., Arlington, Texas)

- Number of lumina available for simultaneous infusion of fluids

Effect: Potentially incompatible fluids can be administered at the same time through the same peripheral line when a dual-lumen catheter is selected (Fig. 2-4)

Considerations when choosing an IV catheter include the size and condition of the vein selected, the viscosity of the fluid to be infused, the patient's age, and the type and duration of therapy. Consult the following list when selecting a catheter gauge:

16 gauge—major surgery, trauma, obstetric emergency

18 gauge—blood and blood products, administration of viscous medications

20 gauge—most patient applications

22 gauge—most patient applications, especially children and elderly patients

24 gauge—pediatric patients, neonates, and elderly patients

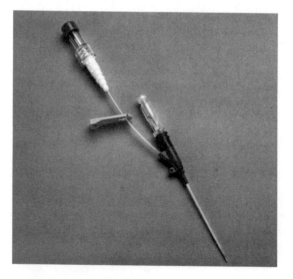

Fig. 2-4
Arrow dual-lumen catheter.
(Courtesy Arrow International, Inc., Reading, Pa.)

CLINICAL ALERT: Choose the shortest catheter with the largest gauge (smallest bore) appropriate for the type and duration of the infusion. The larger the gauge number, the smaller the bore of the catheter.

Insertion Technique
Vein Location

To locate a suitable vein, the practitioner should find a comfortable position in a well-lighted area and apply a tourniquet 4 to 6 inches above the proposed site. The tourniquet should be tight enough to stop venous blood flow but not arterial flow. If the radial pulse cannot be felt, the tourniquet is too tight. To encourage vein distension, the practitioner should ask the patient to clench and unclench his or her fist several times. When venous fill is difficult to achieve, placing the arm in a dependent position or applying warm packs may help alleviate the problem. The vein should be stabilized by holding the skin taut because stabilization of the vein before sticking is a key to atraumatic catheter insertion.

If the patient has a great amount of hair on the arm, the hair should be clipped before venipuncture rather than shaved because shaving may nick the skin and create a potential site for infection. The refill capacity of the vein should be assessed by running a finger along the vein. If the refill is sluggish, the vein will be prone to collapse. If a bifurcation exists below a desired site, the practitioner should enter the skin 2 to 3 cm below the bifurcation and proceed up into the main branch.

Guidelines
Catheter Insertion

1. Use meticulous handwashing.
2. Select the best available vein.
3. Cleanse the skin from the center outward with an approved solution (povidone-iodine, tincture of iodine, or 70% alcohol), and allow it to dry.
4. Apply a flat, soft tourniquet 4 to 6 inches above the site (Fig. 2-5).
5. Put on gloves; cleanse the insertion site with antiseptic (Fig. 2-6).

Some people are extremely anxious about the pain of an IV catheter insertion. For children, patients with a history of difficult IV starts, or those in whom some probing for vein location may be

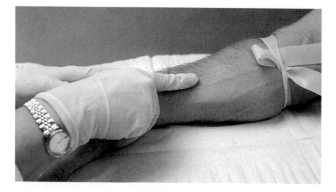

Fig. 2-5
Selection of vein with tourniquet applied.
(From Perry AG, Potter PA: *Clinical nursing skills and techniques,*
ed 4, St Louis, 1998, Mosby.)

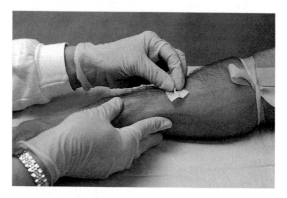

Fig. 2-6
Cleanse insertion site with antiseptic.
(From Perry AG, Potter PA: *Clinical nursing skills and techniques,*
ed 4, St Louis, 1998, Mosby.)

necessary, chances for a successful first needlestick can be
improved if lidocaine cream ointment or an intradermal lidocaine
wheal is used to numb the IV insertion site. Neither lidocaine
ointment nor the lidocaine wheal can be used in patients who are
allergic to lidocaine.

The following technique should be used to create an intradermal lidocaine wheal through which the IV catheter may be inserted:

1. Hold a tuberculin syringe filled with 0.1 ml of 1% lidocaine bevel up at a 5-degree angle to the skin.
2. Insert only the bevel into the subcutaneous tissue.
3. Aspirate to be sure the needle is not in a vein.
4. Slowly inject the lidocaine solution.
5. Wait a few seconds for the lidocaine to take effect and insert the IV catheter through the wheal.
6. Anchor the vein; place your thumb over the vein to prevent movement and to stretch the skin taut against the direction of insertion.
7. Puncture the vein; hold the flash chamber of the catheter, not the hub. For a direct approach, place the needle bevel up at a 30- to 45-degree angle from the patient's skin (Fig. 2-7). Insert it in the direction of venous flow; and enter the vein. You may feel a "pop" and see a blood flashback. For an indirect method, enter the skin beside the vein and then direct the catheter to enter the side of the vein until you see a blood flashback (Fig. 2-8).
8. Lower the needle until it is almost flush with the skin.
9. Advance the catheter into the vein an additional ¼ to ½ inch before removing the stylet; release skin tension, hold the stylet, and advance the catheter (Fig. 2-9).
10. Release the tourniquet and remove the stylet.
11. Apply primed tubing or an intermittent injection cap.
12. Tape the IV catheter and tubing into place (Fig. 2-10).
13. Apply a sterile dressing.
14. Label the site with date and time of insertion (Fig. 2-11).

CLINICAL ALERT: When a stick is unsuccessful, use a new catheter for a second attempt. Insert most catheters with one continuous forward motion until the hub of the catheter is flush with the patient's skin. If the catheter is not advanced to the hub, dislodgment and infection occur more easily.

Securing and Taping Peripheral IV Sites

Procedures for securing a peripheral IV cannula vary among agencies and institutions as well as among nurses. The basic standards to be observed include the following:

- Secure the site so that early signs of phlebitis or infiltration can be observed.

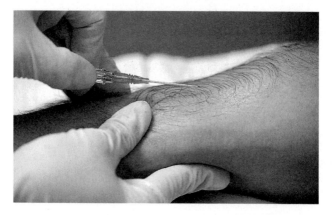

Fig. 2-7
Puncturing of skin with the over-the-needle catheter.
(From Perry AG, Potter PA: *Clinical nursing skills and techniques,*
ed 4, St Louis, 1998, Mosby.)

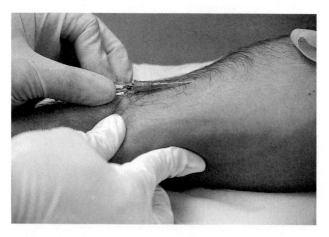

Fig. 2-8
Entering with bevel up.
(From Perry AG, Potter PA: *Clinical nursing skills and techniques,*
ed 4, St Louis, 1998, Mosby.)

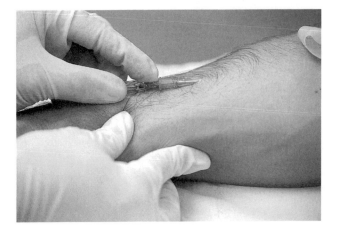

Fig. 2-9
Advance catheter off stylet using one-handed technique.
(From Perry AG, Potter PA: *Clinical nursing skills and techniques,*
ed 4, St Louis, 1998, Mosby.)

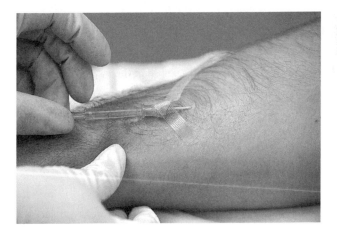

Fig. 2-10
Taping the over-the-needle catheter to skin.
(From Perry AG, Potter PA: *Clinical nursing skills and techniques,*
ed 4, St Louis, 1998, Mosby.)

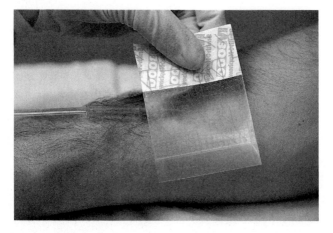

Fig. 2-11
Apply transparent dressing over IV site of catheter; label site.
(From Perry AG, Potter, PA: *Clinical nursing skills and techniques,*
ed 4, St Louis, 1998, Mosby.)

- Place tape above the catheter, neither directly over the
  catheter insertion site nor around the entire extremity;
  otherwise, blood flow may be impeded.
- Use a minimum amount of tape.
- Anchor the cannula hub flush with the skin to prevent
  movement of the catheter within the vein. Movement can
  cause mechanical phlebitis.
- Loop the IV tubing close to the cannula and secure with tape
  independently of the cannula, to prevent kinking or pulling.
- Frequently monitor the devices used to immobilize a hand or
  arm, such as splints and arm boards, to ensure that the vein
  or skin has not been constricted.
- Label the site completely (see Fig. 2-11).

Patency

Patency of the IV site is indicated by blood return. One factor that
may influence the rapidity of the blood return is the catheter gauge.
For sites that have been in place, patency can be evaluated by
observing for blood return in the IV tubing when the solution is
lowered below the level of the IV site. Infiltration is indicated by

coolness, pallor, and swelling at the site. Warmth, erythema, and/or pain at the site indicate phlebitis.

Site Care

A sterile dressing is required at the peripheral IV cannula entrance site. The dressing should be changed whenever it becomes soiled, wet, or loose. Several types of dressings, including bioclusive dressings, sterile Band-Aids, gauze dressings, and tape, are acceptable as long as sterility is maintained. Povidone-iodine and antibiotic ointments have not been shown to decrease infection, and they obscure site visualization.

Site Rotation

Venipuncture sites need to be changed on a planned basis to reduce the potential of phlebitis and infiltration. The frequency of site rotation depends on the catheter material. Catheters of Teflon or Vialon need to be changed every 48 to 72 hours. Aquavene catheters can remain in place for extended periods. A new site is always required if erythema, tenderness, or infiltration occurs. If the device remains in place longer than 72 hours because of limited vein selection, the reason should be documented in the patient's record. A new site is selected by moving up the patient's arm or in a proximal direction from the previous site.

Peripherally Inserted Central Venous Catheters

Peripherally inserted central venous catheters are available for insertion by nurses with advanced IV therapy skills as an alternative to physician-placed central venous catheters. These Silastic catheters may vary in length, gauge, and number of lumina. Refer to Chapter 4 for catheter procedures and maintenance.

Venipuncture for Laboratory Sampling

Blood samples are most commonly drawn from an antecubital vein using vacuum collection devices. The antecubital vein is selected because these veins are large and have thicker walls than the veins that are lower in the arm and hand. When antecubital veins are not available, samples are drawn using a butterfly needle attached to a syringe because the vacuum containers collapse the smaller veins.

   CLINICAL ALERT: Obtain blood samples from the arm without an IV whenever possible because laboratory values may be altered by the IV fluids. If laboratory samples are drawn from the arm with an IV catheter, stop the infusion for 1 to 2 minutes before drawing the blood sample.

◎ Troubleshooting Tips for Venipuncture of Difficult Veins

With difficult veins, remember that systematic preparation is the key to a successful stick. The patient should be in a comfortable position with the arm lowered. The practitioner should assume a confident attitude while reassuring the patient and urging him or her to relax.

Several techniques may increase the visibility of difficult-to-find veins:

- Wipe the skin with alcohol and tap it with the fingers to make the vein more prominent.
- Place warm packs over the arm for several minutes.
- Transilluminate the vein with a fiberoptic light source or designated vein Doppler device.

Additional tips are offered in Table 2-1.

Infection Control Practices
Patient Protection

Infection at the venipuncture site is usually caused by a break in aseptic technique during the procedure. The following measures reduce patient risk:

1. Wash hands before starting an IV infusion or working with the IV equipment.
2. Use an approved antiseptic to clean the patient's skin.
3. Clip hairs at the venipuncture site.
4. Do not reuse a catheter or needle.
5. Apply a sterile dressing to the site.

If an infection occurs at a venipuncture site, such as purulent drainage or cellulitis, the following intervention is recommended.

1. Culture the drainage before removing the catheter.
2. Remove the catheter by holding the hub to avoid touching the portion of the catheter under the skin.
3. Hold the catheter over a sterile container and use sterile scissors to cut the distal portion of the catheter so that it drops directly into a sterile container (Fig. 2-12).
4. Label the container and send it to the laboratory.
5. Restart the IV infusion using all new supplies, including the tubing and solution.

◎   Table 2-1   Troubleshooting tips for venipuncture of
difficult veins

Nursing Assessment	Nursing Intervention
Obese patient; unable to palpate or see veins	Create a visual image of the venous anatomy; select a longer catheter.
Fragile skin and veins; infiltration occurs after stick	Use minimal tourniquet pressure; if pulse is bounding, do not use tourniquet.
Vein rolls with attempted stick	Anchor vein with thumb while sticking.
Patient in shock or has minimal venous return	Leave tourniquet on to promote venous distension; use 16- or 18-gauge catheter.

Nurse Protection

Both human immunodeficiency virus (HIV) and hepatitis virus are blood borne. When performing the venipuncture procedure, the nurse must adhere to the Centers for Disease Control and Prevention guidelines for invasive procedures. Recommended practices for nurses involved with IV therapy include the following:

1. Consider IV needles potentially infective. Do not recap needles after use. Have a puncture-resistant container at the bedside for disposal of used needles.
2. Wear gloves when inserting IV needles or handling tubings.
3. Wash hands thoroughly and immediately if they are accidentally contaminated with blood.
4. If a needlestick or a blood splash occurs, you should be evaluated as soon as possible after exposure and periodically thereafter. Each professional needs to be acquainted with new information related to epidemiology, modes of transmission, and prevention of HIV infection and other blood-borne diseases. Furthermore, the nurse should incorporate into daily practice universal precautions concerning blood, body fluid, and secretions.

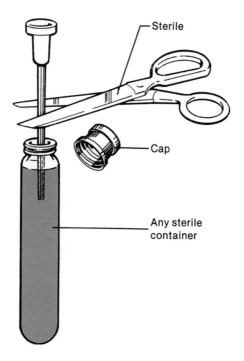

Fig. 2-12
Culturing the IV catheter.

5. Handwashing is the *single* most important action for the health care professional, the patient, and the patient's family and visitors. The Centers for Disease Control and Prevention (CDC) reports approximately 70% to 80% of nosocomial infections could be prevented with prudent handwashing. The importance of adequate handwashing using warm, running water; soap; and friction cannot be overemphasized. The health care professional must use good handwashing before and after any contact with direct patient care, IV therapy equipment, supply, and/or dressing. Gloves are not to be used as a substitute for good handwashing.

Documentation Recommendations

Record the following information on the patient's dressing:

- Nurse's initials
- Date and time of procedure
- Catheter or needle gauge

Document the following information in the patient's medical record according to agency policy:

- Date and time of venipuncture
- Number of attempts required
- Site/vein location
- Catheter gauge and length
- All IV supplies used
- IV fluids and flow rate, if infusion initiated
- Presence of any complications and actions to correct the problem
- Patient teaching and a reflection of understanding

Nursing Diagnoses

- Skin integrity, impaired: potential related to catheter insertion
- Infection, potential for, related to break in skin, contamination of supplies, or break in sterile technique at time of venipuncture
- Anxiety related to invasive procedure
- Altered comfort: pain associated with procedure or complications at insertion site

Patient/Family Teaching for Self-Management

Patients who are receiving IV therapy need information that will enable them to protect their IV site and alert them to report complications to the nurse. Information should include the following:

1. Movement restrictions
2. Information to be reported
   - Redness, induration, swelling, or discomfort at site
   - Blood in tubing
   - Moisture on the dressing
   - IV fluid not infusing or infusion device alarms
3. Changing of the IV site (every 48 to 72 hours or immediately if complications occur)
4. How to bathe with the IV site

Geriatric Considerations

Arm muscles become less firm with aging. There is a loss of dermal skin thickness, which leads to paper-thin skin. Anchor catheters carefully to avoid skin tear and IV infiltration. Loss of subcutaneous fat makes tendons and veins prominent. The catheter should be inserted without use of a tourniquet if the skin is fragile and veins are visible and palpable. Vascular disease and dehydration may limit venous access.

Resources

Clinical Competency

	Yes	No	NA
Venipuncture Procedure			
1. Wear gloves while performing venipuncture and other vascular access procedures.			
2. Wash hands immediately after gloves are removed.			
3. Wash hands or other skin surfaces immediately and thoroughly if contaminated with blood or other body fluids.			
4. Place used sharps, such as needles or scalpels, in the biohazard needle box.			
5. Do not purposely bend, break, or recap needles.			
6. Do not overfill needle container.			
7. Place disposable wastes and articles contaminated with blood or large amounts of body fluids in impervious containers for a trash pickup.			
8. Verify physician order.			
9. Verify appropriate laboratory data.			
10. Verify allergy data.			
11. Calculate flow rate.			

Clinical Competency—cont'd

	Yes	No	NA
12. Select and set up appropriate equipment: solution, set, and venipuncture device.			
13. Wash hands.			
14. Correctly label IV site with patient name, IV additives, and rate of administration.			
15. Introduce self to patient.			
16. Verify patient identification.			
17. Explain procedure to patient and answer patient questions appropriately.			
18. Select appropriate vein: location, size, and condition.			
19. Apply tourniquet without occluding arterial flow.			
20. Cleanse area according to agency policy.			
21. Perform venipuncture according to accepted procedure using no more than two attempts.			
22. Attach tubing to IV cannula and establish flow of solution.			
23. Anchor needle and apply dressing to venipuncture site according to accepted procedure.			
24. Label venipuncture site with date, catheter gauge, catheter length, and nurse's initials.			
25. Set flow rate according to prescribed rate.			
26. Observe and monitor for infiltration.			
27. Place IV pole on same side of bed as IV site.			
28. Record procedure in patient medical record according to agency policy.			

Study Questions

1. Veins commonly used for peripheral IV therapy include the following:
   a. Basilic, cephalic, femoral
   b. Basilic, cephalic, metacarpal
   c. Cephalic, cubital, basilic
   d. Cubital, basilic, metacarpal

2. When selecting a vein to start an IV infusion, all the following are true *except:*
   a. Use proximal veins first.
   b. Avoid areas of flexion.
   c. Catheter size should be based upon size of vein.
   d. Blood flow around a catheter is an important consideration.

3. Which of the following is characteristic of veins?
   a. Blood flows away from the heart.
   b. A single vein supplies a given area.
   c. Blood return is rapid.
   d. Valves are present at points of branching.

4. The anatomic location of the basilic vein is the:
   a. Radial side of forearm
   b. Lateral aspect of forearm
   c. Ulnar side of forearm
   d. Antecubital area of the forearm

5. Clinical features that distinguish basilic veins from cephalic veins include that basilic veins are:
   a. Found on the radial side of the forearm, are larger, and curve more on the ascent up the arm
   b. Found on the ulnar side of the forearm, are smaller, and run up the anterior side of the arm
   c. Found on the radial side of the forearm, are larger, and ascend along outer region of the arm
   d. Found on the ulnar side of the forearm, are larger, and run up the posterior or back of the arm

6. Considerations for IV catheter selection include:
   a. Selecting the longest catheter with a larger gauge
   b. Selecting the longest catheter with the smallest gauge

    c. Selecting the shortest catheter with a larger gauge

    d. Selecting the shortest catheter with the smallest gauge

7. Successful venipuncture tips for patients who are in shock or who have minimal venous return include:

    a. Selecting a 14- to 16-gauge catheter; releasing the tourniquet to promote venous relaxation

    b. Selecting a 16-to 18-gauge catheter; leaving the tourniquet in place to promote venous distension

    c. Selecting a 18- to 20-gauge catheter; releasing the tourniquet to promote venous relaxation

    d. Selecting a 20- to 22-gauge catheter; leaving the tourniquet in place to promote venous distension

8. Nursing interventions for infection (cellulitis, purulent drainage) at a venipuncture site include:

    a. Culturing the drainage after removing the catheter; sending the catheter in a sterile container for analysis

    b. Culturing the drainage before removing the catheter; sending the catheter in a sterile container for analysis

    c. Culturing the drainage during removal of the catheter; sending the catheter in a sterile container for analysis

    d. Culturing the drainage before and after removal of the catheter; sending the catheter in a sterile container for analysis

9. Common practice for a scheduled frequency of venipuncture site rotation includes:

    a. A new site every 24 hours

    b. A new site every 48 hours

    c. A new site every 72 hours

    d. A new site every 96 hours

10. All the following information should be documented on the IV site dressing *except:*

    a. Name of specific vein

    b. Catheter or needle gauge.

    c. Date and time of the procedure

    d. Initials of nurse who started the IV infusion

Answers   1. b   2. a   3. d   4. c   5. d   6. c
7. a   8. b   9. c   10. a

Central Venous Catheters

3

Objectives

1. Compare and contrast the types and features of central venous access devices.

2. Describe techniques for maintenance of central venous access devices: heparinization, dressing, and blood sampling.

3. Identify the major complications associated with central venous access devices: air embolus, fibrin sheath, occlusion, sepsis, and superior vena cava syndrome.

4. Discuss issues to be considered in patient/device selection.

5. Summarize the patient and family education needs associated with daily, weekly, and/or monthly maintenance of central venous access devices.

Long-term venous access without repeated venipuncture is required for many patients with various medical diagnoses. Catheters, implantable ports, or both may be placed for continuous or intermittent infusions, simultaneous infusion of incompatible drugs, administration of viscous or high-volume fluids or blood products, blood sampling, parenteral nutrition, apheresis, hemodialysis, central venous pressure monitoring, or high-flow administration in trauma or urgent situations. Central venous access devices are commonly used to administer fluids for hydration and medications such as antimicrobials, analgesics, chemotherapy, and thrombolytic agents.

In clinical practice settings such as acute care, ambulatory care, clinics, extended care, and home care, the nurse is primarily responsible for drug or fluid administration, monitoring of the venous access and infusate, and the patient. Nurses involved with the care of venous access devices must be able to recognize complications and initiate appropriate interventions. Procedures for care and maintenance of the device may vary from agency to agency, and the numerous central venous access devices now available are posing additional challenges. Therefore safe and prudent nursing care is necessary to ensure successful catheter/port use and longevity. (See Table 3-1 for types and characteristics of central venous catheters.)

Text continued on p. 58

Table 3-1   Central venous catheters

Types of Catheters	Characteristics
Subclavian catheter: single and multilumen (dual-, triple-, or quadruple-lumen catheters available)	Short-term use (<60 days)
	Polyurethane and Silastic material
	Added mechanical barrier available
	VitaCuff or SureCuff with antimicrobial activity, placed at or near insertion site
	Catheters with new antiseptic surface; for example, antimicrobial agents silver-sulfadiazine and chlorhexidine, both antimicrobial agents, reduce incidence of catheter-related infection
	Sutured in place
	Volume 0.5 to 0.6 ml/lumen
	Sterile dressing required for duration of catheter placement
	Allows simultaneous administration of potentially incompatible medication and fluids (applies to the multilumen catheter only)
	Requires heparinization of each lumen every 12 hours
	Can be repaired if damaged

Continued

Table 3-1   Central venous catheters—cont'd

Types of Catheters	Characteristics

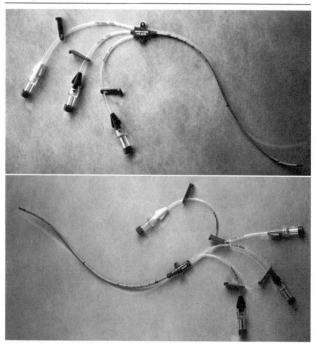

Multilumen subclavian catheters.
(Courtesy Arrow International, Reading, Pa.)

Tunneled catheters: single, dual, or triple lumen, such as Hickman and Broviac catheters	Long-term use (1-2 years)
	Silastic material
	Subcutaneously tunneled in place
	Dacron cuff
	Volume 1.8 ml/lumen uncut adult catheter
	Sterile environment until exit site healed (usually 14-21 days); dressing optional
	Requires scheduled flushings with heparinized saline when not in use
	Repair kits available

Table 3-1   Central venous catheters—cont'd

Types of Catheters	Characteristics

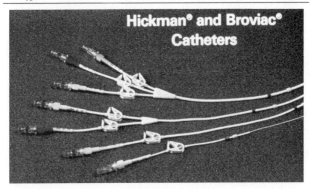

Hickman and Broviac catheters.
(Courtesy Bard Access Systems Inc., Salt Lake City, Utah.)

Types of Catheters	Characteristics
Central venous catheter with three-position valve and closed distal tip, such as Groshong catheter	Same as tunneled catheter except it requires scheduled flushings with normal saline when not in use *Note:* Always vigorously flush the Groshong catheter; do not clamp catheter following flushing Repair kits available

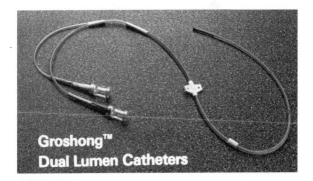

Groshong dual-lumen catheter.
(Courtesy Bard Access Systems Inc., Salt Lake City, Utah.)

Continued

Table 3-1 Central venous catheters—cont'd

Types of Catheters	Characteristics

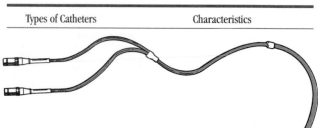

Types of Catheters	Characteristics
Implantable ports: venous placement single and dual lumen	Long-term use (1-2 years)
	Metal (stainless steel or titanium) or plastic portal chamber with silicone septum connected to Silastic/silicone catheter
	Self-sealing dense silicone septum allows up to 2000 punctures
	Portal chamber sutured and catheter tunneled in place
	Requires Huber needle in place for port access
	Volume 2 ml port and lumen (adult)
	Maintain sterile environment when port accessed; change Huber needle and extension at least every 5-7 days when port is accessed for continuous infusion therapy
	Port requires at least monthly heparinization
	Minimal self-care requirements
	Nurse and patient instructional material available from manufacturers
	Does not require a dressing when not in use

Continued

Table 3-1   Central venous catheters—cont'd

Types of Catheters	Characteristics

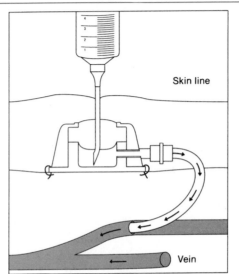

Cross-section of implantable port with needle access.
(Courtesy SIMS Deltec, Inc., St. Paul, Minn.)

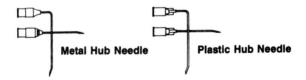

Huber needles.
(Courtesy SIMS Deltec, Inc., St. Paul, Minn.)

CLINICAL ALERT: The implantable port is also available for epidural, intraarterial, and intraperitoneal placement. Administer IV fluids only through the *venous* port. Use other sites only for infusions of medications or fluids specific to that placement site. Be sure to check the product information accompanying each port for instructions and use (Fig. 3-1).

Continued

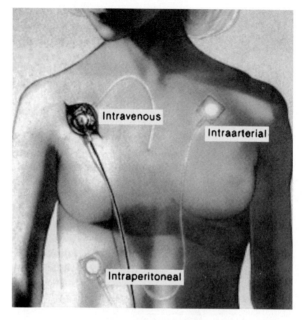

Fig. 3-1
Placement of IV, intraarterial, and intraperitoneal ports.
(Courtesy SIMS Deltec, Inc., St. Paul, Minn.)

Table 3-1 Central venous catheters—cont'd

Types of Catheters	Characteristics
Peripheral venous assess system: PAS port (Fig. 3-2)	Long-term use (1-2 years)
	Titanium portal chamber with silicone system connects to Silastic catheter
	Self-sealing silicone septum allows up to 2000 punctures
CathLink 20 (Fig. 3-3)	May be implanted in the chest or forearm
	System portal usually implanted under the skin in forearm or chest; catheter inserted into major arm vein until tip positioned in superior vena cava and then connected to the portal

Continued

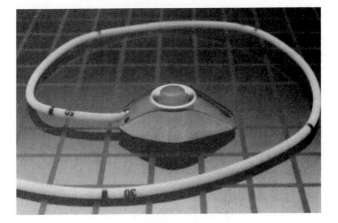

Fig. 3-2
Peripheral implantable venous access system port.
(Courtesy SIMS Deltec, Inc., St. Paul, Minn.)

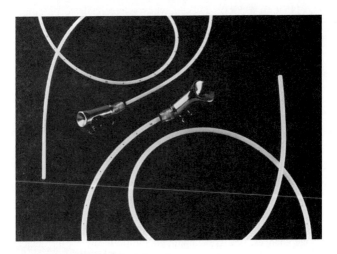

Fig. 3-3
Cath Link 20.
(Courtesy Bard Access Systems Inc., Salt Lake City, Utah.)

Table 3-1   Central venous catheters—cont'd

Types of Catheters	Characteristics
CathLink 20—cont'd	Requires 20- to 22-gauge ½-inch Huber needle to access PAS port; may be accessed via over-the-needle IV catheter (minimum 20-gauge; 1¾-inch length) into the funnel-shaped entrance until resistance is felt; catheter advanced into port while needle simultaneously withdrawn
	Volume 1-2 ml port and lumen (adult)
	Maintain sterile environment when port accessed
	Port requires at least monthly heparinization
	Minimal self-care requirements
	Nurse and patient instructional material available from manufacturer
	Does not require dressing when not in use

CLINICAL ALERT: *Do not* withdraw blood from or infuse medication into the arm in which the implant is located unless you are using the portal. Otherwise, an inadvertent puncture of the catheter could occur, which may result in catheter damage. Do not attempt to measure the patient's blood pressure on the arm in which a peripheral catheter has been placed, because catheter occlusion or other damage to the catheter could occur.

Device Selection

Selection of the vascular access device requires a collaborative effort with input from the physician, nurse, pharmacist, patient, and caregiver. Because many devices are now available, the type, purpose, and duration of therapy need to be considered.

In addition, patient considerations with regard to lifestyle, body image changes, and most important, ability to care for the device need to be a part of the decision process. The patient should be counseled about the following: job function/duties (e.g., clean working environment or environment with a potential for infection); recreational activities (e.g., hunting) (avoid portal septum placement on the side of the chest that receives pressure from a weapon), swimming, or contact sports; hand or arm dominance to assess the patient's ability to self-care for the catheter/device; and body image changes regarding clothing type and style preferences. Financial implications of the device choice are also an important consideration (e.g., total cost of the device and the placement procedure; cost of supplies used in maintenance functions; and costs related to ongoing therapy).

Catheter and Implantable Port Composition

Catheters and implantable ports have become more versatile in their composition and design. The material selected for a catheter or port often depends on the type of the device and insertion procedure for that catheter or port. Polyurethane is commonly used for short-term percutaneously placed catheters. It is a material stiff enough to allow percutaneous insertion that then softens after insertion in response to body temperature. The softening makes the catheter more biocompatible once placed within the vein. In addition, polyurethane has a tensile strength that permits the catheter to be constructed with thinner walls and smaller external diameters. This decreases the volume of foreign material within the vein. A polyurethane catheter is now available (Arrowguard, Arrow International, Reading, Penn). This catheter has been bonded with colonization-resistant surface-treated antiseptic agents, silver sulfadiazine and chlorhexidine, along the entire indwelling length of the catheter. A randomized, comparative trial of 405 central venous catheters showed that catheters with an antiseptic-treated surface were two times less likely to be colonized and four times less likely to produce catheter-related bloodstream infection than were noncoated catheters.

Most tunneled central venous catheters and implantable port catheter lumens are constructed of Silastic or other silicone material. Other features available are bonding of the anticoagulant agent heparin on the catheter lumen surface; a patented, three-position, pressure-sensitive Groshong valve located at the catheter tip; and a Dacron Cuff/SureCuff/VitaCuff/Vita Guard attached to a specific portion of the catheter and designed to provide protection against infections related to vascular access devices.

Implantable ports contain a reservoir that leads to the catheter and a self-sealing silicone septum for access to the reservoir. The reservoirs may be composed of titanium, plastic, stainless steel, or a combination of these materials. The various ports differ in size and profile, single- or dual-lumen structure, place of implantation, and port access (Fig. 3-4). Most implantable ports have septums that lie perpendicular to the skin so that they may be accessed from the top with a Huber needle. The CathLink 20 (see Fig. 3-3) implanted port has a patented funnel-shaped entrance for port access and uses a standard over-the-needle intravenous (IV) catheter (minimum length ¾ inch).

Many low-profile peripherally inserted implantable ports are available for various infusate therapies. These low-profile portal septums are usually implanted in the patient's forearm. Although peripherally inserted and placed implantable ports have the advantage of placement in an ambulatory care or clinic setting versus the conventional chest-placed devices, their use for blood sampling and blood product infusions is limited.

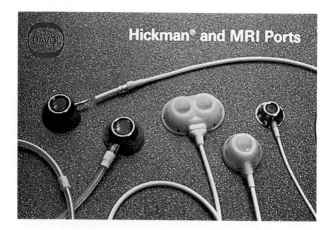

Fig. 3-4
Hickman and MRI ports.
(Courtesy Bard Access Systems Inc., Salt Lake City, Utah.)

Insertion

A physician usually performs catheter insertion using a local anesthetic. Sterile technique is maintained during the procedure. The catheter is inserted via percutaneous placement or a venous cutdown procedure. It is then threaded into the subclavian or jugular vein or the superior vena cava. A subcutaneous tunneling procedure or suturing of the catheter is used to secure catheter placement. Before administration of IV fluids or drugs, a catheter-imaging radiograph is recommended to confirm catheter/port tip placement.

For the CathLink 20, the system portal is usually implanted under the skin in the patient's forearm or chest. The catheter is inserted into a major arm vein or subclavian vein until the tip is positioned in the superior vena cava. The catheter is then connected to the portal, providing venous access.

WARNING: System flushing recommendations are 10 ml of normal saline after infusion of medication and 20 ml of normal saline after infusion of blood, total parenteral nutrition (TPN), or known incompatible medications.

Hemodialysis and Apheresis Catheters

Apheresis catheters are specifically designed for prolonged vascular access for hemodialysis, harvesting peripheral blood stem cells, or apheresis therapy via the jugular or subclavian vein. Occasionally, these catheters are placed in the femoral vein. The catheters are composed of polyurethane, Silastic material, or a combination of both; they may have a Dacron Cuff to facilitate tissue growth and are inserted similarly to the way venous access tunneled catheters are inserted. Hemodialysis/apheresis catheters are divided into two separate lumens by a septum, allowing a blood exchange process (Fig. 3-5). The catheter lumen is usually 12 to 14 gauge to allow for exceptional pressurized flow rates (300 to 400 ml/min) or high-volume viscous infusion/apheresis.

Care and maintenance of hemodialysis and apheresis catheters include the following:

1. A physician directive that the catheter is not to be used for any purpose other than the prescribed therapy.
2. Sterile technique for access and site care.
3. Daily monitoring of the catheter integrity and exit site.

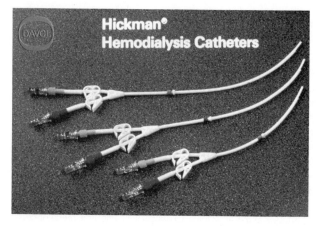

Fig. 3-5
Hickman hemodialysis catheters.
(Courtesy Bard Access Systems Inc., Salt Lake City, Utah.)

4. Maintenance of catheter patency between therapies by the creation of a heparin lock in each lumen of the catheter.
   a. Inject 5000 units of heparin/ml into each lumen, *equal* to the priming volume of each lumen (e.g., arterial volume is 1.3 ml; venous volume is 1.4 ml). *The volume of heparin may vary according to catheter design, lumen gauge, and prescribed patient therapy.*
   b. Ensure that each lumen is totally filled, then vigorously inject the flush solution and clamp the extension tubing while exerting positive pressure (e.g., maintain your thumb on the syringe plunger as you withdraw the syringe/needleless device from the extension tubing).
   c. Attach a sterile injection cap to each clamping extension.
   CLINICAL ALERT: The heparin solution must be aspirated out of both lumens immediately before use of the catheter to prevent systemic heparinization of the patient.

Critical Elements of Nursing Management of Central Venous Catheters
Aseptic Technique

Strict aseptic technique is required to maintain venous integrity and to prevent serious infection. A needleless, Luer-Lok injection cap is used to provide a sterile closed system when the catheter/port is not directly connected to IV tubing. This cap must fit securely to prevent any air embolus, contamination, or loss of blood. All tubing, needleless junctions, or injection caps must be prepared with povidone-iodine before syringe or IV tubing insertion to prevent introduction of microorganisms into the catheter.

Infection Control

Nursing management of central vascular devices encompasses many patients with the potential for multiple infectious diseases and/or complications. The nurse is the primary person who accesses the devices, obtains blood samples, and infuses the drugs or fluids and therefore has a high risk for a blood-related injury from contaminated devices. Recommendations for nurses' protection against infection include disposing of syringes or blood-contaminated injection caps and tubings into puncture-resistant containers, wearing gloves during catheter management procedures such as blood sampling, and washing hands thoroughly and immediately after accidental contamination with blood.

Catheter Maintenance Procedures and Guidelines

Catheter maintenance procedures may vary according to the specified patient therapy, clinical practice setting, and individual manufacturer's recommendations. Heparinization of venous access devices varies in heparin solution concentration, volume, scheduled frequency, type of catheter/port, and patient's age, weight, and specified therapy. The nurse should consult with the physician managing the patient's care and the agency for the nursing management protocol regarding heparinization of central venous catheters/implantable ports. For the patient with an alteration in coagulation factors or heparin allergy/intolerance, the nurse should consider the frequency of the intermittent device use. These patients may require a low concentration (e.g., 10 units of heparin/ml) or alternative flushing solution (e.g., sodium citrate 1.4% solution).

The specific protocol for each device should be consulted before use. Tables 3-2 and 3-3 summarize the recommended nursing management for central venous catheters for adults and children, respectively. The suggestions outlined thereafter are within the guidelines of requirements for each product.

Site Care

1. Site cleansing: All preparation solutions should be applied with friction, working outward from the insertion site. Typical products used include povidone-iodine with three swabs, 70% isopropyl alcohol with three swabs, and hydrogen peroxide to remove crusting. Alternative products include chlorhexidine in place of povidone-iodine or application of ointment to the site at the physician's discretion.
2. Change the gauze dressing every 24 hours.
3. Change the Bioclusive dressing every 3 to 5 days or more frequently to maintain an occlusive seal. Consider the moisture permeability of dressing. Consider the patient's status (e.g., diaphoresis, secretions, and myelosuppression).
4. With all types of dressings, the dressing should be changed in conjunction with any extension set change. Dressings should be adapted to catheter location (e.g., jugular vein catheter site). Consideration should be given to the use of sterile gloves and mask when performing dressing changes (e.g., to prevent catheter/port infection or patient myelosuppression).
5. Coil a tunneled catheter and tape it securely to the skin when the catheter is not in use.

Cap Change (Depends on the Frequency of Catheter Access)

1. Change the cap on a subclavian catheter every 72 to 96 hours.
2. Change the cap on a tunneled catheter every 72 to 96 hours or every 7 days in the home care setting.
3. Change caps when rubber coring occurs.
4. Change the cap at the time of dressing change or catheter heparinization.

Huber Needle and Tubing Change for Implantable Port

1. Change the sterile needle and tubing for each new bolus access.
2. Change the sterile needle and tubing for continuous infusion every 5 to 7 days.

Text continued on p. 71

Table 3-2   Adult central venous catheters: recommended nursing management

Type	Heparinization	Dressing	Blood Sampling
Central Venous Catheters			
Short-term use			
Subclavian			
Single lumen	After each use, flush *each* lumen with 5 ml normal saline (NS) then heparinized saline 2 ml (100 units/ml). For catheter *NOT* in use, flush each lumen with heparinized saline 2 ml (100 units/ml) every 12 hr.	Daily sterile dressing change at the site for duration of catheter placement. Change Luer-Lok injection caps every 72-96 hr.	Shut off all IVs for 1-3 min. Withdraw 5 ml blood. Discard. Withdraw blood sample. Flush lumen with 5 ml NS, then heparinize or resume IV. *For TPN:* Shut off IV for 10 min.
Dual lumen			
Triple lumen			
Long-term use			
Tunneled catheters	After each use, flush *each* lumen with 5 ml NS, then heparinized saline 2 ml (100 units/ml). For catheter *NOT* in use, flush each lumen with heparinized saline 2 ml (100 units/ml) daily/biweekly.	Daily sterile dressing change at the exit site for initial 14-21 days. Thereafter, cleanse exit site daily (Betadine/alcohol). Apply clean dressing. Change Luer-Lok injection caps weekly.	Shut off IVs for 1-3 min. Withdraw 5 ml blood. Discard. Withdraw blood sample. Flush lumen with 5 ml NS, then heparinize or resume IV. *For TPN:* Shut off IV for 10 min.
Single, dual, and triple lumens			
Hickman			
Quinton			
Raaf			

Continued

Table 3-2   Adult central venous catheters: recommended nursing management—cont'd

Type	Heparinization	Dressing	Blood Sampling
Long-term use—cont'd			
Groshong			
Single lumen Dual lumen Triple lumen	Does not require heparin to maintain* catheter patency. Use force when flushing. Flush each lumen with 5 ml NS after each use—except for TPN, then flush with 30 ml NS. For catheter *NOT* in use, flush with 5 ml NS weekly.	Daily sterile dressing change at the exit site for initial 14-21 days. Thereafter, cleanse exit site daily (Betadine/alcohol). Apply clean dressing. Change Luer-Lok injection caps weekly.	Shut off all IVs for 1-3 min. Withdraw 5 ml blood. Discard. Withdraw blood sample. Flush lumen with 30 ml NS *vigorously*, then resume IV or apply injection cap. *For TPN:* Shut off IV for 10 min.
Implantable Vascular Access Devices			
Davol Port Infuse-A-Port Life Port Omega Port Port-A-Cath	After each use, flush *each* port with Huber needle—10 ml NS, followed by 3-10 ml heparinized saline (100 units/ml).*† For port *NOT* in use, flush *each* port with 3-10 ml heparinized saline (100 units/ml) every 30 days (venous placement).‡	Sterile Bioclusive dressing when port accessed. Sterile strips at new incision site for 3 days. When incision site is healed and port is not accessed, no dressing is required. Change Huber needle access tubing every 5-7 days for continuous access of port.	Shut off all IVs for 1-3 min. Withdraw 5 ml blood. Discard. Withdraw blood sample. Flush with 20 ml NS, followed by 3-10 ml heparinized saline (100 units/ml)* or resume IV. *For TPN:* Shut off IV for 10 min.

Peripherally Inserted Catheter

Longline PICC§	After each use, flush lumen with 2 ml NS, then 1 ml heparinized saline (100 units/ml). For catheter *NOT* in use, flush lumen with 1 ml heparinized saline (100 units/ml) every 12 hr.	Sterile dressing change after first 24 hr, then every 72 hr. Change Luer-Lok injection caps every 72-96 hr.	Shut off all IVs for 1-3 min. Withdraw 2-3 ml blood. Discard. Withdraw blood sample. Flush lumen with 2-5 ml NS; then heparinize or resume IV. *For TPN:* Shut off IV for 10 min.

*Some oncologists use 2 to 5 ml of heparinized saline (100 units/ml).

†Check manufacturer's specific recommendations regarding volume. Oncologists use 10 ml of heparin (100 units/ml).

‡Assess patient, disease, and platelet count with frequency/volume/concentration of heparinization schedule.

§Use 5 ml or larger syringes when flushing and/or blood sampling from PICCs.

Table 3-3 Pediatric central venous catheters: recommended nursing management

Type	Heparinization	Dressing	Blood Sampling
Central Venous Catheters			
Short-term use			
Subclavian	After each use, flush *each* lumen with 2 ml normal saline (NS), followed by 1 ml heparinized saline solution (10 units/ml), after each use or at least bid.	Daily sterile dressing change at site for duration of catheter placement. Gauze dressing change every 24 hr. Change Luer-Lok injection caps every 24 hr.	Shut off all IVs for 1-3 min. Withdraw 3 ml blood. Discard. Withdraw blood sample. Flush lumen with 2 ml NS, then heparinize or resume IV. *For TPN:* Shut off IV for 10 min.
Single lumen			
Multilumen			
Long-term use			
Tunneled catheter	After each use, flush the lumen with 2 ml NS, then 1 ml heparinized saline (10 units/ml). For catheter *NOT* in use, flush the lumen with 1 ml heparinized saline (10 units/ml) daily.	Daily sterile dressing change at the exit site for initial 14 days. Gauze dressing change every 24 hr. Thereafter, cleanse exit site daily with Betadine. Apply sterile 2×2 gauze dressing. Change Luer-Lok injection caps weekly.	Shut off all IVs for 1-3 min. Withdraw 3 ml blood. Discard. Withdraw blood sample. Flush lumen with 2 ml NS, then heparinize or resume IV. *For TPN:* Shut off IV for 10 min.
Broviac			

Implantable Vascular Access Devices

Port-A-Cath

After each use, flush the port with Huber needle—5 ml NS followed by 2 ml heparinized saline (100 units/ml). For port *NOT* in use, flush port with 2 ml heparinized saline (100 units/ml) every 30 days (venous placement).

Sterile Bioclusive dressing when port accessed. Sterile strips at new incision site for 3 days. When incision site is healed and port is not accessed, no dressing is required. When port is accessed for continuous infusion, change needle and extension tubing every 5-7 days.

Shut off all IVs for 1-3 min. Withdraw 3-5 ml blood (depending on size of child). Discard. Withdraw blood sample. Flush with 5 ml NS, then heparinize or resume IV. *For TPN:* Shut off IV for 10 min.

Peripherally Inserted Catheter

Longline PICC
Single lumen
Dual lumen
(Use gentle pressure on syringe plunger for PICCs)

Use 3-5 ml or larger syringe. After each use, flush lumen. *For pediatrics:* 2 ml NS in 5-ml syringe or larger, followed by 1 ml heparinized saline (10 units/ml) after each use or at least bid.

Sterile dressing change after first 24 hr, then every 72-96 hr. Change Luer-Lok injection caps every 72 hr.

Shut off all IVs for 1-3 min. Withdraw 1-2 ml blood. Discard. Withdraw blood sample. Flush lumen with 2.5 ml NS, then heparinize or resume IV. *For TPN:* Shut off IV for 10 min.

Continued

Table 3-3   Pediatric central venous catheters: recommended nursing management—cont'd

Type	Heparinization	Dressing	Blood Sampling
	For special care nursery (neonates): 0.5 ml NS, preservative free, in 5-ml syringe or larger, followed by 0.5 ml heparinized saline (4 units/ml). Intermittent flush schedules every 4-8 hr—consult physician orders.		

Blood Sampling

1. To ensure a pure blood sample from multilumen catheters, *turn off all IV fluids for 1 to 3 minutes* (TPN solutions, 10 minutes) before withdrawing blood or discarding fluid.
2. The recommended discard for laboratory samples should equal three times the volume of each catheter lumen (for most adult catheter lumens, approximately 1 ml/lumen); therefore the blood discard will range from 2 to 5 ml for all the adult central venous catheters.
3. Obtain laboratory samples with a Vacutainer or syringe.
4. Immediately flush the catheter lumen with normal saline or heparin solution.
5. Resume previous catheter function or heparin lock on the device. Note specific instructions on blood sampling for a peripheral PAS port and CathLink 20.

Heparinization

The heparin volume, solution concentration, and scheduled frequency of heparinization vary with the catheter/port, lumen size, and patient's age, weight, and specified therapy.

Volume

1. The volume of the heparinized saline flush should be equal to two times the volume capacity of the catheter lumen/implantable port.
2. Use between 1 and 2 ml per catheter/lumen (child) for a tunneled catheter and implantable port.
3. Use approximately 2 ml per catheter/lumen (adult) for tunneled and subclavian catheters and peripherally inserted central catheters (PICC) lines.
4. Use approximately 5 ml for an implantable port (adult).

NOTE: The amount of heparin and the frequency of flush should be such that the patient's clotting factors are not altered. It is helpful to standardize the heparin volume and concentrations used to flush the various central venous access devices to decrease confusion in trying to remember the flushing protocol for each device. Fig. 3-6 shows a sample of a physician's orders for an adult standard flush protocol.

DATE	TIME	PHYSICIAN ORDER SET	NOTE: specify route of administration on Medication Orders
		Generic or therapeutic substitutions (as deemed appropriate by the Pharmacy and Therapeutics Committee) may be made unless the physician writes "NO SUBSTITUTION" on EACH medication order.	

☐ OUTPATIENT PROCEDURE   ☐ OBSERVE AS OUTPATIENT   ☐ ADMIT AS INPATIENT

DOES NOT APPLY TO HEMODIALYSIS CATHETERS

ADULT STANDARD FLUSH PROTOCOL ORDERS

Per physician discretion, Normal Saline or low dose heparin (eg. 10u/ml) is indicated for a flush when intermittent medications are administered more than qid and a continuous infusion is not maintaining the patency. 1.4% Sodium Citrate solution is an alternative to heparin in the following situations: Heparin Allergy or Intolerance; Heparin Induced Thrombocytopenia; Leukemic Patients with low platelet counts, eg. 20,000 or less.

(Check the box indicating the appropriate Protocol.)

1. **Peripheral IV Lock:**
    ☐ 2ml Normal Saline after each use or at least q-12 hours. 8am-8pm.
2. **Peripheral Inserted Long Line Catheter: (circle type)**   Single lumen   Dual lumen
    (circle lumen gauge)   23ga   20ga   19ga   18ga   16ga   other
    ☐ 2ml Normal Saline (5ml syringe or larger) followed by 1 ml heparin 100u/ml in <u>each</u> lumen after each use or at least q 12 hours. 8am-8pm
    (See Standard Flush Protocol Orders for Sodium Citrate if Indicated.)
3. **Central Venous Catheter:** (circle type)   Single lumen   Dual lumen   Triple lumen   Quad lumen
    (circle type)   Hickman   Quinton-Raff   Subclavian   Other: _____
    (circle hub color)   white   red   blue   brown   grey   other
    ☐ 5ml Normal Saline followed by 2ml heparin 100u/ml in <u>each</u> lumen after each use or at least daily for catheter not in use. 8am. (<u>Arrow Subclavian Catheter</u> - Flush each lumen q 12 hours. 8am-8pm)
    (See Standard Flush Protocol Orders for Sodium Citrate if Indicated.)

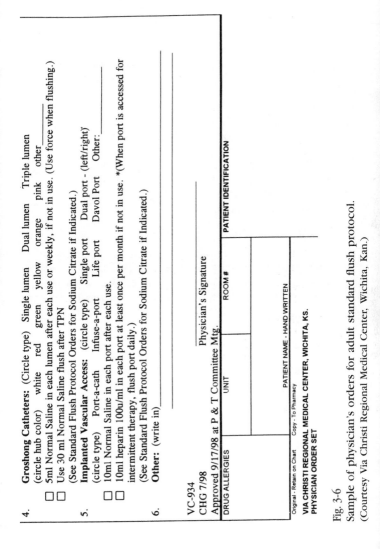

4. **Groshong Catheters:** (Circle type)   Single lumen   Dual lumen   Triple lumen
    (circle hub color)   white   red   green   yellow   orange   pink   other _____
    ☐ 5ml Normal Saline in each lumen after each use or weekly, if not in use. (Use force when flushing.)
    ☐ Use 30 ml Normal Saline flush after TPN
    (See Standard Flush Protocol Orders for Sodium Citrate if Indicated.)

5. **Implanted Vascular Access:** (circle type)   Single port   Dual port - (left/right)
    (circle type)   Port-a-cath   Infuse-a-port   Life port   Davol Port   Other: _____
    ☐ 10ml Normal Saline in each port after each use.
    ☐ 10ml heparin 100u/ml in each port at least once per month if not in use. *(When port is accessed for
    intermittent therapy, flush port daily.)
    (See Standard Flush Protocol Orders for Sodium Citrate if Indicated.)

6. **Other:** (write in) _____

VC-934
CHG 7/98
Approved 9/17/98 at P & T Committee Mtg.

_____
Physician's Signature

DRUG ALLERGIES	UNIT	ROOM #	PATIENT IDENTIFICATION

PATIENT NAME - HAND WRITTEN

Original - Retain on Chart   Copy - To Pharmacy

VIA CHRISTI REGIONAL MEDICAL CENTER, WICHITA, KS.
PHYSICIAN ORDER SET

Fig. 3-6
Sample of physician's orders for adult standard flush protocol.
(Courtesy Via Christi Regional Medical Center, Wichita, Kan.)

Concentration of heparin (10 to 1000 units/ml)

1. Per physician discretion, normal saline or low-dose heparin (e.g., 10 units/ml) is indicated for heparinization when intermittent medications are administered more than four times daily and a continuous infusion is not maintaining line patency. Sodium citrate 1.4% solution is an alternative to heparin for patients with heparin allergy or intolerance, heparin-induced thrombocytopenia, or low platelet counts (e.g., 20,000/mm^3 or less).

2. Individualized adjustments in the solution concentration for heparinization are indicated for pediatric patients who approach adult sizes (e.g., 50 kg).

Frequency

1. Subclavian catheters and PICC lines: every 12 to 24 hours
2. Tunneled catheters: daily to weekly
3. Implantable ports: monthly

Heparin lock

To ensure a heparin lock, maintain a positive pressure (keep a forward motion on the syringe plunger as needleless is removed from cap or port) while injecting the heparin solution into the catheter to prevent a backflow of blood into the catheter tip.

Catheter Repair

Most subclavian and tunneled catheters have product repair kits designated by the manufacturer.

1. Obtain the recommended repair kit specific to the lumen gauge of the catheter (Fig. 3-7).
2. Maintain a sterile environment during the catheter repair procedure.
3. Clamp the desired catheter lumen to be repaired before cutting or splicing the lumen.
4. Follow the manufacturer's guidelines for inserting the new lumen link or connector and repairing the catheter step by step.
   a. Use of adhesive product
   b. Cutting of the damaged catheter
   c. Use of a splicing device
   d. Use of suture material
   e. Use of protective splice material

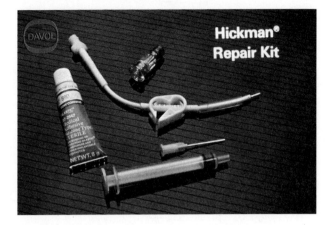

Fig. 3-7
Hickman repair kit.
(Courtesy Bard Access Systems Inc., Salt Lake City, Utah.)

    f. Splinting and stabilization of the catheter repair section
    g. Limitations on catheter use after repair
  5. Use caution when cementing the new catheter lumen connector; for example, avoid getting the cement inside the catheter lumen.
  6. Flush the repaired catheter lumen with heparinized saline solution per physician request.
    Note: Some tunneled catheter repair kits have restrictions limiting use of the repaired catheter lumen for 8 to 24 hours after catheter repair.
  7. Document the catheter repair procedure results in the patient's medical record.

Accessing an Implantable Port

Because the portal septum is located beneath the skin surface, the specific boundaries for each device and the resilience of the silicone septum need to be known before needle access. This procedure requires aseptic technique using sterile supplies.
  1. Wash hands and apply gloves.
  2. Cleanse the portal site with povidone-iodine swabs, starting over the portal and moving outward in a spiral motion to cover an area 5 inches wide.

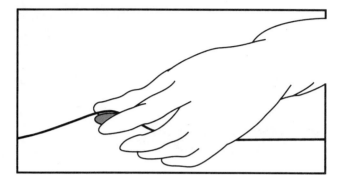

Fig. 3-8
Palpating the implantable port.
(Courtesy SIMS Deltec, Inc., St. Paul, Minn.)

3. Attach tubing with a Huber needle to a syringe filled with saline.
4. Locate the portal septum by palpation (Fig. 3-8).
5. Insert the needle perpendicular to the septum and push it slowly but firmly through the skin and portal septum until it comes to rest at the bottom of the portal chamber.
6. Aspirate for a blood return; flush the system with normal saline to confirm that fluid flows through the system (Fig. 3-9).
   a. Note any unusual resistance to flow or any swelling around the injection site. Either may be a sign of insufficient needle penetration, incorrect needle placement, catheter blockage, or a leaking portal system, catheter, or connection. During all syringe or tubing connections and disconnections, ensure *clamping of extension tubing* to prevent occurrence of an air embolus.
   b. For bolus injection of medication, remove the empty saline syringe, replace it with the drug-filled syringe, and administer the medication. At the completion of the

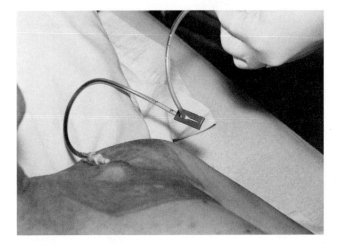

Fig. 3-9
Aspirating blood return.
(From Perry AG, Potter PA: *Clinical nursing skills and techniques,*
ed 4, St Louis, 1998, Mosby.)

injection, flush the catheter with normal saline and then
heparin lock the device while withdrawing the needle
from the portal septum (Fig. 3-10).

c. For a continuous infusion, remove the empty saline
syringe, replace it with IV infusion tubing, and secure
the tubing. Because the Huber needle remains in the
portal chamber during the infusion, secure the needle
to prevent inadvertent dislodgment by placing a 2×2
gauze dressing underneath the needle and applying
antibacterial ointment around the needle site. Finally,
apply a semipermeable occlusive dressing over the
entire area. Secure extension tubing to minimize needle
dislodgment (Fig. 3-11).

CLINICAL ALERT: Use the Huber needle at a 90-degree bend
for continuous infusion. Use only a 20- to 22-gauge ½-inch
90-degree bend needle to access the peripherally inserted ports of
the PAS port system.

Table 3-4 provides troubleshooting tips and Table 3-5 lists
potential complications.

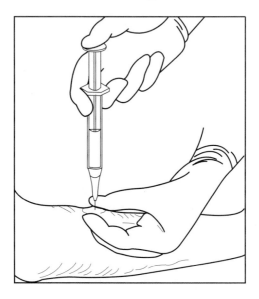

Fig. 3-10
Bolus injection into an implantable port.
(Courtesy SIMS Deltec, Inc., St. Paul, Minn.)

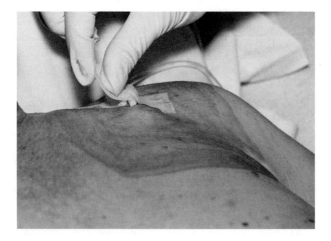

Fig. 3-11
Securing a Huber needle.
(From Perry AG, Potter PA: *Clinical nursing skills and techniques*,
ed 4, St Louis, 1998, Mosby.)

◎ Table 3-4   Troubleshooting tips—central venous catheters

Nursing Assessment	Nursing Interventions
Deeply implanted port	Note portal chamber scar.
Unable to palpate port	Use deep palpation technique or seek assistance of second person to locate port.
Do not feel needle stop against portal chamber	Use 1½- or 2-inch Huber needle.
Unable to obtain blood return	Try to change catheter alignment by raising the patient's arm on same side as catheter.
	Roll the patient to opposite side.
	Ask the patient to cough, sit up, and take a deep breath.
	Try infusing 10 ml of normal saline into catheter.
	Reaccess catheter or implantable port with new sterile needle.
Unable to inject fluid or medication	Follow steps to obtain blood return.
	If unable to inject fluid or obtain blood return, notify physician.
	Determine catheter placement by radiographic examination.

Documentation Recommendations

- Daily assessment of port or exit site, skin or catheter integrity, and catheter placement
- Procedure access for each catheter or device
- Heparinization or normal saline flush—drug, concentration, dose, volume, date, and time
- Injection cap or extension tubing changes
- Site care management
- Patency of catheter, blood sampling, and infusion of medications or fluids
- Patient symptoms related to catheter malfunction or potential complications associated with central venous catheter
- Patient and family education regarding understanding (verbalized or return demonstration) of device selection and insertion and catheter/port self-care management

Text continued on p. 86

Table 3-5 Potential complications—central venous catheters

Nursing Assessments	Nursing Interventions
Air Embolus	
May occur during connections or disconnections of syringes and IV tubing	Clamp central line.
	Instruct patient to lie on left side with head down; Trendelenburg position.
Sudden onset of symptoms	Notify physician.
Chest pain	Monitor vital signs.
Cyanosis, anxiety	Remain with patient.
Increased pulse and respirations	Administer O_2.
Decreased blood pressure	Initiate peripheral IV access.
Catheter Dislodgment	
Medication or fluid leaking from catheter or exit site	Note presence or absence of suture in securing subclavian catheter or Dacron cuff protruding from exit site of tunneled catheter.
	Report finding to physician.
	Secure catheter and extension tubing with tape.
Catheter Migration	
Unable to inject fluid or medication	Notify physician to determine catheter placement.

Catheter Occlusion

Unable to inject fluid or medication

Gently flush catheter with appropriate normal saline flush. *Do not use force* (catheter may rupture).

Notify physician; there is a potential need for injection of fibrinolytic agent.

Inject urokinase 1 ml (5000 units/ml) into catheter port using a 5-ml syringe.

After 10 min, try to aspirate the clot.

If necessary, repeat aspiration at 5-min intervals for 30 min. Declotting procedure may be repeated using two doses of the fibrinolytic agent; wait 1 hr between procedures.

Hydrochloric acid (HCl) has been used to restore patency of catheters obstructed by drug precipitate including etoposide, calcium salts plus sodium bicarbonate, parenteral nutrition solution, or heparin plus an incompatible antibiotic (amikacin or vancomycin). Instill 0.2-1 ml solution (0.1 M HCl) into obstructed catheter. One to several hours may be required to restore total patency. HCl is proposed to work by lowering pH, which increases the solubility of these agents.

Continued

Table 3-5   Potential complications—central venous catheters—cont'd

Nursing Assessments	Nursing Interventions
	Upon establishing catheter patency, withdraw 5 ml fluid and discard before flushing catheter lumen with normal saline; resume previous catheter function or heparin lock the device.
	For TPN and lipid solutions, if urokinase does not clear the blockage, a 70% ethanol solution may be instilled and left in place for 1 hr. Follow procedure for urokinase instillation. This may help clear the catheter of lipid material deposition.
	An effective alternative to urokinase for occluded central venous catheters is alteplase (Activase). The usual dose is 2 mg (1 mg/ml) over a 2-hr dwell time for restoring catheter patency. Once reconstituted with sterile water for injection USP to a concentration of 1 mg/ml, the alteplase solution should be used within 8 hr.
Catheter Sepsis	
Inflamed, reddened, painful catheter exit or port site	Culture catheter exit site, port site, and extension tubing, and obtain a blood sample from peripheral site.
Purulent exudate	Notify physician.
Elevated temperature, chills	Administer appropriate prescribed antibiotics.
May or may not be able to aspirate or infuse antibiotics	*Do not access* an inflamed port site.

Catheter/Port Drug Extravasation

Possible causes:

Catheter misplaced out of vessel into soft tissue

Catheter has rupture secondary to vigorous flushing

Implantable port—Huber needle dislodged from port
septum because of anatomical location, excess
adipose tissue, or movement or activity of patient

"Pinch-off sign"—compression of catheter between
clavicle and first rib

Thrombus or fibrin sheath formed at the distal end of
the catheter

Symptoms:

Stinging/burning pain and swelling along catheter site
infusion

Redness

Warmth

Leaking of fluid at catheter site or at Huber needle
insertion site

Stop the infusion.

Do not use the catheter/implantable port.

Notify the physician.

Determine the cause of extravasation.

May need a chest x-ray study or venogram to determine
catheter placement.

Remove a ruptured catheter.

Continued

Table 3-5   Potential complications—central venous catheters—cont'd

Nursing Assessments	Nursing Interventions
Catheter Pinch-Off Syndrome	
Resistance to flushing, infusion, or aspiration	Roll shoulder or raise arm on ipsilateral side (same side of body) for immediate relief of problem. May require observing catheter under fluoroscopy.
Fibrin Sheath	
Partial or total occlusion at the tip of the catheter forming platelet aggregation and fibrin deposition; results in a one-way valve effect and diminishes withdrawal of blood Symptoms: *Retrograde flow* of infusate back up the length of the catheter *Ability to infuse* fluids but not aspirate (partial occlusion) *Reverse ball effect:* fibrin or precipitate deposits accumulate within the port reservoir around the port/catheter outlet—aspiration is possible but on attempt to flush the catheter, the obstruction lodges against the port/catheter outlet, totally occluding the flow	Notify physician—potential exists for administration of lytic agent (urokinase) or prophylactic oral anticoagulant; radiograph of catheter for position, tip location, catheter integrity, and thrombosis formation; change in catheter flushing solution or frequency.

Superior Vena Cava Syndrome

Possible causes: mediastinal tumor growth (lung, breast, esophageal, head and neck, and lymphoma) or growth secondary to central venous access placement

Symptom: progressive upper extremity, neck, and facial edema with dilation of the superficial veins of the chest, neck, and arms

Stop the infusion.
Do not use the catheter/implantable port.
Notify the physician.
Monitor the patient.
Initiate oxygen through nasal cannula.
Administer treatment as ordered for fibrinolytics or anticoagulants.
May require immediate treatment for tumor (chemotherapy/radiation therapy).

Vessel Thrombosis

May be related to diameter of catheter in relation to patient's vessel size

Symptoms:

Edema and tenderness of neck, shoulder, and arm on the same side as catheter

Shortness of breath, cough, cyanosis of face and upper extremities

Notify the physician to determine catheter placement via radiograph.

Nursing Diagnoses

- Skin integrity, impaired: potential related to erosion of skin at exit site or frequent implantable port access
- Injury, potential for, related to venous obstruction, catheter dislodgment, catheter migration, or catheter occlusion
- Infection, potential for, related to contamination of supplies, break in sterile technique when managing catheter, performing site care, accessing catheter, or changing dressings
- Knowledge deficit regarding ongoing self-management of catheter
- Self-concept, disturbance: body image, related to placement of venous access device

Patient/Family Teaching for Self-Management

- Assess the patient's ability and willingness to learn, availability of caregiver, home environment, and previous experience or expectations.
- Describe the purpose and function of the catheter or device. (See "Device Selection" on page 58 and "Resources" on page 87 for patient information on caring for the venous access device.)
- Instruct the patient regarding insertion procedure, radiograph for catheter tip placement, and physician follow-up evaluation.
- Explain self-care management issues. Completing site care, changing the injection cap, and flushing the catheter with heparin solution or normal saline require demonstration with return demonstration to facilitate learning and integration of necessary skills.
- Review symptoms related to each potential complication with emergency self-management techniques and reporting of that information immediately to the physician.
- Reinforce the "Helpful Hints" (p. 97) related to potential catheter malfunctions with appropriate intervention strategies.
- Provide information on obtaining, storing, and disposing of supplies and availability of a 24-hour hotline for problems (e.g., keeping supplies and equipment used for catheter management in a secure place). Schedule daily or intermittent catheter flushings at the same time every day to coincide with the patient's activities of daily living.

Geriatric Considerations

The nurse must consider neuromuscular and sensory deficits that may be present, such as visual and hearing losses and arthritic joints. Individualized self-care teaching of catheter maintenance should be planned. Printed materials may require large print for reading ease. Return demonstration techniques may require more simplistic steps to facilitate ease in use of the supplies. The nurse should assess the abilities of the patient and caregiver and determine whether additional resources, such as a home care agency, are needed to provide self-care catheter maintenance.

Resources
Patient/Caregiver Education—Venous Access Devices
Caring for Your Venous Access Device
What is a venous access device?

Your physician has recommended a *venous access device* because your treatment requires frequent administration of intravenous fluids, drugs, and blood products or frequent taking of blood samples.

These medications or fluids can be delivered directly into the bloodstream by inserting one end of a *catheter* (thin tube) or accessing a *port* into a large vein or artery. The other end of the catheter or port extends from a small incision in the skin. Drugs or fluids can then be injected, via a syringe or tubing, through the external end of the catheter/port.

Where is the venous access device placed?

Your physician will insert the device while you are receiving local or general anesthesia. The following illustration shows some of the most common locations for catheter and port placement.

What does a venous access device look like?

Following are pictures of some common venous access devices. Your physician has selected the device that is most appropriate for your type and duration of therapy.

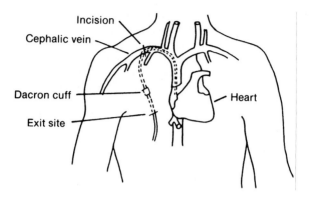

Multilumen Subclavian Catheter

This catheter is composed of pliable polyurethane material and allows easy access to your vascular system (bloodstream). Because of its unique design (three separate ports), more than one medication or IV fluid can be given at one time. The catheter is used for short-term situations (usually 2 to 8 weeks) to give medication or to take blood samples. It is inserted by a physician using sterile technique and local anesthesia. Catheter placement is usually verified by getting a radiograph at the end of the procedure. The catheter is held in place by sutures securing the small wing-tip device next to the skin. It is important to keep this area free of germs.

Groshong Catheter

This catheter is composed of a transparent silicone rubber material and allows easy access to your vascular system (bloodstream). Because of its unique design (a patented two-way slit valve next to a rounded, closed tip), it requires minimal catheter care. The catheter may have a single, double, or triple lumen and is usually in place for months to 2 years. It is inserted by a physician using sterile technique and a local anesthetic. Catheter placement is usually verified by getting a radiograph at the end of the procedure. A Dacron fiber cuff is placed below the skin to hold the catheter in place and to prevent infection.

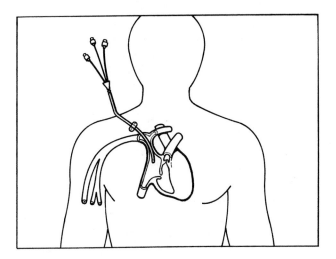

Multilumen subclavian catheter.

Tunneled Catheter

The tunneled catheter, or Hickman catheter, is a flexible silicone tube that gives easy access to your vascular system (bloodstream). The catheter can be used to draw blood for laboratory samples or to give chemotherapy drugs and/or other medications, IV fluids, blood or blood components, and nutritional support. The catheter is inserted using a local anesthetic—you cannot feel it inside your body. With the aid of a radiograph fluoroscope, the catheter is placed into your upper chest and directed into the superior vena cava (a very large vein in your chest). After insertion, the catheter is anchored in place by a Dacron fiber cuff placed below the skin that also minimizes your potential for infection. When you no longer need the catheter, your physician or nurse can remove it.

Implantable Venous Access Devices (Ports)

An implantable venous access device (port) has two major parts: a catheter and a small chamber called a *portal*. In the center of the

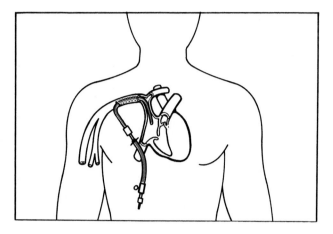

Grushong catheter.

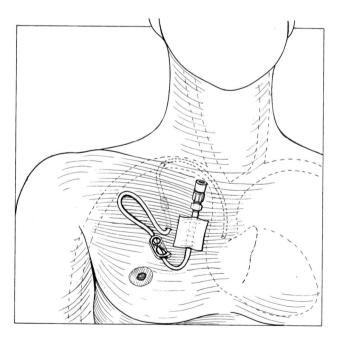

Tunneled catheter.
(Courtesy Pharmacia Deltec, St. Paul, Minn.)

portal is a self-sealing silicone septum. Some implantable venous access devices have more than one portal, making it possible for more than one medication or fluid to be given through the system at the same time.

A physician, usually in a hospital or outpatient operating room setting, places the implantable venous access device. An anesthetic is used at the insertion site to make the area numb during the placement procedure. The catheter is put through the skin and into a vein in the chest. The tip of the catheter is threaded into the superior vena cava. The other end of the catheter is tunneled under the skin for a short distance. An incision is made and the portal is placed under the skin. The catheter is then attached to the portal. After the incision is closed, the entire device is under the skin.

Peripherally Placed Implantable Venous Access Devices (Peripheral Ports)

A peripherally placed implantable venous access device has two major parts: a catheter and a very small chamber called a *portal*. In the center of the portal is a self-sealing silicone septum.

A physician, usually in an outpatient operating room setting, places the implantable venous access device. An anesthetic is used

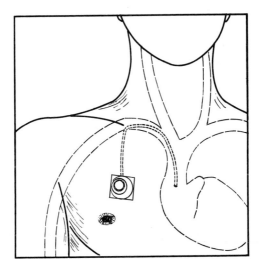

Placement of an implantable venous access device.

at the insertion site to make the area numb during the placement procedure. The catheter is put into a vein in the lower arm. The tip of the catheter is threaded through the vein to the superior vena cava. The other end of the catheter is tunneled under the skin for a short distance. An incision is made and the portal is placed under the skin. The catheter is then attached to the portal. After the incision is closed, the entire device is under the skin.

Peripherally Inserted Central Venous Catheters (PICC Lines)

A peripherally inserted central venous catheter is a very small, flexible, hollow tube with an extension tubing and injection cap on the end. A specially trained nurse in a procedure room in a hospital or ambulatory care setting usually inserts this catheter. The catheter is inserted much like having an IV infusion started in your arm; you will feel a needlestick, the nurse verifies a blood return, and then slowly threads the catheter into the vein until it reaches the desired endpoint placement. An extension tubing with an injection cap is attached to the catheter and a sterile dressing is applied. A radiograph is done to verify catheter tip placement.

Care of the Venous Access Device
Flushing the catheter or port

Flushing the catheter helps keep the catheter clean and prevents it from becoming blocked.

Your catheter should be flushed every _____ hours/days with _____ solution.

What you need

- Normal saline needleless syringes
- Heparin solution needleless syringes
- Alcohol swabs
- Povidone-iodine wipes
- Tape
- Leak-proof, puncture-proof container (for disposal of used injection caps and needleless syringes)

What to do

1. Wash your hands for 10 seconds using warm, soapy water and then rinse.
2. Dry your hands on a clean towel.

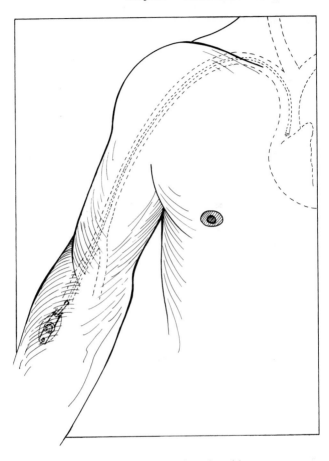

Placement of a peripherally inserted implantable venous access device.
(Courtesy Pharmacia Deltec, St. Paul, Minn.)

3. Prepare heparin and/or normal saline syringe. Examine the syringe for particles.
4. Cleanse the catheter cap with povidone-iodine and then alcohol.
5. Inject heparin or normal saline into the catheter injection cap.
6. Withdraw the syringe, continuing to press down on the plunger with your thumb.

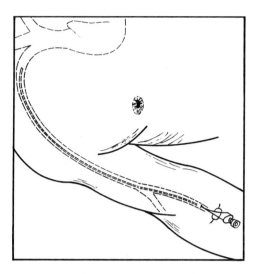

Placement of a peripherally inserted central venous catheter.

7. Discard the needleless syringe in the puncture-proof container.
8. Wash your hands for 10 seconds using warm, soapy water and then rinse.
9. Dry your hands on a clean towel.

Care of the "Exit Site"
Dressing change
The dressing at the exit site needs to be changed regularly to prevent infection and allow you to inspect the catheter exit site. Your dressing change should be done according to the schedule prescribed by your physician or nurse.

Your dressing should be changed times _____ a day/week.

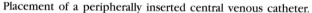

What you need
- Bag for disposal of used items
- Sterile alcohol swabs or povidone-iodine swabs
- Hydrogen peroxide (used if allergic to povidone-iodine)
- Povidone-iodine ointment (use only if prescribed by physician or nurse)

- Sterile disposable gloves
- Sterile cotton-tipped swabs
- Sterile gauze dressing and tape or sterile transparent dressing

Changing the dressing

1. Wash your hands for 10 seconds using warm, soapy water and rinse.
2. Dry your hands on a clean towel.
3. Carefully remove and discard the old dressing (if you have a dressing).
4. Wash your hands for 10 seconds using warm, soapy water and rinse.
5. Dry your hands on a clean towel.
6. Examine the site for redness, swelling, tenderness, or drainage. If you note any, finish changing the dressing and take your temperature. Notify your physician, nurse, or home care agency.
7. Carefully clean the catheter exit site with povidone-iodine swabs, alcohol swabs, and/or hydrogen peroxide. Starting at the exit site, work in a circular motion around and away from the catheter exit site.
8. Allow the area to dry for 10 seconds. Pat the site with a sterile, dry gauze sponge.
9. Clean the catheter/port:
   - Using a sterile alcohol swab, grasp the catheter near the exit site.
   - Use a second alcohol swab to gently wipe the catheter, beginning at the exit site and ending at the catheter injection cap.
10. Prepare the catheter for flushing. If you are flushing the catheter at this time, follow the procedures listed under "Flushing the Catheter or Port" on page 92.
11. Coil the catheter, and tape it in place.
12. Wash your hands for 10 seconds using warm, soapy water and then rinse.
13. Dry your hands on a clean towel.

Changing the Catheter Cap

The catheter injection cap is used for needleless syringe access and needs to be changed regularly.

Your catheter cap should be changed every _____ days.

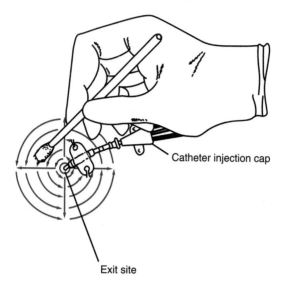

Catheter injection cap

Exit site

Cleansing of the exit site.

What you need

- New sterile injection cap
- Alcohol swabs
- Catheter clamp (attached to catheter)

What to do

1. Wash your hands for 10 seconds using warm, soapy water and then rinse.
2. Dry your hands on a clean towel.
3. Be sure the catheter is securely clamped over the reinforced sleeve. (Do not clamp the Groshong catheter—this catheter does not need a clamp.)
4. Wipe with an alcohol swab around the area where the cap is connected to the catheter.
5. Unscrew the old cap and discard.
6. Pick up the new injection cap by the top and remove the protective covering over its base.
7. Attach the new cap by firmly screwing it onto the catheter.
8. Release the catheter clamp.

9. Follow the directions your doctor or nurse has given you regarding whether to leave the clamp in place.
10. If the catheter requires flushing, follow the procedures listed under "Flushing the Catheter or Port" on page 92.
11. Wash your hands for 10 seconds using warm, soapy water and then rinse.
12. Dry your hands on a clean towel.

When to Contact Your Physician or Nurse

Alert your physician or nurse immediately if any of the following occur:

- Pain
- Shortness of breath
- Bleeding from catheter site
- Redness, swelling, or tenderness at or near the catheter site
- Drainage at or near the catheter site
- Temperature greater than 100° F

For years, catheters have been used safely by many patients. The risk of complications can be minimized with proper care.

Helpful Hints

Don't expect problems, but be prepared if they should occur. Following is a list of potential problems with information about what to do if they occur.

Catheter flushing

If your catheter resists the flushing solution, do not force the solution into the catheter. First, change your body position; take a deep breath, exhale, or cough. If your catheter still resists the flushing solution, stop and call your physician or nurse.

Catheter damage

Keep sharp objects away from your catheter. If the catheter is accidentally cut or punctured, clamp the catheter or tubing by folding the catheter back onto itself. Secure it with a rubber band. Report catheter damage to your physician or nurse immediately.

Blood in catheter/tubing

Follow catheter-flushing steps.

Pump malfunction

Check and if necessary replace the battery or electrical plug; check the start and stop function; check for clamped tubing.

Bleeding or irritation at exit site

If you note pain, redness, swelling, or oozing at the exit site, you should call your physician immediately. These signs may indicate an infection. Avoid possible infections by following your physician's instructions regarding activity.

Infection

Call your physician if you experience fever or chills. Infection may also cause you to note a foul odor, feel pain or heat, or observe swelling or oozing at the exit site. To prevent infection, wash your hands before beginning any procedure, wear a mask if you have a cold, avoid persons who are ill, and perform your procedure in a well-ventilated but draft-free place.

Other Questions

How will I know if something is wrong?

If you are unable to inject your medication, the filter may be clogged or you may have a catheter obstruction. Try changing the filter. If this does not help, call your physician.

If you notice redness and swelling at the catheter exit site or have a low-grade temperature (98.6° to 100° F) or if you have a feeling of general discomfort that lasts more than 24 hours, this may indicate the beginning of an infection.

If your temperature spikes (goes higher than 100° F), this may also indicate an infection.

Contact your physician as soon as you suspect that something is wrong.

May I bathe or swim?

You should ask your physician this question. The answer will depend on your health and risk for infection. It will also depend on how long you have had the catheter in place. If your physician approves swimming, the catheter and exit site must be covered with an appropriate waterproof dressing. When finished, you will need to cleanse and dress the exit site.

Does the exit site always need a dressing?

This depends on how long the catheter or port has been in place. Check with your physician or nurse to see if you should keep your incision or exit site covered with a dressing or bandage.

What if I get a cold?

If you have a cold, your physician may instruct you to wear a mask when you are caring for the catheter, especially during the filter and cap change procedure.

What happens if the catheter is damaged?

If the damage is far enough away from the exit site, it can be repaired. If there is too little catheter to work with, you may need to have the catheter replaced. Clamp the catheter above the damaged area, then contact your physician or nurse immediately.

What do I do if I run out of supplies?

Call the company, pharmacy, physician, or nurse that is providing your supplies. You should always have extra supplies on hand so that you will not run out.

What happens if the catheter gets pulled out?

The catheter is anchored with sutures underneath your skin. Therefore it is unlikely to get pulled out. The catheter may stretch a bit and may seem like it has slipped out. If you think your catheter is slipping out, do not try to test it by pulling on it. Call your physician.

What if I become allergic to the povidone-iodine or tape?

There are many choices for antiseptic solutions and tape. Check with your physician or nurse if you think you are having an allergic reaction. He or she can determine which tapes and antiseptics are best for you.

Should someone else learn the procedure?

Having another person available who has been trained in all of the necessary procedures is important. If you become too ill to perform a procedure, the other person could perform it for you.

Can some chemicals hurt the catheter?

Some chemicals can damage the catheter, so it is important not to use anything on or near the catheter unless you consult with your physician or nurse.

Acetone, which is found in nail polish remover and tape removers, is especially harmful and should not be used on or around the catheter.

How long can the catheter or port stay in place?

The catheter or port is designed to stay in place for lengthy periods (e.g., months to 2 to 3 years), but each patient's situation is unique. The better you take care of your catheter, the longer it will last.

What support services can I access?

Your physician and other members of your health care team are available to answer your questions about your venous access device while you are in the medical center. They can also help you make arrangements for supplies and home care nursing after you go home.

You will be in charge of caring for your venous access device when you are at home. If you have questions at any time, call and ask for the nursing staff for the unit you were on during your hospital stay or call your home care agency staff.

Clinical Competency—Central Venous Catheters

	Yes	No	NA
Patient Education and Preparation			
1. Participates in device selection and preparation for device insertion procedure.			
2. Provides nursing assessment/ intervention information regarding device care (access, blood sampling, catheter repair, drug/infusion solution, heparinization, management of potential complications, e.g., air embolus, fibrin sheath, occlusion, sepsis, and/or catheter repair) and self-care			

Clinical Competency—Central Venous Catheters—cont'd

	Yes	No	NA
Patient Education and Preparation—cont'd			
maintenance procedures (heparinization, injection cap change, exit site care, obtaining supplies, catheter/port malfunctions to promptly report to physician/ nurse, and clinical symptoms re pain, bleeding, fever, and/or shortness of breath).			
Nursing Assessment and Interventions			
1. Washes hands before and after all procedures.			
2. Maintains strict aseptic technique and sterile, Luer-Lok supplies for access; blood sampling; heparinization; dressing, injection cap, and tubing changes; drug/ solution infusion; exit site care; and catheter repair, occlusion, and/or fibrin sheath management.			
3. Follows prescribed physician protocol for catheter/port heparinization regarding volume, concentration, and scheduled frequency and catheter occlusion and repair.			
4. Consults and communicates promptly to the physician regarding any catheter/port malfunction or complication.			
5. Documents all patient/family/ caregiver education, nursing assessment and intervention procedures, consultation with home care agency, and nursing management of catheter/port complications in the medical record.			

Continued

Clinical Competency—Central Venous Catheters—cont'd

	Yes	No	NA
Blood Sampling			
1. Stops infusing solution for 1 to 3 minutes.			
2. Clamps catheter/extension tubing.			
3. Removes and discards at least 5 ml of blood or solution.			
4. Withdraws the prescribed amount.			
5. Flushes/heparinizes catheter/port with prescribed solution/volume.			
Exit Site Care			
1. Selects and prepares appropriate supplies.			
2. Carefully removes old dressing.			
3. Inspects and palpates exit site: erythema, tissue swelling, and leakage.			
4. Cleanses exit site.			
5. Applies appropriate dressing.			
Injection Cap Change			
1. Selects and prepares appropriate supplies.			
2. Clamps catheter/extension tubing.			
3. Cleanses catheter and changes injection cap.			
Catheter Patency: Heparinization or Normal Saline Injection			
1. Selects and prepares appropriate supplies.			
2. Confirms catheter/port placement before initiating therapy.			
3. Cleanses injection cap with povidone-iodine or alcohol.			
4. Verifies catheter/port patency via blood/solution return.			
5. Infuses correct solution: concentration, volume, at prescribed schedule.			

Clinical Competency—Central Venous Catheters—cont'd

	Yes	No	NA
Catheter/Port Access			
1. Selects, prepares, and uses appropriate supplies.			
2. Assists the patient to a comfortable position.			
3. Clamps and unclamps catheter/extension tubing at appropriate times.			
4. Confirms catheter/port placement before catheter/port access.			
5. Verifies catheter/port patency via blood/solution return.			
6. Infuses correct solution: concentration, volume, at prescribed schedule.			
7. Secures catheter/extension tubing to patient's body.			
Catheter/Port Occlusion Management			
1. Verifies occlusion management with physician.			
2. Selects, prepares, and uses appropriate supplies.			
3. Verifies patient drug allergy and platelet count status.			
4. Accesses catheter/port.			
5. Instills urokinase and follows sequential time allotments for incremental injection of urokinase.			
6. Aspirates catheter/port contents.			
7. Follows procedure for heparinization and/or flushing with normal saline.			
Catheter/Port Repair Procedure			
1. Consults with physician and verifies appropriate repair procedure.			
2. Selects, prepares, and uses appropriate supplies.			

Continued

Clinical Competency—Central Venous Catheters—cont'd

	Yes	No	NA
Catheter/Port Repair Procedure—cont'd			
1. Clamps and unclamps catheter/ extension tubing at appropriate times.			
2. Follows designated catheter repair procedure.			
Nursing Management for Potential Complications			
Demonstrates knowledge and skill in assessment and management of the following:			
1. Air embolus			
2. Catheter dislodgement			
3. Catheter/port malfunction			
4. Catheter/port migration			
5. Catheter/port drug extravasation			
6. Catheter/port sepsis			
7. Superior vena cava syndrome			
8. Vessel thrombosis			

Study Questions

1. Patient device selection is based on:
   a. Patient preference, type, purpose, and duration of therapy
   b. Nurse intervention, type, purpose, and duration of therapy
   c. Physician practice, type, purpose, and duration of therapy
   d. Patient, physician, and nurse consultation; type, purpose and duration of therapy

2. Patient/caregiver education for self-care management of catheter/port includes:
   a. Blood sampling, catheter malfunction, catheter occlusion, heparinization
   b. Blood sampling, changing injection cap, exit site care, heparinization
   c. Catheter malfunction, changing injection cap, exit site care, heparinization

    d. Catheter malfunction, catheter complications, catheter repair, heparinization

3. Central venous access devices include all the following *except:*
   a. Implanted ports
   b. Peripheral dual-lumen catheter
   c. Subclavian catheters
   d. Tunneled catheters

4. The Groshong tunneled catheter has unique catheter characteristics that include:
   a. Three-position valve, closed distal tip, no clamps
   b. Three-position valve, closed distal tip, clamps
   c. Three-position valve, closed distal tip, specially designed clamps
   d. Three-position valve, open distal tip, specially designed clamps

5. Catheter occlusion nursing interventions include:
   a. Assessing occlusion, verifying procedure with physician, vigorously flushing with urokinase
   b. Assessing occlusion, vigorously flushing with urokinase, repeating procedure every 24 hours
   c. Assessing occlusion, verifying procedure with physician, injecting urokinase with caution
   d. Assessing occlusion, injecting urokinase with caution, repeating procedure every 24 hours

6. Air embolus clinical features associated with central venous access devices include:
   a. Sudden onset of chest pain, cyanosis, decreased blood pressure and pulse
   b. Sudden onset of chest pain, cyanosis, decreased blood pressure and increased pulse
   c. Sudden onset of chest pain, cyanosis, increased blood pressure and pulse
   d. Sudden onset of chest pain, cyanosis, increased blood pressure and decreased pulse

7. Hemodialysis and apheresis catheters require the following care and maintenance guidelines:
   a. Direction for use, heparin (10 units/ml), aspiration of lumen contents before infusion of medication/solution, secure injection caps and catheter clamps

b. Direction for use, heparin (100 units/ml), aspiration of lumen contents before infusion of medication/solution, secure injection caps and catheter clamps

c. Direction for use, heparin (1000 units/ml), aspiration of lumen contents before infusion of medication/solution, secure injection caps and catheter clamps

d. Direction for use, heparin (5000 units/ml), aspiration of lumen contents before infusion of medication/solution, secure injection caps and catheter clamps

8. Usual heparinization and/or normal saline flushing protocols for central venous access devices include:
   a. Every: day, week, month
   b. Every: hour, day, week
   c. Every: hour, day, month
   d. Every: hour, week, month

9. Common symptoms of partial or total occlusion of catheter tip (e.g., fibrin sheath) are:
   a. Ability to infuse fluids, retrograde flow of infusate, head and neck edema
   b. Ability to infuse fluids, reverse ball effect, edema and tenderness of neck
   c. Ability to infuse fluids, retrograde flow of infusate, reverse ball effect
   d. Ability to infuse fluids, retrograde flow of infusate, facial edema and vessel dilation

10. Catheter repair procedure encompasses the following:
    a. Clean supplies, physician verification, manufacturer dedicated repair kit
    b. Sterile supplies, physician verification, manufacturer dedicated repair kit
    c. Clean supplies, physician verification, assemble own repair kit
    d. Sterile supplies, physician verification, assemble own repair kit

Answers   1. d   2. c   3. b   4. a   5. c   6. b
7. d   8. a   9. c   10. b

Peripherally Inserted Central Catheters

4

Objectives

1. Describe the types and features of the peripherally inserted central catheters (also called *PIC catheters* or *PICCs*).

2. Recognize critical principles for proper insertion and placement.

3. Discuss the procedure for blood sampling, heparinization, and dressing application.

4. Identify the major complications associated with PICCs.

5. List the patient and family education needs associated with device maintenance.

The use of PICCs continues to increase in all health care settings. Advances in catheter technology, diagnostic verification, and clinical nursing expertise in intravenous therapy have had a significant impact on patient care and improved outcomes. PICCs can remain in place from weeks to months to provide multiple infusion therapies such as chemotherapy, hydration, blood products, analgesia, antimicrobials, and/or parenteral nutrition. In addition, the uses of PICCs are increasing because they fill a void between the simple peripheral venous access catheters and long-term indwelling catheters and ports.

Catheter Placement Education Requirements

The PICC can be inserted in a designated procedure room near the patient's bedside or in the home setting by nurses with advanced intravenous (IV) therapy skills as an alternative to physician-placed central venous catheters. Catheter insertion and management of complications require nurses to seek special training and maintain ongoing competency. The initial education course with a competency program should include catheter insertion techniques and nursing management of the PICC.

Selected topics for the educational course and clinical competency are anatomy and physiology of the vascular system, device selection criteria, patient assessment, aseptic technique, procedural technique, suturing technique, product evaluation, and potential complications (emphasizing prevention, recognition, and nursing interventions). Additional ongoing education issues include quality improvement issues, expected and unexpected patient outcomes, and program planning. Clinical competence should be observed in the appropriate patient care setting under the preceptorship of a clinical expert. Protocols for meticulous care and management of the PICC should be in place to facilitate prudent nursing practice guidelines. Some states have specific nurse practice regulations for PICC insertion. It is the responsibility of the institution or agency to establish qualifications within that organization and the responsibility of each nurse to be knowledgeable of both the state's nurse practice regulations and agency policies.

Indications and Contraindications

Currently, the PICC is considered appropriate for IV therapy needed for longer than 7 to 14 days and can remain in place weeks to months. The type and size of the PICC depend on considerations such as the duration and type of therapy, expected catheter uses, desired flow rates, catheter tip placement, and/or patient preferences. There are no limitations for use related to age, gender, or diagnosis. These catheters are particularly advantageous for high-risk groups such as neonatal, pediatric, geriatric, malnourished, and immunocompromised populations. Patients with medical conditions such as an inability to undergo a surgical procedure for vascular access, neurologic conditions contraindicating changes in head positions, and physical disability for positioning, such as kyphosis, may benefit from PICC placement.

Contraindications for use include dermatitis, cellulitis, burns at or about the insertion site, and thromboses of the subclavian, innominate, or superior vena cava veins. The PICC is not suitable for high-volume fluid infusions, rapid bolus injection, hemophoresis, or hemodialysis. The following situations require careful assessment: contractures, mastectomy, existing thrombophlebitis, radiation therapy, pacemaker wires, crutch walking, and potential future use of the extremity for hemodialysis access.

Description of Catheter Products

These catheters are made of a soft, biocompatible silicone elastomer, Silastic, or flexible polyurethane radiopaque material (Fig. 4-1). Like tunneled catheters, PICCs are available in single-lumen or multilumen designs and have an open-ended tip or a valve that closes the catheter tip when it is not in use (Fig. 4-2). They may vary in length (33 to 60 cm) and should be longer than the length measured for the patient to ensure adequate tip placement. The gauge size (23 gauge = French to 14 gauge = French) should be large enough to facilitate the infusion of the prescribed infusates and blood sampling but small enough for the selected vein. (See Chapter 14, Table 14-1, page 471.)

The type of device used for venipuncture, the internal guidewire or stylet, and the catheter material mainly differentiate product designs. Venipuncture device designs (Fig. 4-3) include over-the-

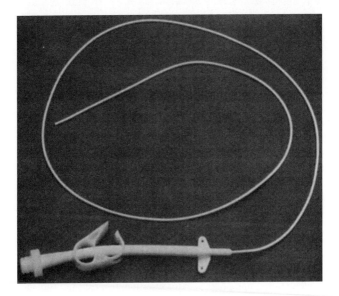

Fig. 4-1
Peripherally inserted central venous catheter.
(Courtesy Cook Incorporated, Bloomington, Ind.)

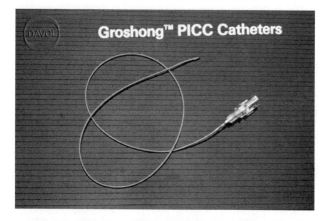

Fig. 4-2
Groshong PICC.
(Courtesy Bard Access Systems Inc., Salt Lake City, Utah.)

needle sheaths that strip away or slide off after insertion of the catheter, a scored butterfly needle that breaks and strips away from the catheter, and a small-gauge needle for an over-the-wire technique. A flexible, blunt-tipped stylet or guidewire positioned within the catheter is important for ease of insertion and to reduce the risk of coiling or reversing direction while advancing the catheter. When the breakable needle is used, the risk of catheter shearing is reduced when internal guidewires or stylets are used, because the stylet or guidewire would be cut before transecting the catheter.

Principles of Catheter Insertion

- Verify the physician's order and obtain the patient's informed consent.
- Identify the appropriate vein for insertion. In most adult patients, the basilic vein is more suitable for cannulation than the cephalic vein because of its larger size and straighter, less tortuous shape. The cephalic, medial cephalic, and medial basilic veins may also

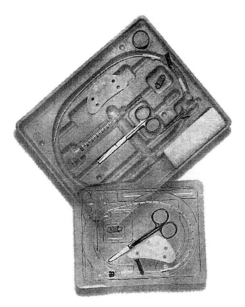

Fig. 4-3
Peripherally inserted central venous insertion set.
(Courtesy Arrow International, Reading, Pa.)

be successfully used for venipuncture. Occasionally, the external jugular vein is selected as the insertion site when the patient has compromised vasculature and/or may need placement of access for hemodialysis. Fig. 4-4 provides vasculature identification and upper extremity vein anthropometric measurements. In infants and neonates, other veins such as the temporal, external jugular, or saphenous can be used for placement.

- Ensure accurate placement by measuring the distance from the insertion site to the catheter tip termination point. Add a predetermined length (5 to 8 cm) to allow sufficient distance for securing the catheter.
- Perform catheter placement with strict aseptic technique, including surgical hand scrub by the nurse; use of hair cover, mask, sterile gown, gloves, and drapes; and appropriate antiseptic preparation of the patient's skin.
- Silastic catheters must remain free of external particular matter before and during insertion. Rinsing the gloved hand with sterile

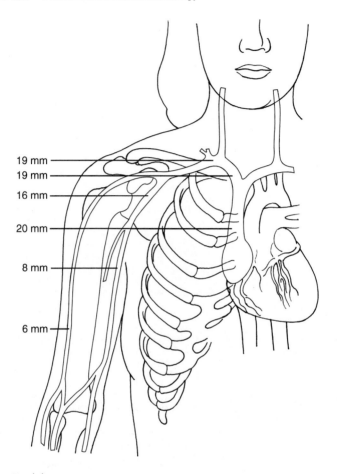

Fig. 4-4
Vasculature identification: upper extremity vein and anthropometric measurements.
(Courtesy Gesco International, Inc., San Antonio, Tex.)

water or saline before handling the catheter prevents glove powder contact with the catheter.
- Place the patient in a comfortable, convenient position. For central venous tip placement, the patient should be lying flat with arm extended at a 90-degree angle to the body. To help prevent

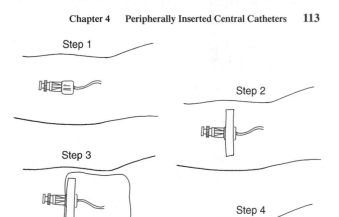

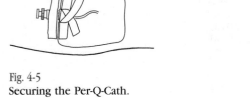

Fig. 4-5
Securing the Per-Q-Cath.
(Courtesy Gesco International Inc., San Antonio, Tex.)

catheter tip migration into the jugular vein, the patient should turn his or her head toward the accessed side and place the chin on chest.
- After the skin preparation and application of the sterile drape, perform the venipuncture.
    1. Advance the catheter to the predetermined length.
    2. Validate blood return.
    3. Flush the catheter with heparinized saline solution.
    4. Attach the injection cap or extension tubing.
    5. Secure the catheter with sutures or sterile strips.
- Refer to the PICC product recommendations or contraindications for catheter suturing. Fig. 4-5 illustrates securing of the PICC with tape and transparent bioclusive dressing.

- Stabilization of the catheter directly at the site reduces introduction of microorganisms with the in-and-out motion of the catheter through the skin.
- Standards of practice recommend that any catheter tip located within the central venous system be verified through radiographic examination to ensure proper location before any infusion.

Placement Technique—PICC

The technique for placement of the PICC will vary according to the product selected.

- *Breakaway needle technique:* Use a specifically designated needle introducer for venipuncture. Advance the catheter to the desired endpoint, and then remove the introducer from the venipuncture site, break it in half, and peel it away from the catheter.

  Advantages: The catheter hub is attached by the manufacturer, which minimizes blood exposure. This is the most popular technique for manufacturers. Multiple products are available.

  Disadvantages: The procedure may be awkward for the clinician, and the potential exists for catheter damage during the insertion procedure.

- *Through-the-cannula technique:* Use a large-gauge angiocatheter for venipuncture. Remove the stylet, thread the catheter to the desired endpoint through the angiocatheter, remove the angiocatheter over the PICC, and attach the hub to the distal end of the PICC.

  Advantages: This technique eliminates the potential for catheter damage during insertion, and the removable catheter hub allows for easier repair. A variety of products are available.

  Disadvantages: This is a slightly more complex insertion procedure, which requires a larger introducer unit. The catheter hub must be attached by the clinician.

- *Guidewire technique:* Use a solid introducer needle to make a venipuncture, and thread a guidewire through the needle and into the vein. Remove the needle, and thread the catheter over the guidewire and into the vein. Advance the catheter into the vein slowly, using a gentle touch to avoid trauma. After threading the catheter to the desired catheter tip placement, remove the guidewire.

Advantages: This technique has a reduced potential for catheter damage during insertion procedure. Multiple products are available.

Disadvantages: This is a more complex insertion procedure, which has the potential for vein wall perforation and increased trauma to vein wall intima.

Guidelines for Catheter Maintenance Procedure

Dressing Change

The practitioner should provide a sterile environment for the duration of the catheter placement; the dressing should be changed at scheduled intervals to coincide with tubing and injection cap changes. The dressing must be removed carefully, the hub stabilized, and then the old dressing gently pulled away from the hub toward the venipuncture site parallel to the skin to prevent pulling the catheter out from the insertion site. The insertion site and surrounding area should be inspected for any signs of infection (e.g., drainage, edema, erythema, pain). If purulent drainage is present, the practitioner should obtain a culture using a sterile swab and send it to the laboratory for evaluation; the incident must be reported to the physician promptly. During all dressing changes, the practitioner should verify that the catheter length remaining outside the patient corresponds with the initial placement measurement to determine if catheter migration has occurred (see Fig. 4-5).

CLINICAL ALERT: The initial dressing (first 24 hours) requires a sterile gauze and tape dressing over the insertion site to absorb any bloody drainage. Change this dressing within 24 hours, and follow agency protocol for the sterile dressing procedure. Monitor the insertion site for hematoma, edema, discoloration, and/or mechanical phlebitis.

Heparinization

The amount of heparinized saline necessary to flush the catheter should be equal to the catheter/extension set volume plus approximately 0.2 ml. The priming volume of catheters varies with catheter gauge and length. Usually, 1 ml/lumen is adequate to maintain patency. Guidelines recommended by the manufacturer may include the following.

- *Adult, intermittent use:* Flush with 100 U/ml heparin every 12 hours and after each use.

- *Child or neonate, intermittent use:* Flush with 10 U/ml heparin every 8 hours and after each use.
- *Home care maintenance:* Flush every 24 hours.

Blood Sampling

Blood sampling may be obtained from the infant or adult PICC with proper technique. For consistently good blood sampling, a larger catheter, greater than 3 French, should be used. The pliable soft walls of the catheter may collapse if a strong vacuum is applied; instead, a 5-ml syringe should be used with a push/pull technique rather than a Vacutainer to obtain the blood sample specimen. Normal saline (10 to 20 ml) should be used for catheter flushing after blood sampling. Refer to the product manufacturer's guidelines regarding contraindications related to the small size of catheter for blood administration and blood sampling. See Chapter 3, Tables 3-2 and 3-3, pages 65 and 68.

Catheter Declotting

The PICC may be cleared by using urokinase according to the product manufacturer's recommendation with a physician's order. The small volume of the PICC must be taken into consideration as well as the potential for catheter rupture. The practitioner should use at least a 5-ml or larger volume syringe for the catheter declotting procedure. After successful catheter declotting, the practitioner should flush the catheter lumen with normal saline. Fig. 4-6 illustrates a recommended declotting procedure.

CLINICAL ALERT: Never apply excessive force or pressure when flushing the PICC or when encountering severe resistance because of the danger of dislodging a clot or rupturing the catheter.

Catheter Removal

1. Place the patient in a supine position and remove the dressing; position the patient's arm at a 45- to 90-degree angle to the body.
2. Apply gloves.
3. Slowly pull the PICC out, using a gentle hand-over-hand technique. This process should take about 60 seconds.
4. Examine the site, note any abnormalities, and apply a small sterile pressure dressing to the insertion site.
5. Measure and examine the PICC to make sure the entire catheter has been removed.

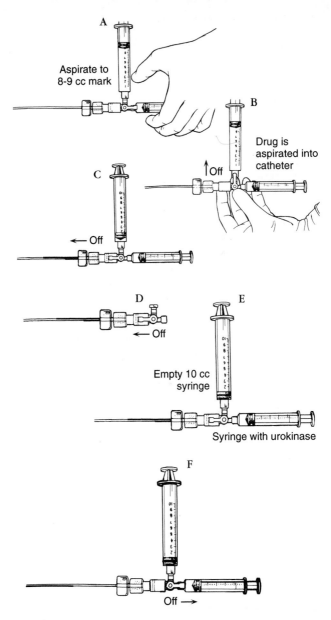

A Aspirate to 8-9 cc mark

B Drug is aspirated into catheter

↑Off

C ← Off

D ← Off

E Empty 10 cc syringe

Syringe with urokinase

F Off →

Fig. 4-6
Declotting PICCs.
(Courtesy Gesco International Inc., San Antonio, Tex.)

6. Compare its length with the length documented in the insertion procedure.

Catheter repair or exchange: Refer to the PICC manufacturer's guidelines for catheter repair options and kits. Only personnel skilled in the procedure should perform PICC exchange.

Precautions for Syringes and Infusion Pumps

- *Syringes:* All PICC product manufacturers recommend a minimum syringe size of 5 ml for any PICC maintenance procedure. Small-diameter syringes, such as tuberculin syringes, can create very high pressure (120 to 150 psi). If the catheter becomes occluded, the small syringe could rupture the catheter or force whatever is causing the occlusion downstream into the patient.
- *Infusion pumps:* Large-volume, small-volume, volumetric, linear, and rotary peristaltic pumps have all been used successfully with PICCs. When infusion pumps are used to administer infusates, the mechanism's alarm feature must not exceed 15 psi.

Troubleshooting Tips/Potential Complications

Refer to Table 4-1 for troubleshooting tips for PICCs and to Table 4-2 for potential complications.

Documentation Recommendations

- For catheter insertion, record the following: brand of catheter, gauge/size, lot number, and insertion site; location of tip placement; length of PICC inserted and length of external segment; date, time, and any problems encountered during insertion; radiograph confirmation of PICC tip placement; the type of dressing; patient and caregiver education regarding understanding of catheter self-care management; and heparin or normal saline flush—drug, concentration, dose, volume, date, and time.
- For the duration of PICC placement, record the following: assessment of insertion site; length of external segment of PICC; dates and description of sterile dressing and cap changes; presence and quality of blood return or blood sampling; heparin or normal saline flush—drug, concentration, dose, volume, date, and time; any infusion problems and interventions.

Table 4-1   Troubleshooting tips for peripherally inserted central catheters

Nursing Assessment	Nursing Intervention
Accidental catheter removal	Apply pressure dressing at the insertion site for at least 5 minutes, and notify physician. Assess the source of catheter removal, and measure the catheter length to determine if measurements coincide with catheter insertion measurements.
Fluid leak at insertion site	May be related to a hole or tear in the catheter or a loose connection between catheter and connection tubing. Follow agency guidelines for catheter repair or exchange. Use sterile technique and apply new connection/extension tubing. *Never use scissors to remove tape or dressing.*
Inability to aspirate blood	May be due to catheter occlusion or a PICC too small for blood sampling. Follow flushing protocol, reposition the patient's arm, and use push/pull technique with a 5-ml syringe. Venipuncture may be required to obtain a blood sample.
Mechanical phlebitis	Related to sensitivity of PICC insertion. Elevate extremity; apply warm compresses qid for 72 hours. Consult with physician for potential catheter removal.
Pain, redness, drainage at insertion site	May be related to movement of the PICC, skin or suture irritation, or infection. Reposition the catheter hub, remove sutures if skin is healed, apply sterile dressing, monitor skin irritation or infection, and obtain cultures. Consult with physician for potential catheter removal.

Continued

◎ Table 4-1   Troubleshooting tips for peripherally inserted
                central catheters—cont'd

Nursing Assessment	Nursing Intervention
Pain in arm, ear, shoulder	May be due to thrombosis of the superior vena cava, misplacement of the PICC in the internal jugular vein, or internal PICC leak. Notify the physician: need radiograph, venogram, or ultrasound to determine PICC placement. Consider catheter removal.
Pump occlusion alarm	Assess for kink in IV tubing or in PICC at dressing site and for occlusion in catheter. Palpate the IV tubing and catheter with hand to detect kinks and reposition tubing and catheter; for suspected occlusion use the catheter-flushing protocol. If unable to obtain catheter patency, notify the physician. Potential exists for declotting PICC.
"Stuck catheter"	Catheter will appear to be firmly held within the vessel—potential causes are vasospasm, vasoconstriction, and thrombophlebitis. Remove the PICC dressing, apply moderate tension on the catheter with tape below the insertion site, and apply a sterile dressing. Apply warm compresses, and attempt catheter removal in 8, 12, and 24 hours.

$\overset{n}{d_x}$ Nursing Diagnoses

- Injury, potential for, related to venous obstruction, catheter dislodgment, catheter migration, or catheter occlusion
- Infection, potential for, related to contamination of supplies, break in sterile technique when managing the catheter, performing site care, accessing catheter, or changing dressings
- Knowledge deficit regarding ongoing self-management of catheter

Table 4-2   Potential complications for peripherally inserted central catheters

Nursing Assessment	Nursing Interventions
Air embolus Symptoms: Chest pain, dyspnea, air hunger, tachycardia, hypotension, confusion, restlessness	Immediately place patient into a left-lateral, steep Trendelenburg position. Notify physician, initiate O_2, and remain with the patient.
Arterial puncture Symptoms: Bright red color blood flashback, pulsatile blood flow	Withdraw cannulation immediately, apply pressure at venipuncture site, and observe for hematoma. *Know venous anatomy* before inserting the device; observe dark red blood flashback/nonpulsatile flow on venipuncture for venous *access*.
Bleeding	Excessive bleeding more than 24 hours after PICC insertion requires further evaluation for coagulation status. Obtain physician orders for prothrombin time/partial thromboplastin time, apply moderate pressure dressing, and change sterile dressing when applicable.
Cardiac arrhythmia Symptom: Irregular heart rate	Potential need to reposition PICC tip to middle to lower third of superior vena cava to allow normal arm movements. Securing/suturing catheter at the insertion site prevents internal and external catheter migration.
Catheter embolism Symptoms: Catheter shear, "pinch off syndrome"	Related to catheter product or catheter insertion technique. Apply a tourniquet proximal to the site to prevent catheter fragment migration into central veins. Notify the physician, obtain a radiograph, and prepare for catheter fragment removal.

Continued

Nursing Assessment	Nursing Interventions
Catheter malposition or migration Symptom: Referred pain in jaw, ear, teeth, or shoulder	During catheter placement, the risk of entry into the internal jugular vein can be reduced by turning the patient's head toward the same side, while advancing the catheter. Spontaneous migration may occur during coughing, sneezing, or vomiting; Periodic PICC tip verification by radiograph may be required with long-term PICC placement.
Catheter occlusion Symptoms: Resistance to flush or fluid infusion, inability to perform blood sampling	Follow agency guidelines for flushing, blood sampling, and declotting catheter.
Cellulitis Symptoms: pain, tenderness, erythema at insertion site and/or surrounding subcutaneous tissue	Notify the physician. Remove the catheter, administer prescribed antimicrobials, and observe insertion site.
Nerve damage Symptoms: numbness, tingling, or weakness in area of insertion site	Notify the physician. Remove the catheter, reposition the extremity, and use sterile technique to apply a new dressing.
Thrombosis/ thrombophlebitis Symptoms: pain, erythema, and tenderness at insertion site; slowing of infusion rate	Observe and note osmolarity of infusate. Notify the physician and initiate prescribed therapies.
Sepsis Symptoms: elevated temperature, pain, tenderness, chills	Notify the physician. Administer prescribed therapies. Potential exists for catheter removal. Use sterile technique for catheter insertion, care, and maintenance.

Patient/Family Teaching for Self-Management

- Assess the patient's or caregiver's ability and willingness to learn, the availability of the caregiver, the home environment, and previous experience or expectations.
- Describe the purpose, function, and potential duration of placement for the catheter. (See "Patient/Caregiver Education" in Chapter 3 on pages 87 and 92.)
- Instruct the patient on the insertion procedure.
- Explain self-care management issues: site care, dressing and injection cap changes, flushing of the catheter with heparin or normal saline, and disposal of used supplies in an appropriate container.
- Review the symptoms related to each potential complication, teach emergency self-management techniques, and emphasize the need for prompt reporting of that information to the physician or nurse.
- Reinforce the troubleshooting tips related to potential catheter malfunctions with appropriate intervention strategies.
- Provide information on obtaining, storing, and disposing of supplies and the availability of professional care.
- Suggest that the patient carry a medical-alert card identifying the PICC type, tip location, insertion and external catheter length, and date of insertion.

Geriatric Considerations

The practitioner should consider age-related physiologic changes such as loss of subcutaneous tissue, fragile skin, neuromuscular and/or sensory deficits, visual and hearing losses, and arthritic joints. The patient's and caregiver's abilities to provide catheter site care, dressing changes, and catheter heparinization should be assessed. Individualized self-care teaching of catheter maintenance using demonstration and return demonstration techniques should be planned. The practitioner should consider large print for educational materials.

Resources

Clinical Competency

	Yes	No	NA
Peripherally Inserted Central Catheters			
Refer to Chapter 3, pages 87-100, for Patient Education and Preparation, Nursing Assessment and Interventions, and Nursing Management for Potential Complications. The remainder of this section refers to catheter insertion and management.			
1. Acquires approved PICC education; completes posttest requirement.			
2. Attains skill and competency for catheter insertion, under clinical preceptorship.			
3. Maintains skills and competency for catheter insertion and management via scheduled educational and clinical opportunities.			
4. Catheter insertion technique:			
▪ Verifies informed consent.			
▪ Reviews patient's allergy and laboratory values status.			
▪ Obtains appropriate supplies.			
▪ Explains the procedure to the patient.			
▪ Washes hands.			
▪ Assists patient to position of comfort for catheter insertion and prevention of catheter insertion complications.			
▪ Assesses catheter insertion site: basilic, medial basilic/cephalic, or external jugular vein.			
▪ Measures and records catheter length distance from insertion to desired endpoint placement.			

Clinical Competency—cont'd

	Yes	No	NA
Peripherally Inserted Central Catheters—cont'd			
■ Prepares patient's skin with bactericidal skin cleanser.			
■ Prepares sterile supplies for catheter insertion, flushing, and dressing procedures.			
■ Applies sterile protective coverings and gloves.			
■ Prepares catheter insertion site with sterile supplies.			
■ Measures and prepares PICC (e.g., primes catheter with sterile normal saline, trims catheter, beveling tip).			
■ Applies tourniquet and performs venipuncture.			
■ Validates blood return: dark red blood flashback, nonpulsatile flow.			
■ Threads catheter through introducer needle, with sterile gloved fingers or *nontooth forceps,* as appropriate to advance catheter.			
■ Inserts catheter to desired catheter tip placement.			
■ Stabilizes catheter and removes introducer.			
■ Flushes catheter to verify catheter patency.			
■ Cleanses catheter insertion site.			
■ Connects designated extension tubing with clamp and injection cap.			
■ Applies sterile "wick gauze dressing" for initial 24 hours, then changes to sterile transparent occlusive dressing at prescribed frequency.			

Continued

Clinical Competency—cont'd

	Yes	No	NA
Peripherally Inserted Central Catheters—cont'd			
■ Documents procedure in the patient's medical record: PICC brand, gauge, lot number, catheter length inserted and external length, insertion site, number of attempts, insertion difficulties, patient's tolerance of procedure, and patient/caregiver instructions regarding self-care maintenance.			
■ Verifies, communicates, and records evidence of radiograph procedure for desired catheter tip placement.			

Study Questions

1. Knowledge and clinical competency for PICC insertion include:
   a. Initial education, attain and maintain skill by clinical practice
   b. Initial education and clinical competency by post-test procedure
   c. Initial education, attain competency under preceptorship, maintain clinical skills
   d. Initial education, attain and maintain competency by designated practice

2. The vein of choice for PICC insertion is:
   a. Axillary
   b. Basilic
   c. Median carpal
   d. Innominate

3. Contraindications for PICC insertion include:
   a. Geriatric or neonate, requiring antimicrobial or blood product infusion

b. Geriatric or neonate, requiring hydration therapy or parenteral nutrition

c. Adult or pediatric patient with cellulitis or burns near the insertion site

d. Adult or pediatric patient requiring analgesia or chemotherapy administration

4. Confirmation of PICC tip placement is attained by:
   a. Aspiration of dark-red blood, nonpulsatile flow
   b. Infusion of normal saline to confirm patency
   c. Measurement of catheter internal and external length
   d. Radiograph confirming tip placement in the subclavian and/or superior vena cava vein

5. Patient/caregiver instructions for catheter self-care management include:
   a. Procedure for heparinization, problems to promptly report to physician or nurse
   b. Procedure for blood sampling, problems to promptly report to physician or nurse
   c. Procedure for catheter removal, problems to promptly report to physician or nurse
   d. Procedure for catheter repair, problems to promptly report to physician or nurse

6. Steps to take immediately for accidental catheter removal by patient include:
   a. Notifying the physician, applying sterile dressing, discarding the old catheter
   b. Notifying the physician, applying pressure dressing, measuring the catheter length
   c. Notifying the physician, applying a warm compress, measuring the catheter length
   d. Notifying the physician, applying pressure dressing, discarding the old catheter

7. Referred pain in the jaw, ear, teeth, or shoulder on the catheter insertion side may be attributed to:
   a. Catheter malposition or migration
   b. Catheter embolism
   c. Catheter occlusion
   d. Catheter sepsis

8. To minimize resistance in a prescribed PICC removal, you should:
   a. Remove the dressing, apply tension to the catheter with tape, vigorously flush the catheter
   b. Remove the dressing, apply tension to the catheter with tape, apply cold compresses
   c. Remove the dressing, apply tension to the catheter with tape, slowly flush the catheter
   d. Remove the dressing, apply tension to the catheter with tape, apply warm compresses

9. Nursing assessment and intervention for PICC sepsis include:
   a. Notifying the physician, obtaining a radiograph for tip placement, administering antimicrobials
   b. Notifying the physician, following the declotting procedure, administering antimicrobials
   c. Notifying the physician, culturing the purulent drainage, administering antimicrobials
   d. Notifying the physician, heparinizing the catheter, administering antimicrobials

10. Critical elements for PICC insertion documentation include:
    a. Insertion site, catheter length inserted, catheter brand and gauge, and physician permission to insert catheter
    b. Insertion site, catheter length inserted and external length, catheter brand and gauge, and radiograph verification tip placement
    c. Insertion site, catheter brand and gauge, radiograph verification tip placement and physician permission to insert catheter
    d. Insertion site, external length of catheter, catheter brand and gauge, and physician permission to insert catheter

Answers   1. c   2. b   3. c   4. d   5. a   6. b
7. a   8. d   9. c   10. b

IV Fluids

5

Objectives

1. Name the two major fluid compartments in the body.

2. Discuss the processes by which fluid balance is maintained.

3. Identify important measures of electrolyte balance.

4. Summarize the differences between isotonic, hypotonic, and hypertonic solutions.

5. Recognize clinical features for fluid volume deficit and fluid volume excess.

The body's fluid and electrolyte needs are altered by a variety of diseases and conditions (e.g., impaired cardiac, hepatic, or renal function). When individuals experience prolonged vomiting or diarrhea, abnormalities can occur in their fluid and electrolyte balance. Intravenous (IV) therapy is usually prescribed to restore previous losses of body fluids, maintain daily body fluid requirements, or replace present losses of body fluids. It is essential for the nurse to recognize the importance of fluid and electrolyte metabolism and how to provide therapeutic interventions for patients in all clinical settings.

Fluid Balance
Fluid Compartments

Although a small amount of body fluid is transcellular, it is primarily intracellular or extracellular. Intracellular fluid (ICF)—fluid within the cells—accounts for approximately 25 L of fluid

129

Table 5-1   Comparison of electrolyte values for ICF, ECF, and serum values on laboratory reports

Electrolytes	ICF	ECF	Normal Laboratory
Sodium	2-10 mEq/L	138-142 mEq/L	135-145 mEq/L
Potassium	135-155 mEq/L	3.8-5 mEq/L	3.5-5 mEq/L
Chloride	4-10 mEq/L	92-105 mEq/L	100-110 mEq/L
Calcium	< mg/dl trace	<5 mg/dl	8.5-10.5 mg/dl
Magnesium	80 mg/dl	1-2 mg/dl	1.7-3.4 mg/dl

ICF, Intracellular fluid; *ECF,* extracellular fluid.

and 40% of the body weight in an average-size adult. Extracellular fluid (ECF) is found in the spaces between cells (interstitial space) and in the intravascular fluid or plasma and represents 15% of body weight. Approximately 15 L of fluid are contained in the ECF—12 L in the interstitial space and 3 L in the plasma or intravascular space. ECF values are similar to chemistry laboratory values (Table 5-1).

Fluids shift from one compartment to the other as the concentration of electrolytes (solutes) is altered in the body. Fluids always move from the compartment with the lowest concentration of solutes to that with the greatest concentration. *Dehydration,* or body fluid loss, leads to *greater* concentrations of electrolytes in the *extracellular* compartment. This is treated with the administration of IV fluids. Fluid retention in the ECF compartment is treated with sodium restriction and restriction of fluid volumes.

Losses of ECF may be difficult to assess if the patient has pooling of fluids in the bowel, peritoneum, or intestinal spaces, as may occur with intestinal obstruction, peritonitis, hepatic failure, and/or burns. These areas are sometimes referred to as a *third space.* During surgery, pooling in the third space occurs and reabsorption is seen by an increased urine output 48 to 72 hours after the operation. This can often be anticipated, and fluids are adjusted accordingly. As fluid from the third space is reabsorbed into the circulation, the patient is monitored for fluid overload.

CLINICAL ALERT: Headache and confusion may indicate ICF volume changes. Thirst and nausea may indicate ECF volume changes. Noninvasive assessments of plasma volume include examining jugular veins, assessing pulse and respiratory rate, and obtaining blood pressure.

Water Balance

Water is essential for life; people can live several weeks without food but only a few days without water. Water maintains blood volume, regulates temperature, transports electrolytes and nutrients to and from cells, and is a part of many biologic reactions. Chemically, water and electrolytes work in concert to maintain water balance. Water intake is regulated through the sensation of thirst; water and electrolytes are continuously lost and replaced. Water balance is maintained primarily by the kidneys' response to the concentration of solutes present in the filtered body water.

Actual body water content depends on variables such as age, weight, sex, body composition, and disease processes. Adults are composed of approximately 60% water and infants of approximately 77%. Women have slightly lower water content than men because of a larger amount of body fat. There is an inverse relationship between body water and adipose tissue (fat): the more adipose tissue, the less body water. Many disease processes alter body water; examples are renal failure, congestive heart failure, and gastrointestinal dysfunction. These abnormal conditions alter the concentration of electrolytes present in the ICF and ECF and cause a shift in fluid between compartments.

Water balance is monitored through body weight. An otherwise unexplained weight change of 1 kg (2.2 pounds) represents a gain or loss of 1 L of body water. An individual's average daily water intake and water output is approximately 2500 ml (Table 5-2).

Nursing assessments with clinical findings of fluid imbalances (fluid volume deficit or fluid volume excess) are provided in Table 5-3—Evaluation for fluid balance.

CLINICAL ALERT: Major alterations in fluid balance can occur before clinical signs and symptoms are present. Approximately 3 days after major abdominal or thoracic surgery, fluid can move rapidly from the abdominal cavity and interstitial space to the intravascular compartment, creating fluid overload. Expect a significant change in the patient's urine output at this time.

Electrolyte Balance

Attaining and maintaining electrolyte balance are critical components of IV therapy because imbalances can be fatal. Electrolytes

Table 5-2   Normal fluid intake and loss in an adult eating 2500 calories per day*

Intake		Output	
Route	Amount of Gain (ml)	Route	Amount of Loss (ml)
Water in food	1000	Skin	500
Water from oxidation	300	Lungs	350
Water as liquid	1200	Feces	150
		Kidney	1500
Total	2500	Total	2500

From Phipps WJ, Cassmeyer VL, Sands JK, Lehman MK: *Medical-surgical nursing: concepts and clinical practice,* ed 6, St Louis, 1999, Mosby.
*Approximate figures.

are related to at least four fundamental physiologic processes: water distribution in the ICF and ECF, neuromuscular irritability, acid-base balance, and maintenance of osmotic pressure.*[1] IV therapy is directed at restoring lost electrolytes; once the electrolytes are replaced, the metabolic acid-base balance corrects itself. There are respiratory acid-base disturbances that cannot be corrected with IV therapy alone, such as hyperventilation, which causes increased pH secondary to blowing off CO_2, or hypoventilation with CO_2 retention, which results in decreased pH or acidosis. The primary regulation of fluid and electrolyte status is determined by renal function. Proximal tubules of the kidney are responsible for reabsorption, filtration, and secretion of electrolytes.

CLINICAL ALERT: Elderly patients are at particular risk for compromised fluid and electrolyte status. Arteriosclerosis, heart failure, cardiomyopathy, diabetes, hypertension, and many other chronic conditions place patients at risk for diminished renal

---

Osmotic pressure refers to the pull or force created by random movements in a compartment or area. Fluids always flow from areas of lesser concentration of solute to areas of greater concentration. Concentration in the blood plasma is largely determined by serum proteins, such as albumin. The osmotic influence (osmolality) of an IV fluid is a key consideration when determining which type of IV fluid to administer in a particular situation.

Table 5-3   Evaluation for fluid imbalance

Nursing Assessment	Clinical Features
Blood pressure	*Fluid deficit:* Fall in systolic blood pressure (BP), decreased pulse pressure, and postural hypotension *Fluid excess:* Increased BP, no postural changes
Pulse	*Fluid deficit:* Weak, thready pulse *Fluid excess:* Bounding pulse; increased pulse rate; tachycardia may be present with either fluid excess or deficit
Jugular vein	*Fluid deficit:* Flat neck veins *Fluid excess:* Vein distension visible; pulsation higher than 2 cm above sternal angle when head of bed raised 45 degrees
Respirations	*Fluid deficit:* Rare crackles and wheezes; dry, thick secretions *Fluid excess:* Crackles and wheezes; moist secretions
Edema	*Fluid deficit:* Infrequent edema *Fluid excess:* First found in dependent parts, such as sacral edema in persons on bed rest; pedal edema in ambulatory persons
Skin turgor	*Fluid deficit:* Loose, toneless skin; skin tense when lifted with two fingers; inaccurate assessment in elderly persons related to loss of adipose tissue *Fluid excess:* Good skin turgor
Intake and output	*Fluid deficit: Output* greater than *intake;* sluggish urine output; high specific gravity *Fluid excess: Intake* greater than *output;* rapid urine output; low specific gravity
Weight	*Fluid deficit:* Weight loss *Fluid excess:* Weight gain

function and renal failure. Monitor renal function by closely monitoring intake and output records and changes in the serum creatinine level.

The electrolytes of greatest importance in fluid therapy are discussed in the following sections.

Sodium

The main role of sodium is to control the distribution of water throughout the body and to maintain a normal fluid balance. Because sodium attracts water, it is the primary factor determining the volume of extracellular space. Sodium is administered intravenously as sodium chloride. Sodium disorders are considered extracellular volume disorders. High sodium concentrations in the plasma (hypernatremia) result from conditions such as an impaired sense of thirst, hyperventilation, fever, head injuries, decreased secretion of antidiuretic hormone (ADH), diabetes insipidus, and the inability of the kidneys to respond to ADH.

Low sodium concentrations in the plasma (hyponatremia) involve an increase in the proportion of water to salt in the blood. Hyponatremia results from a disturbance in the ADH secretory mechanism, such as a head injury or severe physiologic and psychologic stress (this disturbance is called *SIADH*—syndrome of inappropriate ADH secretion). Additional patient-related factors such as excessive sweating combined with a large intake of water by mouth (salt is lost and fluid increased) may result in reduced sodium concentration. Hyponatremia may also occur when excessive amounts of nonelectrolyte fluids (e.g., hypotonic solutions) are administered to such patients at a time when ADH secretion is excessive.

Hypernatremia	Hyponatremia
Serum sodium >145 mEq/L	Serum sodium <145 mEq/L
Hypotension	Hypertension, increased intra-cranial pressure
Hypervolemia	Hypovolemia
Dry, sticky mucous membranes	Abdominal cramps
Urine volume <30 ml/hr	Low urine specific gravity
Altered mental status (e.g., irritable, disorientation)	Altered mental status (e.g., confusion, insomnia, combative)
Seizures	Seizures, coma, and death

CLINICAL ALERT: *Hypernatremia* is corrected slowly—over 48 hours or more—because rapid treatment can produce serious consequences, including loss of consciousness and death. Use normal saline to correct hypernatremia because normal saline is less concentrated than the serum of a patient with severe hypernatremia. *Hyponatremia* is treated with IV infusion of hypertonic 3% to 5% sodium chloride solutions in conjunction with diuretics that will result in the loss of more water than sodium. *Always* infuse these solutions via an infusion pump cautiously while monitoring closely neurologic, cardiovascular, and renal status.

Potassium

Potassium—the major electrolyte of the ICF—is required to maintain osmotic balance and cell membrane electrical potential and to move glucose into the cell. Dehydration, vomiting, gastric suction, diarrhea, polyuria, steroid therapy, blood pH, and diuretic therapy influence plasma potassium or the potassium found in the ECF measured by laboratory testing. When potassium balance between the ICF and ECF is altered, cellular metabolism is affected along with the cardiovascular, renal, respiratory, and neuromuscular systems.

Elevated serum potassium levels are referred to as *hyperkalemia;* reduced serum potassium levels are called *hypokalemia. Acidosis* drives potassium out of cells, resulting in *hyperkalemia; alkalosis* drives potassium into cells, resulting in *hypokalemia.*

Hyperkalemia	Hypokalemia
Serum K^+ >5 mEq/L	Serum K^+ <3.5 mEq/L
Cardiac arrhythmias	Ectopic cardiac activity
Electrocardiogram (ECG): peaked T wave, widened QRS, lengthened PR	ECG: flattened T wave, depressed ST segment
Diarrhea, abdominal pain	Decreased bowel sounds, ileus
Neuromuscular irritability (e.g., paresthesia)	Muscle cramps
Oliguria or anuria	Polyuria
Irregular or slow heart rate	Postural hypotension

Potassium is administered intravenously as potassium chloride (KCl). Hypokalemia is treated with oral or IV administration of KCl. A potassium deficit is corrected slowly to prevent the development of transient hyperkalemia. Treatment of hyperkalemia depends on the rate at which the potassium level increased. Immediate treatment measures may include IV administration of calcium gluconate, sodium bicarbonate, glucose, or insulin. In mild states of hyperkalemia, oral and IV intake of potassium is restricted.

CLINICAL ALERT:

1. Correction of hydration deficits before potassium administration is critical to prevent renal complications. Urine output of at least 30 ml/hr should be verified before initiating IV potassium medications or solutions.
2. If the IV administration rate exceeds 20 mEq/hr, cardiac monitoring is recommended.
3. Potassium chloride should never be administered directly in a concentrated form by IV bolus because of the danger of cardiac arrest.
4. KCl should be thoroughly mixed when adding to an IV infusion bag to prevent layering of potassium at the bottom of the bag.
5. A small dose of lidocaine may be added to the KCl solution to diminish the burning sensation patients often complain of when IV infusions contain potassium greater than 40 mEq/L.

Chloride

Chloride is the major electrolyte in the ECF. Chloride levels in blood are passively related to those of sodium, so when serum sodium increases, chloride also increases. Factors causing losses or gains of chloride often affect sodium levels. Increased chloride levels are caused by dehydration, renal failure, or acidosis. Decreased chloride levels result from fluid losses in the gastrointestinal tract (nausea, vomiting, diarrhea, and gastric suction).

Chloride Excess	Chloride Deficit
Serum Cl⁻ >110 mEq/L	Serum Cl⁻ <100 mEq/L
Dehydration	Fever
Hyperventilation	Nausea and vomiting
Urine output less than 30 ml/hr	Tissue wasting (burns)

Chloride is always administered intravenously in conjunction with sodium and potassium.

Calcium

Calcium, the most abundant electrolyte in the human body, is stored primarily in the skeleton. More than 99% of skeletal calcium is unavailable for day-to-day electrolyte regulation. Calcium is present in the blood in two forms: free, ionized calcium, which is circulating, and calcium that is bound to protein. The bound form attaches to the plasma protein (albumin) and other complex substances such as phosphates. For this reason, it is important to correlate the serum calcium concentration with the serum albumin level.

Calcium levels have an effect on neuromuscular function, cardiac status, and bone formation. Disturbances in calcium balance result from alterations in bone metabolism, secretion of parathyroid hormone, renal dysfunction, and altered dietary intake.

Hypercalcemia	Hypocalcemia
Serum Ca^{++} >10.5 mEq/L	Serum Ca^{++} <8.5 mEq/L
Lethargy, fatigue	Bone pain
Polydipsia, polyuria	Neuromuscular irritability, seizures
Muscle weakness	Muscle tremors, cramps
Anorexia, constipation	Diarrhea

Acute symptoms of hypocalcemia are treated with IV administration of calcium gluconate or calcium chloride. Oral calcium supplements are used for chronic hypocalcemic states.

Hypercalcemia treatment includes supportive measures to lower the serum calcium level and to correct the underlying cause. Sodium chloride infusion and the administration of thiazide diuretics, usually furosemide (Lasix), are given to enhance the body's excretion of calcium. IV administration of calcitonin, pamidronate (Aredia), and zoledronate (Zometa) may be given to inhibit bone resorption in bone-destructive conditions.

Magnesium

Magnesium is normally obtained from dietary intake. Magnesium is excreted through the kidneys. Hypomagnesemia is far more common than hypermagnesemia. Conditions associated with magnesium deficits include prolonged malnutrition or starvation, alcoholism, and long-term IV therapy without magnesium supplementation. Symptoms are potentiated by hypocalcemia. Hypermagnesemia occurs most often in patients with renal failure, those with diabetic ketoacidosis, and those who use excessive amounts of antacids or laxatives.

Magnesium Excess	Magnesium Deficit
Serum Mg^{++} <3.4 mEq/L	Serum Mg^{++} >1.7 mEq/L
Lethargy	Disorientation
Absent deep tendon reflexes	Hyperactive reflexes
Hypotension	Tremors, tetany
Depressed respirations	Mood changes

Magnesium sulfate solutions can be administered intravenously to correct deficits, although monitoring is required to prevent cardiac effects. Magnesium excess may be treated with the IV administration of calcium gluconate, which reverses the action of magnesium. Glucose or insulin may be given to enhance the renal excretion of magnesium.

Fluid and Electrolyte Loss

The major components of body fluids are water and electrolytes. Water losses occur when water leaves the body through the kidneys, lungs, skin, and gastrointestinal tract. Kidneys are the organs principally responsible for regulating the volume and concentration of all body fluids. When given optimal amounts of water and electrolytes, a normally functioning kidney can maintain water and electrolyte balance. However, during serious illness, the kidneys are sometimes unable to make the final adjustments for fluid and electrolyte balance.

Water loss from the lungs and skin increases with elevated temperatures in the environment, fever, rapid respiratory rate, and a loss of skin covering. Examples of situations resulting in skin-covering loss are surgical procedures, burns, and wounds. Gastrointestinal losses increase when vomiting and diarrhea are present. Fluid and electrolyte losses are replaced through the intake of food and water. Nursing assessments with clinical findings of fluid and electrolyte balance are listed in Table 5-4.

IV Fluids

IV fluids are classified as isotonic, hypotonic, or hypertonic solutions, depending on the effect a fluid has on the ICF and ECF compartments (Table 5-5, p. 140).

Table 5-4   Nursing assessment with clinical findings of fluid and electrolyte balance

Nursing Assessment	Clinical Findings
Compare total fluid intake and total fluid output.	Intake should be approximately the same as output.
Compare daily weight obtained at approximately the same time on the same scale.	A gain of 1 kg of body weight corresponds to 1 L of fluid.
Review serum electrolyte laboratory values (sodium, potassium, chloride, magnesium).	*Fluid excess:* Electrolyte level is diluted; thus serum electrolyte values are decreased. *Fluid deficit:* Electrolyte levels are concentrated; serum values are increased.
Observe clinical features.	Condition of mucous membranes and skin, heart rate, presence of thirst, and mental alertness.

Isotonic Solutions

Isotonic solutions are used to expand ECF volume. Fluid initially stays in the intravascular compartment. These solutions contain the same concentration of solute to fluid as that in body fluid and exert the same osmotic pressure as ECF in a normal, steady state. Isotonic fluids are indicated for intravascular dehydration.

Normal saline, or 0.9% NS; lactated Ringer's solution; and 5% dextrose and water all function as isotonic solutions. If an isotonic solution is infused into the intravascular system, fluid volume increases. One liter of isotonic solution expands the ECF by 1 L. Three liters of isotonic fluid is required to replace 1 L of blood loss.

Hypotonic Solutions

Hypotonic solutions exert less osmotic pressure than the ECF. Infusion of excessive hypotonic fluids can lead to intravascular fluid depletion, hypotension, cellular edema, and cell damage. Because these solutions can cause serious complications, the patient and the infusion should be monitored closely. The hypotonic solutions of 0.45% sodium chloride and 0.3% sodium chloride provide free water, sodium, and chloride to aid the kidneys in the excretion of solutes. Hypotonic solutions are administered for cellular dehydration.

Table 5-5   IV fluids: hypotonic, hypertonic, and isotonic

Fluid and Tonicity	Comments
Saline Solutions	
0.33% sodium chloride hypotonic	Extremely hypotonic; used only with close observation.
	Does not supply calories.
0.45% sodium chloride hypotonic	Does not supply calories.
0.9% sodium chloride isotonic	Used to expand plasma volume; provides sodium and chloride in excess of plasma levels; given primarily with blood transfusions and to replace large sodium losses, as in burns, gastrointestinal fluid loss; *contraindicated* in congestive heart failure, pulmonary edema, renal impairment, sodium retention.
	Does not supply calories.
3% sodium chloride hypertonic	Correction of severe sodium depletion.
	Does not supply calories.
5% sodium chloride hypertonic	Maximum daily amount should not exceed 400 ml; can result in fluid volume excess and pulmonary edema.
	Does not supply calories.
Dextrose in Water Solutions	
5% dextrose in water isotonic	Used to maintain fluid intake or to reestablish plasma volume; does not replace electrolyte deficits; aids in renal excretion of solutes; *contraindicated* in head injuries; may increase intracranial pressure.
	Supplies 170 calories/L.
10% dextrose in water hypertonic	Used for peripheral nutrition.
	Supplies 340 calories/L.
20% dextrose in water hypertonic	Irritating to veins; acts as a diuretic; may increase fluid loss; central venous access is required.
	Supplies 680 calories/L.

Table 5-5   IV fluids: hypotonic, hypertonic,
and isotonic—cont'd

Fluid and Tonicity	Comments

Dextrose in Water Solutions—cont'd

50% dextrose in water hypertonic	Must be administered via central venous access. Supplies 1700 calories/L.
70% dextrose in water hypertonic	Used to provide calories to persons with compromised renal and cardiac status; central venous access is required. Supplies 2400 calories/L.

Dextrose in Water and Saline Solutions

5% dextrose and 0.2% NaCl isotonic	Supplies 170 calories/L.
5% dextrose and 0.3% NaCl isotonic	Supplies 170 calories/L.
5% dextrose and 0.45% NaCl hypertonic	Used to treat hypovolemia and to promote diuresis in dehydration; used to maintain fluid intake; maintenance fluid of choice if no electrolyte abnormalities. Supplies 170 calories/L.
5% dextrose and 0.9%NaCl hypertonic	Supplies 170 calories/L.
10% dextrose and 0.9%NaCl hypertonic	Supplies 340 calories/L.

Multiple Electrolyte Solutions

Ringer's solution isotonic	Electrolyte concentrations of sodium, potassium, calcium, and chloride similar to normal plasma levels. Supplies calories only when mixed with dextrose.

Continued

Table 5-5　IV fluids: hypotonic, hypertonic,
and isotonic—cont'd

Fluid and Tonicity	Comments
Multiple Electrolyte Solutions—cont'd	
Lactated Ringer's solution isotonic	Electrolyte concentrations similar to plasma levels; lactate for correction of metabolic acidosis; used to replace fluid losses due to bile drainage, diarrhea, and burns; fluid of choice for acute blood loss replacement; *contraindicated* in congestive heart failure, renal impairment, head injury, liver disease, respiratory alkalosis. Does not supply calories.
5% dextrose and lactated Ringer's solution hypertonic	Used to replace gastric fluid losses; not to be given with blood products; *contraindicated* in congestive heart failure, renal impairment. Supplies 170 calories.
5% dextrose and electrolyte #2 hypertonic	Electrolyte maintenance solution. Supplies 170 calories.

CLINICAL ALERT: Never administer sterile distilled water intravenously except when using it as a drug diluent, because plain distilled water has an extremely hypotonic effect on red blood cells and can lead to lysis of the red blood cells.

Hypertonic Solutions

Hypertonic solutions exert greater osmotic pressure than ECF. These solutions are used to shift ECF into the blood plasma by diffusing fluid from the tissues to equalize the solutes in the plasma. Rapid administration of a hypertonic solution can cause circulatory overload and dehydration. Hypertonic IV fluids include 5% dextrose in 0.9% saline, 5% dextrose in lactated Ringer's solution, and dextrose and water solutions of 10% dextrose and greater.

Documentation Recommendations

1. Volume and composition of all administered fluids
2. Fluid intake and output
3. Fluid deficit

a. Eyes: dry conjunctiva, reduced tearing, sunken appearance
b. Mouth: dry, sticky mucous membranes; dry, cracked lips
c. Skin: diminished turgor
d. Neurologic: reduced central nervous system activity
e. Cardiac: Narrowed pulse pressure, lowered blood pressure
f. Weight: loss
g. Other: fever, source, and amount of any body fluid loss
4. Fluid excess
a. Eyes: orbital edema
b. Skin: warm, moist; edema in dependent areas
c. Cardiac: bounding pulse, vein distention
d. Respiratory: dyspnea, crackles, wheezes, increased rate, pulmonary edema
5. Electrolyte imbalance
a. Sodium excess: urine volume and patient temperature
b. Sodium deficit: increased viscosity of saliva, increased urine volume, all mental status changes, and signs and symptoms of increased intracranial pressure, such as headache and increased blood pressure
c. Potassium excess: irregular heart rate, diminished urine volume, ECG changes
d. Potassium deficit: muscle weakness, cardiac arrhythmias

Nursing Diagnoses

- Fluid volume deficit, related to excessive fluid loss from abnormal routes (vomiting, diarrhea, indwelling tubes), diuretic therapy, burns, trauma, and surgical procedures
- Fluid volume deficit, related to inability to receive or absorb fluids, such as in hypermetabolic states (fever), head injury, coma, and electrolyte imbalance
- Fluid volume excess related to excess fluid or sodium intake

Patient/Family Teaching for Self-Management

- Emphasize that IV fluids do not provide sufficient calories to meet basic energy needs, and when indicated, encourage small, frequent meals.
- Teach signs and symptoms of fluid excess and deficit, such as significance of weight gain, edema, shortness of breath, dyspnea on exertion, and recognition of gastrointestinal losses.
- Teach measurement of fluid intake and output so patients and family members can participate in record keeping.

Guidelines for Home Care Infusion Therapy

Successful home infusion therapy depends on patient motivation, disease stability, and the availability of venous access. A knowledgeable and competent caregiver must be present in the home during the infusion to monitor patient changes.

- Instruct patients and caregivers to monitor weight gains and losses and to report significant findings.
- Reinforce the need to report all abnormal findings to the physician, such as shortness of breath, dyspnea on exertion, edema, and elevated temperature; discuss an emergency plan with the patient and caregiver.
- Monitor electrolytes status on a planned basis; ideally, electrolytes should be obtained within 24 hours of initiating infusion therapy; obtain results of recent blood urea nitrogen (BUN), creatinine, blood glucose values, and any other tests relevant to the patient's condition.
- Plan oral fluid electrolyte supplements with the physician.
- Clearly document all education provided.

Geriatric Considerations

Many older individuals experience diminished homeostasis as a result of the reduced capacity of various body systems. Nurses caring for elderly patients should carefully monitor the patients' clinical status, laboratory results, vital signs, weight gain or loss, and intake and output.

- Common alterations in fluid and electrolytes affecting the cardiovascular patient include hypovolemia, hypervolemia, potassium and calcium imbalance, heart failure, and arrhythmias. Correction of imbalances and prevention of serious complications caused by the imbalances lead to increased survival rates.
- Obstructions of the urinary tract are likely to result in fluid and electrolyte imbalances. Removal of the obstruction results in diuresis, which can significantly alter fluid and electrolyte status.
- In acute or chronic renal failure, patients have a tendency to develop hypervolemia, hyperkalemia, hypocalcemia, and metabolic acidosis. Sodium is generally retained.
- Postoperatively and especially after intestinal surgery, elderly

patients are at high risk for fluid and electrolyte imbalances, particularly fluid overload and sodium and potassium imbalances.

Resources

Clinical Competency—IV Fluids

	Yes	No	NA
1. Verify physician order for date, time, rate, infusion solution, and composition.			
2. Verify appropriate laboratory data.			
3. Verify allergy data.			
4. Calculate flow rate.			
5. Select an appropriate infusion solution and composition with designated IV tubing.			
6. Correctly label with patient name, IV additives, and rate of administration.			
7. Wash hands.			
8. Verify patient identification.			
9. Use aseptic technique to set up gravity flow and/or infusion pump, prime IV tubing, and adjust rate.			
10. Verify correct flow rate via gravity flow and/or infusion pump.			
11. Document in the medical record solution volume and composition, rate, infusion pump use, fluid intake and output, fluid deficit and/or fluid excess status clinical features, electrolyte imbalance clinical features, and patient teaching regarding signs and symptoms to report.			
12. Observe and monitor the patient on a scheduled frequency.			

Study Questions

1. Approximately 40% of the body weight is in which space?
   a. Intracellular
   b. Extracellular
   c. Transcellular
   d. None of the above

2. Dehydration leads to increased electrolyte concentration in which space?
   a. Intracellular
   b. Extracellular
   c. Transcellular
   d. None of the above

3. An otherwise unexplained weight change of 1 kg (2.2 pounds) represents:
   a. 0.25 L of body water
   b. 0.50 L of body water
   c. 1.0 L of body water
   d. 2.0 L of body water

4. Critical serum (mEq/L) laboratory values depicting within-normal-limits serum electrolyte values include:
   a. Sodium 135-145; potassium 0.5-3.5; chloride 100-110; calcium 8.5-10.5; magnesium 1.7-3.4
   b. Sodium 135-145; potassium 3.5-5.0; chloride 110-120; calcium 8.5-10.5; magnesium 1.7-3.4
   c. Sodium 135-155; potassium 3.5-5.0; chloride 100-110; calcium 7.0-10.5; magnesium 1.7-3.4
   d. Sodium 135-145; potassium 3.5-5.0; chloride 100-110; calcium 8.5-10.5; magnesium 1.7-3.4

5. Serum electrolyte values in a patient experiencing fluid volume deficit are expected to be:
   a. Decreased
   b. Increased
   c. Unchanged
   d. Reflected via intake and output

6. Fluid volume excess clinical features include:
   a. Tachycardia, flat jugular vein, infrequent edema

    b. Tachycardia, distended jugular vein, toneless tense skin

    c. Tachycardia, distended jugular vein, good skin turgor

    d. Tachycardia, distended jugular vein, output greater than intake

7. Before administering IV potassium to an adult, verify that urine output is at least:

    a. 30 ml/hr

    b. 40 ml/hr

    c. 50 ml/hr

    d. 60 ml/hr

8. Isotonic solutions are often used to expand the ECF column, these common solutions are:

    a. 0.9% sodium chloride, 5% dextrose/lactated Ringer's, 5% dextrose and water

    b. 0.33% sodium chloride, 0.45% sodium chloride, 5% dextrose/0.2% sodium chloride

    c. 3% sodium chloride, 5% dextrose/0.45% sodium chloride, 10% dextrose and water

    d. 0.9% sodium chloride, 5% dextrose and water, lactated Ringer's

9. Hyponatremia and hypernatremia treatment corrections are administered as follows:

    a. Infuse the solutions and/or medications quickly to correct deficits, use gravity flow process, and monitor cardiac, neurologic, and renal status.

    b. Infuse the solutions and/or medications quickly to correct deficits, use infusion pumps, and monitor cardiac, neurologic, and renal status.

    c. Infuse the solutions and/or medications slowly to correct deficits, use gravity flow process, and monitor cardiac, neurologic, and renal status.

    d. Infuse the solutions and/or medications slowly to correct deficits, use infusion pumps, and monitor cardiac, neurologic, and renal status.

10. Documentation recommendations for IV fluids include:

    a. Electrolyte imbalance, fluid deficit and excess, fluid intake and output, solution composition

    b. Electrolyte imbalance, fluid deficit and excess, fluid intake and output, solution volume

  c. Electrolyte imbalance, fluid deficit and excess, fluid intake and output, solution volume and composition

  d. Electrolyte imbalance, fluid deficit and excess, fluid intake and output, laboratory serum electrolyte values

Answers   1. a   2. b   3. c   4. d   5. b   6. c
7. a   8. d   9. d   10. c

IV Medication Administration

6

Objectives

1. Verbalize the sequential steps for patient drug administration.

2. Identify critical elements of therapeutic drug monitoring.

3. List immediate actions to be taken in the event of an adverse drug reaction.

4. Discuss the advantages and disadvantages of various routes of intravenous (IV) drug administration.

5. Describe features that differ among IV infusion pumps.

More medications are being administered intravenously than before, and nurses are assuming greater responsibilities related to IV medication administration. With increased usage has come a greater understanding of the benefits and risks of this treatment modality. Many technical improvements have been made in equipment, and innovative and time-saving measures have been developed to increase the efficacy of this practice. This chapter addresses principles of IV medication administration, methods of delivering drugs intravenously, and information on select drugs.

General Principles
Indications for IV Drug Administration

IV drug administration is beneficial for several reasons:

1. Assurance that effective concentrations of the drug are achieved rapidly

2. Control over onset of peak serum drug concentrations

3. Production of a biologic effect when a drug cannot be absorbed by the oral route

4. Administration of drugs to patients who are unable to take oral medications

Drug Dose Calculations

Because drugs for IV medication administration are injected directly into the vascular system, IV doses are often lower than those administered through other routes. Although the doses of many drugs administered intravenously are calculated according to the patient's weight, dosages are adjusted also according to drug distribution and the patient's absorption ability, metabolism and excretion, and observed signs and symptoms.

Serum albumin levels are important to drug distribution because drugs bind to receptor sites on plasma proteins (especially albumin) and tissues. Only a drug that is not bound to a plasma protein or to a tissue is able to exert a therapeutic effect, so patients with low serum albumin levels have more adverse effects. This occurs because more free (unbound) drug is available to exert a therapeutic effect. Drug binding influences both drug effectiveness and the duration of the effect.

Drug metabolism and excretion are the two components involved in drug elimination from the body. *Metabolism* refers to the transformation of the drug to a water-soluble form that allows excretion to occur. Metabolism occurs mainly in the liver, and most drugs are excreted by the kidneys. Patient age and underlying disease affect elimination. Elderly people usually have diminished liver and kidney function and less muscle mass than younger persons. Any disease process that alters hepatic or renal function also can cause a prolonged drug effect and increase the likelihood of adverse drug effects.

A drug's *half-life* is the time required for plasma levels of the drug to fall to half of the original level. Drug half-life is influenced by both metabolism and excretion rates. In addition, the half-life determines the frequency of doses that must be administered to maintain a steady drug state. Some drugs, such as heparin, must be administered continuously to effectively maintain blood levels. However, antibiotics and various other drugs may be given intermittently. When a new drug is given, loading doses are often required to reach therapeutic plasma concentrations rapidly. Therapeutic blood plasma levels are altered by increasing or decreasing the drug dose or by changing the amount of time between doses.

CLINICAL ALERT: Because the kidney and the liver are the major organs involved in drug excretion, the half-life of a drug is extended in patients with renal or liver disease and in elderly patients.

Therapeutic Drug Monitoring

Therapeutic drug monitoring (TDM) is an important tool that is used to adjust drug dosages when drugs that have a narrow therapeutic range are administered or when patients with complex conditions receive drugs that are known to cause toxic responses. TDM is expected when giving aminoglycosides, immunosuppressants, and selected cardiovascular drugs.

Some goals of therapeutic drug monitoring include the following:

- Reducing drug toxicity
- Improving the effectiveness of therapy
- Reducing the incidence of therapeutic failure
- Providing documentation for careful use of potentially toxic medications

To monitor drug dosages closely, blood is drawn to measure periodic drug peak and trough levels. Accurate laboratory analysis of peak and trough drug levels depends on accurate communication of the time of drug administration and of the time of the blood sampling. Trough levels are measured before administration of a subsequent dose, and peak levels are measured within 30 minutes of the completion of a dose. The intensity of monitoring depends on the clinical circumstances. In relatively low-risk situations, only the steady-state concentration is measured. Medium monitoring includes analysis of two blood levels before steady state and the steady-state level. Maximal monitoring, used with very unstable patients, involves measuring the drug level immediately after a loading dose is given, as well as at least two levels before steady state and the steady-state levels. Trough levels greater than $2~\mu g$ are associated with increased toxicities (see Table 6-1 for a listing of some IV peak and trough levels).

To effectively conduct therapeutic drug monitoring, the laboratory needs the following information:

- Drug name
- Daily or intermittent dose

Table 6-1 Serum drug level monitoring

Drug	Trough	Peak
Aminoglycosides (gentamicin, tobramycin, amikacin)	Within ½ hr of next dose Serum level: <2 μg/ml	½ hr after end of 30-min infusion, or 15 min after end of 1-hr infusion Serum level: <2 μg/ml
Vancomycin	Within ½ hr of next dose Serum level: <10 μm/ml	1 hr after end of infusion Serum level: 20-40 μg/ml
Digoxin IV	5-24 hr after last dose, just before next dose preferred Serum level: 0.82 μg/ml	Do not draw
Aminophylline	Just before dose Serum level: 10-20 μg/ml	1 hr after dose Serum level: 10-20 μg/ml
Dilantin IV	Just before dose Serum level: 10-20 μg/ml	½ hr after end of infusion

- Time and amount of last dose
- Time blood sample was drawn
- Route of drug administration
- Patient age
- Patient diagnosis—pertinent to multiple drug therapies (e.g., anticoagulants)

Combination Drug Therapy

Combination therapy refers to intended drug interactions. Drugs are often administered in combination to potentiate a desired effect that is enhanced by the interaction of two or more drugs; for example, metoclopramide hydrochloride (Reglan) and dexamethasone sodium phosphate (Decadron) for mild to moderate antiemetic management of emesis-induced chemotherapy.

Potential Complications of IV Drug Administration

Every complication that may develop with IV therapy is present when drugs are administered intravenously, including infiltration, phlebitis, and the potential for embolism or infection. Some drugs may damage surrounding tissue if an infiltration or extravasation occurs. Adverse or unplanned effects such as diminished drug potency and toxicities can occur often when multiple drugs are administered. Mild adverse effects are called *side effects;* serious adverse effects are called *toxicities.*

Adverse Drug Reactions

Adverse drug reactions (ADRs) can range from expected side effects of a drug to hypersensitivity reactions and death. According to the U.S. Food and Drug Administration, an adverse reaction is any undesirable experience associated with the use of a medical product in a patient. ADRs are more narrowly defined by agencies and institutions, so it is necessary to be aware of agency policy for reporting ADRs. Hypersensitivity reactions, drug incompatibilities, and unexpected reactions are common examples of reportable ADRs.

Almost any drug can produce hypersensitivity (allergic) reactions in susceptible patients. Unless a person has had a previous allergic episode, there is no way to predict who may experience this medical emergency. Hypersensitivity reactions occur more quickly when drugs are given intravenously than when given by other routes. At high risk are very young patients and elderly patients who have altered renal and hepatic function, patients with a history of multiple allergies, patients receiving investigational drugs, and those receiving more than one drug at a time.

The onset of a reaction is usually sudden, although reactions may be delayed as long as 30 to 60 minutes. Usually, a more rapid onset correlates with a more severe reaction. The extent of a reaction is related to the dose of drug administered and the patient's degree of hypersensitivity. Mild reactions include urticaria, pruritus, and erythema. Sudden onset of inflammation and itching is the most common hypersensitivity reaction. The drug should be stopped and the patient treated symptomatically with antihistamines such as diphenhydramine HCl (Benadryl).

More severe reactions may include laryngeal edema, broncho-spasm, and hypotension. Signs and symptoms of anaphylaxis include angioedema (swelling of the mouth, tongue, extremities, and area around the eyes), respiratory distress (wheezing, cyano-sis), skin reactions (itching, blotchy skin wheals), and symptoms of circulatory collapse (rapidly falling blood pressure, weakness, thready pulse, and vertigo). Patients feel fear, panic, and a sense of impending doom. Suffocation resulting from laryngeal edema is the most common cause of death after an anaphylactic reaction. Many people have a recurrence of anaphylaxis within 24 hours. The following steps should be taken when reactions are identified:

1. Stop the medication immediately.
2. Maintain or initiate patent IV access.
3. Observe the patient's respiratory status; if the patient has respiratory difficulty, keep him or her in an upright position if possible while summoning help.
4. Notify the physician.
5. Prepare to administer emergency medications.
6. Monitor vital signs.
7. Initiate resuscitation if a respiratory or cardiopulmonary arrest occurs.

CLINICAL ALERT: Epinephrine (Adrenalin) followed by di-phenhydramine (Benadryl) is the combination of choice for treating anaphylaxis. Other drugs that may be given include hydrocortisone (Solu-Cortef) and aminophylline (Theophylline).

The following drugs and categories of drugs have the potential for adverse reactions: anticoagulant, antimicrobial, antifungal (amphotericin B), antineoplastic (asparaginase, bleomycin), corti-costeroid, dextran, digoxin, lidocaine, phenytoin (Dilantin), and dyes used for diagnostic testing.

Drug Incompatibility

Potential incompatibility of medications is a concern whenever patients receive multiple IV regimens. Information on drug stability and compatibility is complex and changes frequently as adminis-tration systems and solutions change. New research and additional experience result in changes in drug treatment recommendations. Because of conflicting literature studies and the complexities involved with compatibility information, absolute statements are difficult to make and consultation with a pharmacist is important.

Drug stability is affected by temperature. Refrigeration improves stability, and higher temperatures reduce stability. Always follow the manufacturer's recommendations for drug diluent to ensure drug stability.

Compatibility is most influenced by pH. Drugs with similar pH are compatible; those with significantly differing pHs are incompatible and should not be administered together. Although compatibility charts are helpful tools, they should be used judiciously because conflicting information is often presented as a result of varied study conditions.

Incompatibility occurs when either two drugs or a drug and an IV solution are mixed to make a product that is unsuitable for safe administration. Physical, chemical, and therapeutic changes in the drug result from incompatibility. These changes result in loss of drug activity, unexpected adverse reactions, precipitate formation, and adverse clinical changes in the patient such as anaphylaxis, multiple pulmonary infarctions, and platelet aggregation.

Physical changes in the drug are the most common and the easiest to detect visually. These may be a change in color or precipitate formation. A precipitate formation is often determined by the concentration of the drug, the pH of the solutions, the sequence of additives, and the amount of standing time since admixture. Precipitation can occur immediately, hours later in the tubing or filter, or later in the IV catheter, thus causing occlusion. Visual inspection cannot detect very small precipitates.

Chemical changes result in irreversible drug degradation. The product resulting from chemical change is less active than expected, and therefore the therapeutic effect is altered. Chemical effects are often not detected with a visual inspection.

Therapeutic changes occur when two or more drugs combine to produce an effect that is pharmacologically antagonistic or synergistic, an effect usually considered adverse.

IV Drug Administration Rate

The IV drug administration rate is determined by the amount of drug that can be given over 1 minute. When the administration rate is not known, an IV medication should be administered at the rate of 1 mg/min.

CLINICAL ALERT: Always refer to the package insert or a reference text when administering an unfamiliar drug.

Routes of IV Medication Administration

IV drugs may be given using a variety of techniques. The route chosen depends on the desired effect and the available supplies and equipment. When selecting a route, the clinician should consider the following variables that can affect serum levels of drugs: flow rate, location of injection site, drug volume, and fluid volume of the tubing. Descriptions of various routes follow.

IV Push (Bolus)

High concentrations of medication are administered directly into an IV lock or through an injection port to achieve rapid and predictable serum levels. The IV injection is usually given over 5 minutes or less. This method of drug administration is designed to administer bolus doses. See Box 6-1 for a review of the procedure for administration of bolus doses of drugs.

CLINICAL ALERT: Flush IV tubing after administering a drug to ensure that the complete dose is delivered; otherwise a portion of the drug may remain in the port or may layer in the IV tubing. Administer the flush at the same rate as the medication bolus because the flush pushes medication from the tubing into the patient's vein.

IV Piggyback

IV piggyback is a type of intermittent drug infusion. IV medication is diluted in a small bag or syringe of dextrose 5% in water (D_5W) or normal saline and administered as a drip over approximately 30 minutes. The administration time varies according to the volume of solution intended for infusion. When medication is attached to a primary IV line with a secondary set, the primary line requires a one-way or back-check valve. See Box 6-2 for a review of the procedure for IV piggyback administration of drugs.

Intermittent Infusion

The drug is prepared in the same manner as an IV piggyback solution. Instead of a secondary IV line being attached to the existing infusion, an intermittent infusion is attached directly to an IV lock. See Box 6-3 for a review of the procedure for intermittent infusion of drugs.

Box 6-1 Procedure for IV Drug Administration—Bolus Doses

1. Insert the syringe with medication into the IV lock or through an injection port as close to the IV cannula as possible after cleansing the port with an alcohol swab. (Fig. 6-1, *A* and *B*)

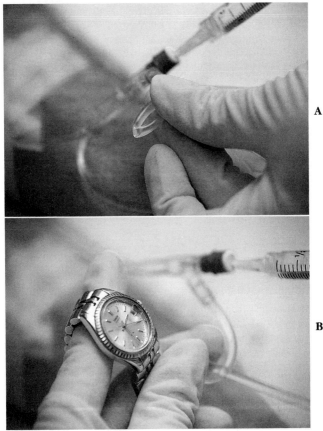

A

B

Fig. 6-1
IV bolus. **A,** Insert tip of syringe containing medication, clamp IV tubing. **B,** Infuse drug, monitor infusion rate.
(From Perry AG, Potter PA: *Clinical nursing skills and techniques,* ed 4, St Louis, 1998, Mosby.)

Box 6-1   Procedure for IV Drug
Administration—Bolus Doses—cont'd

---

2. Clamp off the primary IV line (if applicable).
3. Administer the drug at the prescribed rate.
4. Use a second syringe to administer flush solution.
5. If the medication bolus was given directly into an IV lock, flush the lock with 2 to 3 ml of normal saline or heparinized saline according to policy; continue exerting pressure on the syringe while withdrawing it to prevent a backflow of blood into the IV catheter.

Advantages
- The drug response is rapid and predictable; this method is frequently used in emergency situations.
- The nurse is able to observe the patient throughout the procedure.

Disadvantages
- Adverse effects can be expected at the same time and rate as therapeutic effects.
- The IV push method has the greatest risk of adverse effects and toxicity, because serum drug concentrations are sharply elevated.

Volumetric Chamber

Medication is added to the volume control chamber and diluted with IV fluid. Infusion is generally over 15 minutes to 1 hour. See Box 6-4 for a review of the procedure for administration of medications added to the volumetric chamber.

Continuous Infusion

Medication is added to a large volume of parenteral solution and administered continuously. These infusions are usually regulated with an IV pump or controller to ensure an accurate flow rate. See Box 6-5 for a review of the procedure for continuous infusion of medications.

CLINICAL ALERT: Inadequate drug mixing can result in serious and undesired drug effects. To ensure adequate mixing of

Box 6-2   Procedure for IV Administration—Piggyback

1. Spike the medication container with an IV administration set.
2. Hang the medication container at or above the level of the primary IV (Fig. 6-2).
3. The drug may be administered simultaneously with a compatible IV fluid; if the fluid entering the IV cannula is not compatible with the medication, flush the line with 2 to 3 ml of normal saline before beginning medication infusion and stop the flow of the main solutions; if the primary infusion cannot be interrupted, consider using a dual-lumen catheter or administering the medication through a second site as an intermittent infusion.
4. Infuse the drug at the prescribed rate.
5. After drug administration, the secondary set may remain attached to the IV set or be removed until the next dose; if the line is removed, cap the end of the line with a new needle or cannula.

Advantages
- Incompatibilities are avoided.
- A larger drug dose can be given at a lower concentration per milliliter than would be practical with the IV push method.

Disadvantages
- Administration rate is not controlled precisely unless the infusion is electronically monitored.
- IV set changes can result in the wasting of a drug assumed to have been given.
- Infusion bags are available with only D5W and normal saline solutions.
- The added volume of 50 to 100 ml of IV fluid can cause fluid overload in some patients.

any drug added to an IV solution, do not add a medication to a hanging bag. Follow these guidelines:

1. Use a needleless cannula to infuse drugs into the bag; rotate the bag to evenly distribute the drug contents; otherwise, a concentration of the drug may remain in the port.
2. To assist with mixing, use force when injecting a medication.

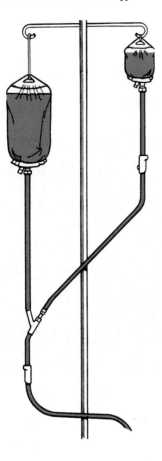

Fig. 6-2
Piggyback IV medication.
(From Perry AG, Potter PA: *Clinical nursing skills and techniques,* ed 4, St Louis, 1998, Mosby.)

(Clinical Alert Continued)

If the added drug is not as dense as the IV solution, the medication floats to the top of the solution; if the drug is more dense than the IV solution, it remains at the bottom of the container. Incomplete mixing of any drug results in drug delivery that is not consistent. Aminophylline is a drug that is less dense than most IV solutions; potassium chloride is more dense than most IV solutions.

Box 6-3 Procedure for Intermittent Infusion

1. Flush IV lock with 2 to 3 ml of normal saline.
2. Insert the infusion into the IV lock and secure the junction with tape.
3. Infuse the drug at the prescribed rate.
4. After drug administration, flush the lock with normal saline or heparinized saline solution; exert a positive pressure on the syringe when withdrawing from the IV lock to prevent a backflow of blood into the IV catheter.

Advantages and *disadvantages* are the same as those for the piggyback method.

Box 6-4 Procedure for Medication Added to the Volumetric Chamber

1. Add medication to the chamber.
2. Add the required amount of IV fluid.
3. Infuse the drug at the prescribed rate.
4. After completion of the drug infusion, resume the IV infusion or flush the IV lock.

Advantages
- Runaway infusions are avoided without the use of electronic equipment.
- This procedure may be used to transport patients without a pump.
- Volume of fluid in which the drug is diluted can be adjusted easily.

Disadvantages
- The drug must travel a long distance before it reaches the patient; there is a significant time delay during very slow infusion rates before the drug dose reaches the patient.
- When the chamber empties and the infusion is slowed, a large amount of the drug can remain in the IV tubing.
- Incompatibilities may develop when the chamber is used for multiple drugs.
- It is necessary to change the labeling on the chamber each time a new solution is added.

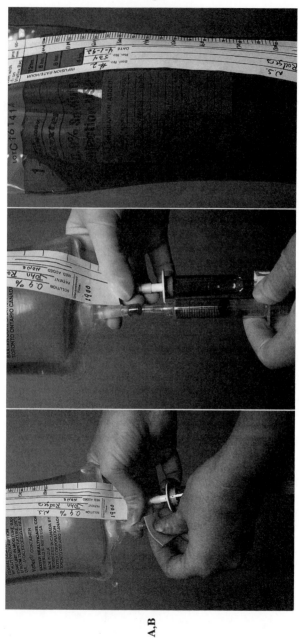

Fig. 6-3
A, Wipe off port or injection site with antiseptic swab; remove needle cap from syringe. **B,** Insert needleless syringe through center of injection port. **C,** Time-tape infusion bag.
(From Perry AG, Potter, PA: *Clinical nursing skills and techniques,* ed 4, St Louis, 1998, Mosby.)

Box 6-5   Procedure for Continuous Infusion

1. Place a time-tape on the bag, even when a pump or controller is used, to verify administration rate.
2. Spike the IV container with an IV administration set.
3. Regulate the flow rate.
4. Observe the patient at least every hour during the infusion; many medications require more frequent patient monitoring (Figure 6-3, *A, B,* and *C*).

Advantages
- Admixture and bag changes can be performed every 8 to 24 hours.
- Constant serum levels of the drug are maintained.

Disadvantages
- When it is not monitored electronically, the administration rate is imprecisely controlled.
- Drug compatibility problems may develop if the line is used to administer piggyback or IV push medications.

Special Drug Manufacturer Packaging

Many innovative premixed and partially mixed medications are available from drug manufacturers. These packages allow medications to be admixed in their original packaging at the time of administration. There is no one best system; however, patient needs may be best met with specialty packages. Use of the medications is convenient and reduces wastage and labor costs. The major disadvantage associated with special packaging is an increase in cost per dose. Consult the manufacturer's directions for procedures related to administration.

Use of Infusion Devices

The volume and complexity of IV drug administration have increased dramatically as a result of rapid improvements in the capabilities of electronic control devices. Device reliability has improved as well as capabilities. Changes will probably continue to occur rapidly as technology improves to meet the challenges of acute care and ambulatory care.

IV pumps and controllers are designed to regulate flow rates precisely and are used widely with IV infusions containing medications. Fluids are delivered at a preselected rate, and most

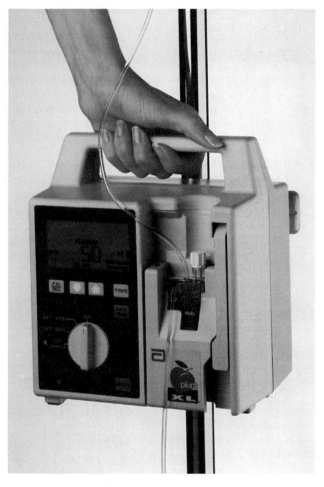

Fig. 6-4
Abbott Plum XL infusion pump.
(Courtesy Abbott Laboratories, Abbott Park, Ill.)

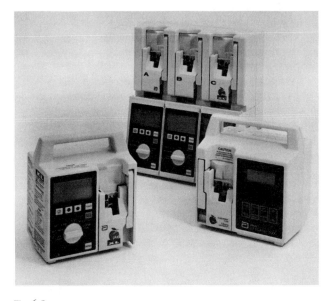

Fig. 6-5
Abbott infusion pumps: Plum XL3; Plum 1.6 With DataPort;
Plum XL.
(Courtesy Abbott Laboratories, Abbott Park, Ill.)

record the amount of fluid infused, automatically prime tubings,
and offer prompts to assist with pinpointing infusion problems.
Most machines are accurate within 2% of the selected rate. They
vary according to ease of use, pressure-monitoring capabilities,
size, programmability, microrate-infusion capability, need for
special tubings, battery life, availability of printouts, and method of
operating.

Devices may administer one to four or more channels
simultaneously and include automatic piggybacking, direct syringe
or vial delivery, back priming and automatic air elimination, dose
calculation, and safeguards against free flow. In the ambulatory
setting, small nonelectronic elastomeric devices are widely used.
Always check the manufacturer's recommendations for specific
device features. See Figs. 6-4 through 6-7.

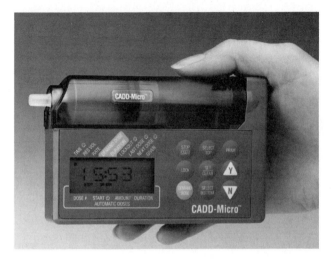

Fig. 6-6
CADD-Micro Ambulatory infusion pump model 5900.
(Courtesy SIMS Deltec Inc., St. Paul, Minn.)

IV Controllers

Controllers deliver fluids with the aid of gravity. The IV fluid container must be placed approximately 36 inches above the IV site to overcome venous resistance and operate properly. A photoelectric eye monitors the flow rate. Controllers are designed to sound an alarm when resistance is detected and thus are useful for the detection of infiltrations.

IV Pumps

Pumps are used to deliver accurate flow rates. Infusion pumps allow concentrated medications and small volumes of fluid to be administered over prolonged periods. Pumps also increase the accuracy of rapid infusions. Pumps provide pressure to fluid delivery when it is necessary to overcome filter resistance, viscous

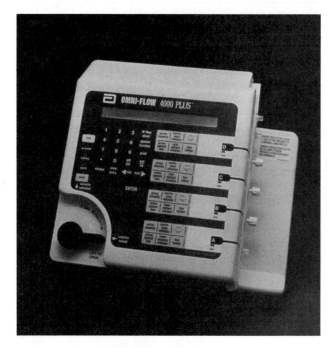

Fig. 6-7
OmniFlow 4000 Plus infusion pump.
(Courtesy Abbott Laboratories, Abbott Park, Ill.)

solutions, small-gauge catheters, and patient activity. When the pump senses resistance, it attempts to maintain the IV flow rate by increasing the pressure of fluid delivery. Many pumps allow the user to set occlusion pressure limits. This is useful if an IV catheter is in an area where it partially occludes with movement (positional IV) or in other situations in which either higher-than-normal or lower-than-normal pressures are desired (e.g., in chemotherapy administration). Select features of IV pumps and related comments are listed in Table 6-2.

Considerations When Working with Pumps and Controllers

If the pump monitors flow with a sensor, follow these guidelines:
1. Fill the administration set's drip chamber to the fill line or

Table 6-2   Selected features of IV pumps

Features	Comments
Operating mechanism	Operate with diaphragm, piston (syringe), or peristaltic mechanism.
Pressure	Maximum pressure applied before occlusion alarm sound varies; some pumps allow variable settings according to desired applications (IV, arterial, epidural).
Programmability	Allows portions of total daily dose to be given at desired times, rates, and intervals; usually able to accommodate at least a 24-hr drug supply for ambulatory patients.
Bolus doses	Pumps designed for patient-controlled analgesia administration have capacity to deliver bolus doses of drug on demand.
Flow rate	Rate can range from 0.1 to 2000 ml/hr according to machine selected.
Variable pressure	Variable pressure settings allow solutions of different viscosity to be administered.
Multiple infusions	One to four solutions may be regulated at different rates by one machine; some have piggyback options.
Alarms	Alarm conditions can include occlusion, machine malfunction, empty container, air in line, door open, and low battery; the number of safety alarms varies according to model.
Tamper-proof settings	Desirable especially for use with children and with opioid infusions.
Energy source	Pumps are designed to operate on electrical or battery power. Many use electrical power and have battery backup. Most ambulatory pumps are battery powered, although some are spring operated or designed for one time use.
Size	Wide range of sizes available; ambulatory pumps are designed specifically to deliver small volumes of 50-100 ml; the pump and a bag are worn by the patient to allow mobility; may have a piston or peristaltic action.
Cost	Wide range according to features; dedicated tubing costs also vary widely according to the manufacturer.

half full to allow the sensor to monitor the drip accurately; most drip sensors are placed at the top of the chamber. Splashes in the chamber may cause inaccurate rates.

2. Most tubing cassettes should be inverted for priming.
3. Verify accurate functioning at regular intervals.
4. Always follow the manufacturer's directions.
5. Do not use tubing clamps with a pump or controller.

CLINICAL ALERT: Some pumps and tubings allow a free flow of IV solution when the pump door is opened or if the IV tubing is removed from the pump. This results in the patient receiving a bolus of a potent medication. Always close the manual clamp on an IV tubing set before opening the pump door.

Avoiding Medication Errors

As in the administration of all medications, the potential for error is a concern. This concern is particularly serious in IV administration because of rapid drug absorption. To minimize the risk of errors, always follow the five "rights" of medication administration:

- Right drug
- Right dose
- Right patient
- Right time
- Right route

In addition, observe the precautions listed in Box 6-6.

Select Drug Information

These drug categories have been compiled to enable the nurse to more effectively and efficiently administer and/or monitor the selected drugs (antimicrobials, anticoagulants, antifungals, antivirals, biotherapy drugs, bronchodilators, hypoglycemic agents, immunosuppressants, and neuromuscular blocking agents). These drugs require special preparation and administration guidelines (e.g., diluent instructions or drug or infusate incompatibility), are administered to patients with potential complex disease disorders, and have potential life-threatening side effects. The nurse should verify the drug, dose, infusion route, and duration with physician's order and patient identification before administering any drug. The manufacturer's recommended guidelines for the drug should be followed; this includes dilution, concentration, and storage; therapeutic monitoring; and comments pertinent to the potential side effects and/or toxicities the patient may experience.

Box 6-6   Guidelines—Avoiding Medication Errors

1. Always read the label on all drugs and verify the medication(s) with the physician's order before administration.
2. Resolve questions about unfamiliar drugs before administration; know the expected dosage ranges, administration rates, incompatibilities, adverse effects and antidotes, and the intended usage of the drugs.
3. Clarify ambiguous medication orders; encourage the use of only approved abbreviations in physician orders.
4. Consider the possibility of drug interactions and take appropriate precautions.
5. If a patient has had an allergic reaction in the past, be cautious, especially when adding a new drug; when starting a new drug, particularly an antibiotic of the same type as one the patient has been allergic to in the past, question the possibility of another reaction.
6. Before administering a drug, check the patient's armband and record for the presence of allergies.
7. Verify dosage calculations with another person to avoid mathematical errors; when possible, refer to calculation tables for medications frequently administered.
8. Document medications immediately after administration to avoid the possibility of administering a repeat dose.
9. To the extent possible, reconstitute drugs so that they can be administered at a rate of 1 mg/min.
10. Encourage the implementation of standardized IV drug dilutions to simplify administration rate calculations.
11. When handwriting is illegible or nonstandard abbreviations are used, confirm the medication order with the physician.

Antimicrobials

Antimicrobial drugs interfere with or inhibit microbial cell wall synthesis, which renders the cell osmotically unstable. Multiple drug therapies may be selected for the varied medical diagnoses. These drugs may be administered prophylactically to decrease the incidence of infection after certain operations, empirically to initiate therapy directed against the most likely infecting organism before receipt of culture and sensitivity reports, or therapeutically. Therapeutic coverage is achieved based on culture and sensitivity reports. Safe administration of antimicrobials includes following the manufacturer's reconstitution guidelines, knowing specific drug incompatibilities, observing and reporting side effects, following therapeutic drug monitoring techniques, and administering the drug in a timely and cost-effective manner. The most common side effects reported include nausea, vomiting, diarrhea, and significant adverse reactions such as anaphylaxis and bone marrow suppression.

The categories of antimicrobial agents most widely used are discussed in the following sections.

Cephalosporins

Cephalosporins are widely used, relatively safe antimicrobials. There is a wide dosage range between toxic drug levels and subtherapeutic drug levels. Adverse effects are similar to those of penicillins; approximately 3% to 5% of individuals who have adverse reactions to penicillin also have adverse reactions to cephalosporins. Those who have had anaphylaxis are most susceptible to an allergic reaction with a cephalosporin. Adverse effects may include hypersensitivity, phlebitis, diarrhea, neutropenia, and altered liver function. Aminoglycosides are chemically inactivated by cephalosporins.

The following target organisms are affected by cephalosporins:

- First generation: most gram-positive organisms and some gram-negative organisms
- Second generation: increased gram-negative action, decreased gram-positive effectiveness
- Third generation: expanded gram-negative coverage, decreased gram-positive coverage

Aminoglycosides

Aminoglycosides are most often used to treat bacteremia, systemic infections, and urinary tract infections. IV administration is always used to achieve a systemic effect because the drugs are not absorbed from the gastrointestinal tract. Target organisms include gram-negative aerobes, staphylococci, and mycobacteria. The mechanism of action is interference with bacterial protein synthesis and replication. One of the major differences among the various aminoglycosides is toxicity incidence.

Adverse effects are a concern when using aminoglycosides

because of the narrow range between therapeutic and toxic effects. To monitor drug dosages closely, the nurse should obtain blood for periodic measuring of drug peak and trough levels. Trough levels are measured before administration of a subsequent dose, and peak levels are measured within 30 minutes of the completion of a dose. Trough levels greater than 2 μg are associated with increased toxicities (see Table 6-1 for a listing of some IV drug peak and trough levels). Adverse effects of aminoglycosides include the following:

- *Nephrotoxicity:* Persons who already have diminished renal function are particularly at risk for developing this effect; when other nephrotoxic drugs are administered, this effect is potentiated.
- *Ototoxicity:* Tinnitus, loss of high-frequency hearing, and altered balance may all result from ototoxicity.

Penicillins

Penicillins act by inhibiting bacterial cell wall synthesis. Most gram-positive organisms and some gram-negative cocci are sensitive to penicillins. Adverse effects can include cutaneous reactions, gastrointestinal symptoms (especially diarrhea), hypersensitive reactions, and renal damage.

Anticoagulants

Anticoagulants alter the patient's coagulation status by preventing conversion of fibrinogen to fibrin and prothrombin to thrombin and by enhancing inhibitory effects of antithrombin III. These drugs are given for various medical conditions—deep vein thrombosis, pulmonary emboli, and disseminated intravascular clotting syndrome—and in open-heart surgery, transfusion, and dialysis procedures. Contraindications to these drugs include hemophilia, peptic ulcer disease, blood dyscrasias, acute nephritis, and thrombocytopenia purpura. Anticoagulants should be used with caution in alcoholic patients, pregnant women, and elderly patients.

Anticoagulation therapy requires drug dose and infusion rate calculation based on the patient's weight. A more accurate dosing guideline can be determined via a designated heparin nomogram (Fig. 6-8, *A* and *B*). The usual components of a heparin nomogram include physician orders for laboratory test frequency (e.g., activated partial thromboplastin time or prothrombin time) and designated bolus and/or continuous heparin administration doses, times, and titration changes based on the patient's response to anticoagulant therapy.

DATE	TIME	PHYSICIAN ORDER SET

NOTE: specify route of administration on Medication Orders

Generic or therapeutic substitutions (as deemed appropriate by the Pharmacy and Therapeutics Committee) may be made unless the physician writes "NO SUBSTITUTION" on EACH medication order.

☐ OUTPATIENT PROCEDURE   ☐ OBSERVE AS OUTPATIENT   ☐ ADMIT AS INPATIENT

HEPARIN NOMOGRAM

Laboratory Monitoring:
1. Draw hemogram (WBC, RBC, Hgb., Hct., Plt. and indices), aPTT, PT, and INR prior to starting heparin, if not already done in prior 12 hours.
2. aPTT 6 hours after initiation of therapeutic heparin.
3. If 6 hour aPTT is 50-75, get an aPTT in 12 hours from initiation of heparin.
4. aPTT 6 hours after any heparin adjustments or boluses, including heparin received in cardiac catheterization lab.
5. Draw hemogram daily during heparin therapy.

Heparin Dosing:
1. Heparin infusion:
   ☐ a. DVT or PE: Patients with recent onset (diagnosed by physician within the past 24 hours) of deep vein thrombosis or pulmonary embolism:
      1a. Initial IV bolus of 80 units/kg. (maximum IV bolus not to exceed 10,000 units, round to the nearest 500 units). If patient has received IV heparin in the previous 2 hours, do not give bolus, but proceed with continuous infusion.
      2a. Initial IV infusion of 20 units/kg/hour (round to nearest 50 units/hr.)
   ☐ b. Cardiac and all other patients:
      1b. Initial IV bolus of 70 units/kg. (maximum IV bolus not to exceed 10,000 units, round to nearest 500 units). If patient has received IV heparin in the previous 2 hours, do not give bolus, but proceed with continuous infusion.
      2b. Initial IV infusion of 15 units/kg/hour, (round to nearest 50 units/hr.)

Additional Orders:
1. Nurse to document all aPTT results, calculations, time of bolus dose, time of infusion changes, time of lab draws and time for future aPTT on the Anticoagulation Flow Sheet.
2. Notify any physician ordering intramuscular (IM) injections or intra-arterial (IA) sticks while the the patient is on continuous heparin infusion that the patient is on intravenous heparin before doing the IM injection or IA stick.
3. Visually monitor urine/stools for blood, report to physician any signs/symptoms of bleeding.
4. Notify physician if heparin drip rate exceeds 2,500 units/hour.
5. Notify physician if aPTT>156 seconds.
6. _____ **PHYSICIAN**, initial this line if you want to be called **ONLY** after 2 consecutive aPTTs>156 seconds.
   (this will nullify order #5, which immediately precedes this order)

VC-046
new 11-97 chg 4/99   **page 1 of 2**

DRUG ALLERGIES	UNIT	ROOM #	PATIENT IDENTIFICATION
	PATIENT NAME - HAND WRITTEN		

Original - Retain on Chart   Copy - To Pharmacy
VIA CHRISTI REGIONAL MEDICAL CENTER, WICHITA, KS.
PHYSICIAN ORDER SET

Fig. 6-8
Heparin nomogram physician order set.
(Courtesy Via Christi Regional Medical Center, Wichita, Kan.)

Continued

Antifungals

Antifungal drugs increase cell membrane permeability in susceptible organisms by binding sterols. Fungal infections such as candidiasis, cryptococcosis, histoplasmosis, sporotrichosis, and aspergillosis are treated with antifungal agents. These drugs are given for infections in patients with the potential for complex disease management. For example, patients with a primary diagnosis (e.g., cancer or organ [heart, kidney, liver] failure) who develop

DATE	TIME		NOTE: specify route of administration on Medication Orders **PHYSICIAN ORDER SET**		
			Generic or therapeutic substitutions (as deemed appropriate by the Pharmacy and Therapeutics Committee) may be made unless the physician writes "NO SUBSTITUTION" on EACH medication order.		

☐OUTPATIENT PROCEDURE   ☐OBSERVE AS OUTPATIENT   ☐ADMIT AS INPATIENT

7. Notify physician for further orders and heparin adjustments if any active bleeding or bleeding complications occur.
8. Daily weight while on heparin therapy.

Heparin Nomogram●

aPTT (seconds)	Bolus Dose*	Continuous Infusion Rate Change (round to nearest 50 units/hr.)	Repeat aPTT	Stop (min.)
<40	50 units/kg	Increase by 4 units/kg/hour	6 hours	0
40-<45	25 units/kg	Increase by 4 units/kg/hour	6 hours	0
45-<50	0	Increase by 2 units/kg/hour	6 hours	0
50-75	0	NO CHANGE	Next AM	0
>75-88	0	Decrease by 1 unit/kg/hour	6 hours	0
>88-113	0	Decrease by 2 units/kg/hour	6 hours	30
>113-156	0	Decrease by 3 units/kg/hour	6 hours	60
>156	0	Decrease by 3 units/kg/hour (Notify physician for an a PTT>156 or as directed by physician in order #6 in "Additional Orders" on page 1)	6 hours	90

*round to nearest 500 units
●This nomogram should only be used at Via Christi Regional Medical Center, because aPTT ranges at other hospitals may be markedly different. The desired range for the aPTT of 50-75 seconds is equivalent to heparin concentrations in plasma of 0.2-0.4 units/ml, based on protamine titration using Actin FSL.

Warfarin Treatment:
1. For patients with DVT or PE: warfarin (Coumadin) _____mg PO at 1600 on first day of heparin therapy.
   Daily PT/INR while on warfarin.
2. Contact physician for initial and daily warfarin doses.

page 2 of 2
VC-046
new 11-97 chg 4/99   PHYSICIAN'S SIGNATURE / DATE

DRUG ALLERGIES	UNIT	ROOM #	PATIENT IDENTIFICATION
		PATIENT NAME - HAND WRITTEN	

Original - Retain on Chart   Copy - To Pharmacy
VIA CHRISTI REGIONAL MEDICAL CENTER, WICHITA, KS.
PHYSICIAN ORDER SET

Fig. 6-8—cont'd
For legend see p. 173.

a fungal infection require astute clinical interventions. The disease and the compromised organ function (bone marrow, heart, kidney, lung) have to be managed in concert regarding the drug toxicity and/or adverse reactions and the patient's organ function. All patients receiving antifungal agents require therapeutic monitoring to prevent or minimize side effects such as anuria, oliguria, acute liver failure, hemorrhagic gastroenteritis, permanent renal impairment, and blood dyscrasias. Other side effects include hypokalemia, nausea, vomiting, anorexia, headache, fever, and chills.

Antivirals

Antiviral drugs interfere with DNA synthesis needed for viral replication. These drugs are used most often for treatment of herpes simplex virus encephalitis, herpes genitalis, and varicella-zoster encephalomyelitis and to immunocompromised persons with herpes simplex virus or cytomegalovirus. These drugs have significant toxicities, dosing guidelines, and hydration requirements. Examples of these drugs include acyclovir, foscarnet, and ganciclovir. Ganciclovir is a mutagenic drug; therefore OSHA guidelines require safe-handling precautions during preparation and administration. Caution should be used for patients with blood dyscrasias, renal and liver disease, and dehydration and for pregnant and lactating patients. Common side effects include nausea, vomiting, anorexia, diarrhea, headache, vaginitis, and moniliasis.

Biotherapy Drugs

Biotherapy drugs augment, modulate, or restore the host's immunologic defense mechanism. Their antitumor activity (cytotoxic and antiproliferative) affects differentiation or maturation of cells and interferes with the ability of the tumor to metastasize. Specific dosing and route (intramuscular, intravenous, or subcutaneous) vary with the patient's disease status and the type, purpose, and goal of therapy. Side effects are related to the dosing principles and usually include flulike syndrome, fever, chills, bone pain, myalgia, and fatigue. Biotherapy drugs may be given in combination with surgery, chemotherapy, radiation therapy, or peripheral blood stem cell (PBSC), and bone marrow and solid organ transplantation, or they may be given as a single agent. They are being used extensively in PBSC and bone marrow and organ transplant protocols to decrease the intensity and duration of the nadir and thereby enhance the patient's recovery process. An additional pertinent use of the colony-stimulating factors is to stimulate stem cells to appear in the peripheral blood. These stem cells are then harvested via apheresis and used in peripheral blood stem cell transplantation.

Bronchodilators

Bronchodilators relax the smooth muscles of the respiratory system by blocking phosphodiesterase, which increases cyclic adenosine monophosphate (cAMP). They are used to treat respiratory diseases such as bronchial asthma, bronchospasm, emphysema, and other obstructive pulmonary disease and to prevent exercise-induced asthma. The nurse should ensure therapeutic drug infusion and monitoring, and observe the patient for potential central nervous system side effects. Common side effects include tremors, anxiety, nausea, vomiting, and throat irritation. Caution should be used in patients with severe cardiac disease, seizure disorders, hypertension, hyperthyroidism, and prostatic hypertrophy and in pregnant and lactating patients.

Hypoglycemic Drugs

Hypoglycemic drugs decrease blood glucose, and the dosage should be adjusted by monitoring blood glucose levels on a scheduled frequency. With intravenous insulin dosing, the nurse must ensure that patient assessment includes blood glucose levels, vital signs, level of consciousness, and intake and output.

Immunosuppressants

Immunosuppressants inhibit the T lymphocytes (responsible for tissue or organ graft rejection and graft-versus-host disease) and are used in multiple immunosuppression regimens. Patients receiving solid organ transplants or donor bone marrow transplants receive these drugs over extended periods. Examples of the drugs include cyclosporine, azathioprine (Imuran), muromonab-CD3 (OKT3), and tacrolimus (Prograf). These drug have significant drug dose preparation and administration guidelines and require prudent patient monitoring for side effects and toxicities. Caution should be used in patients with severe renal or hepatic disease and pregnant patients. Common side effects include nausea, vomiting, candidiasis, tremors, headache, albuminuria, hematuria, proteinuria, and the risk of secondary infection.

Neuromuscular Blocking Agents

Neuromuscular blocking agents are divided into depolarizing and nondepolarizing. They act by inhibiting transmission of nerve impulses by binding with cholinergic receptor sites. Neuromuscular blocking agents are used most often for patients who require endotracheal intubation for general anesthesia or mechanical ventilation. Because of their potential life-threatening side effects (respiratory paralysis, prolonged apnea, bronchospasm, respiratory depression, and bradycardia), they should be administered only by staff knowledgeable and competent in drug administration and patient monitoring. *It is essential the patient be continuously monitored (respira-*

tory, cardiac, and central nervous system) before, during, and after administration of neuromuscular blocking agents.

IV Opioid Infusions

Although opioids may be administered intravenously as a bolus dose for severe pain, the most effective analgesia is achieved when a consistent serum level of narcotic is maintained. IV opioid administration allows predictable drug absorption through the use of an infusion that is titrated to achieve analgesia or with a specialized, programmable pump that allows the patient to administer predetermined doses of the narcotic. The latter method is called *patient-controlled analgesia* (PCA). Opioid infusions prepared as large-volume solutions are regulated by a pump or controller to ensure accurate drug delivery. Patients require frequent monitoring for sedation, respiratory depression, and/or other adverse opioid effects such as nausea and constipation.

PCA doses are individualized for the patient and allow the patient to deliver a drug dose as needed for pain relief by pushing a button connected to the PCA pump. Often, patients use less medication than they are allowed and have accelerated recoveries after surgical procedures. The more consistent the pain control, the greater ease of movement the patient experiences.

Patients with terminal cancer pain are also often candidates for PCA. Often, these patients are cared for at home. A small ambulatory pump is set at a basal level and then programmed to allow intermittent, patient-controlled bolus doses (Fig. 6-9). Successful PCA requires clear patient instructions. The patient should receive a complete explanation of the pump and an explanation of the lockout interval before any clinical use.

PCA pumps are designed with safeguards, such as allowed doses and lockout intervals, to protect against tampering and misuse of the drugs. Physician orders for PCA include the following:

1. *Drug to be administered:* usually morphine
2. *Dose volume:* the amount administered each time the PCA infusor is activated
3. *Time lockout interval:* period during which the pump cannot be activated and no analgesia can be delivered, allowing time for the dose to take effect before the patient receives another; the usual lockout interval is 6 to 10 minutes for postoperative pain, but it may be longer according to patient need
4. *Volume limits:* the maximum volume to be delivered over a prescribed period

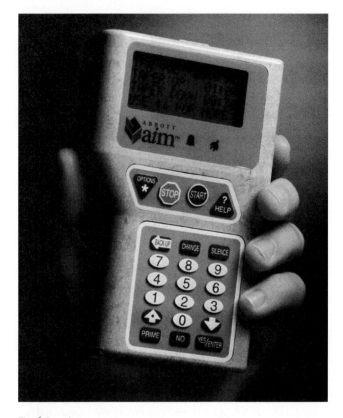

Fig. 6-9
The Abbott AIM pain management.
(Courtesy Abbott Laboratories, Abbott Park, Ill.)

Epidural Analgesia

Epidural analgesia continues to be used for the management of acute and chronic pain (Fig. 6-10). Postoperative patients and oncology, trauma, and chronic pain patients all may benefit from epidural opioids with or without local anesthetics. The discovery of opiate receptors and endorphins has led to the use of morphine in the epidural space for pain control. Opiates such as morphine have a direct spinal effect, acting at receptor sites in the dorsal horn of the spinal cord. The major mechanisms by which morphine is

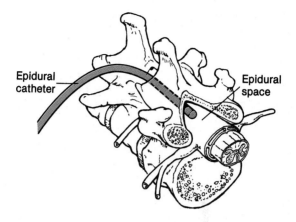

Fig. 6-10
Epidural catheter.

thought to gain entry to the dorsal horn are diffusion into and across the cerebrospinal fluid and venous entry along a nerve root sleeve.

The epidural catheter is placed between the dura mater and the vertebral arch, an area that contains fat, blood vessels, and nerves. Some contraindications to epidural catheter placement include the presence of infection, coagulopathy or current anticoagulation therapy, increased intracranial pressure, allergy to narcotics, and patient refusal.

Epidural analgesia brings the patient longer-lasting pain relief with smaller, less-frequent opioid dosing than the IV route requires. The most intense analgesia is at the level of injection. Analgesia spreads along the dermatomes to provide site-specific pain relief with relatively small morphine doses. Systemic absorption by the epidural vasculature can result in blood levels similar to those provided by an intramuscular injection.

Morphine (Duramorph) and fentanyl citrate are the most common opioids administered. Bupivacaine (Marcaine) and lidocaine (local anesthetics) are often used in drug combinations with the opioids in the management of postoperative pain. Side effects of epidurally administered opioids include respiratory depression, nausea and vomiting, urinary retention, and pruritus. Less commonly, catheter migration to the subarachnoid space can occur, causing profound respiratory depression and hypotension.

CLINICAL ALERT: Clearly label epidural catheters to prevent inadvertent administration of IV medications into the epidural space. *Always* use preservative- and additive-free morphine for epidural analgesia; never administer IV solutions by the epidural route.

Three different systems are used to deliver drugs to the epidural space. The first system is a totally internal system in which an epidural catheter is connected to a reservoir placed in the abdomen. This reservoir's mechanism allows slow, continuous administration of morphine. It must be filled with the desired drug concentration on a weekly or biweekly interval by inserting a Huber needle into the reservoir septum. This system is permanently placed and used most often for the patient requiring long-term pain management.

In the second system, an epidural implantable port with a catheter connected to the portal chamber is anchored to muscle tissue over a bony surface. The catheter is tunneled subcutaneously and then threaded into the epidural space at the desired level, usually L1 or L2. A Huber needle is used to access the septum of the portal chamber, and medication is pumped continuously with an ambulatory, programmable pump. Like the first system, this system is permanently placed and used for the patient who requires long-term pain management.

The third system consists of an externally threaded catheter that is tunneled subcutaneously from the epidural space to an abdominal exit site. It is then connected to an injection cap and a 0.22-μm filter with extension tubing through which morphine can be administered intermittently by an IV infusion pump. This system may be used on a temporary or a permanent basis. Temporary catheters are placed for pain relief after operative procedures such as thoracic, abdominal, orthopedic, and vascular surgery. Temporary catheters may be used also to evaluate the efficacy of this treatment modality before placing a permanent catheter for the management of chronic pain.

Epidural drugs must be free of preservatives and additives and should be prepared under a laminar flow hood. Commercially prepared morphine (Duramorph, Astramorph) is available in the following concentrations: 1, 2, 5, and 25 mg/ml. Preservative-free hydromorphone (Dilaudid) and fentanyl citrate are other medications that may be used for epidural analgesia. Many of the ambulatory infusion pumps can hold a 100-ml infusion bag that allows bag changes every 4 to 5 days for patients who receive epidural infusions for chronic pain management (Fig. 6-11).

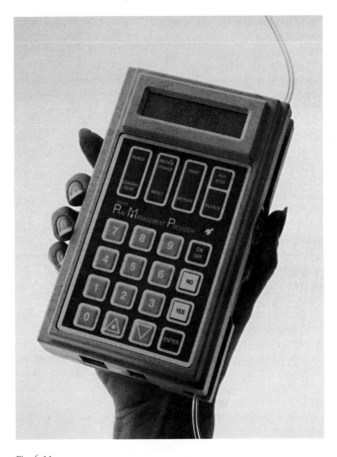

Fig. 6-11
The Abbott Pain Management Provider.
(Courtesy Abbott Laboratories, Abbott Park, Ill.)

Adverse effects associated with epidural analgesia include respiratory depression, urinary retention, pruritus, and nausea and vomiting. These effects are encountered most often with postoperative use of epidural analgesia and may be reversed by an IV naloxone (Narcan) infusion. Patients require ongoing monitoring for pain relief, sedation level, and adverse drug effects, especially respiratory depression. As with all catheters, the site should be assessed for pain or tenderness.

CLINICAL ALERT: Patients receiving epidural analgesia require ongoing observation of their blood pressure and pulse and respiratory rates. Recommended monitoring schedule includes: respiratory rate every hour for the initial 24 hours, then every 4 hours and blood pressure and pulse every 30 minutes for 2 hours and then every 4 hours for duration of short-term (days) epidural analgesia. Sedation status regarding rate, depth, and characteristics of respirations and the presence of swallowing and gag reflex are additional recommended monitoring guidelines.

Guidelines—Conscious Sedation

Combinations of local anesthetics with IV opioids and sedatives are used to produce conscious sedation of patients during diagnostic and minor surgical procedures. Conscious sedation is a depressed level of consciousness during which patients retain the ability to maintain a patent airway and to respond to physical and verbal stimulation. Advantages include maintenance of consciousness and cooperation, elevation of the pain threshold with minimal changes in vital signs, partial amnesia, and rapid recovery after the procedure.

Patient cooperation with the procedure is essential. Restriction of food and liquids before the procedure is based on age (e.g., patients younger than 6 months of age should have nothing by mouth for 4 hours versus adults who should not have food for 6 to 8 hours and clear liquids for 2 to 3 hours). Preprocedural instructions that are given and signed before conscious sedation include diet and food restrictions, procedural information regarding sedation status, and the need for an accompanying adult responsible for transportation home after the procedure.

The patient should be monitored closely during the procedure and during recovery because there is a potential for rapid progression to a state of deep sedation or to general anesthesia. Both experienced personnel and equipment for airway management are essential in all settings where conscious sedation is used. An established and maintained IV access is required throughout the procedure.

A position statement of the Association of Operating Room Nurses requires that the registered nurse managing a patient under IV conscious sedation have no other responsibilities during the procedure. Registered nurses require advanced training before working with conscious sedation and need to follow all procedures carefully when monitoring patients under conscious sedation.

Recommendations for conscious sedation include continuous assessment and documentation within 15-minute periods of the following information:

- Oxygen saturation
- Heart rate and rhythm
- Intermittent respiratory rate
- Intermittent blood pressure
- Responsiveness to commands

The patient is discharged when the following are true:

- Vital signs (respirations, pulse, and blood pressure) return to baseline or presedation levels.
- An adequate airway (able to breathe, swallow, and cough freely), and adequate ventilation (oxygen saturation greater than 90%) are demonstrated.
- The patient is fully reactive (able to move all extremities), can ambulate consistent with developmental stage, is able to retain fluids, had minimal nausea, and is well oriented.
- The patient or caregiver understands the care instructions.

Documentation Recommendations

- Observation of the site before and after infusion or injection of a drug
- Medication name, dose, route, and time of administration
- All supplies used for medication administration
- Name and amount of all flush solutions (normal saline or heparin)
- Any patient complaints of discomfort symptoms experienced in conjunction with the medication; actions taken to alleviate symptoms (report to physician when applicable)
- With opioid infusions: pain relief status, sedation levels, analgesia level, and respiratory rate; with PCA: the total dose delivered since the last notation and the number of doses delivered
- See specific documentation requirements for epidural analgesia and conscious sedation

Nursing Diagnoses

- Infection, risk for, related to a break in sterile technique during drug preparation or administration
- Injury, risk for, related to adverse effect of medication

- Pain, related to infiltration or phlebitis
- Knowledge deficit related to drug and/or analgesia side effects.

Patient/Family Teaching for Self-Management

Education for home IV medication administration is most effective when a standardized content is developed and a standardized approach is taken to patient education. A learning assessment should include the following patient/family information:

- Reading skills
- Motivation
- Prior self-care experience
- Physical limitations that could interfere with the treatment, such as arthritis, neuropathy, or diminished vision

Each skill requires a demonstration and a return demonstration by the patient or the responsible caregiver. Materials sent home with the patient for reference need to be easy to read and should contain pictures of all procedures for nonreaders.

Instructions for Self-Medication

Instructions for self-medication include the following information:

- Name, dose, and frequency of the drug to be administered
- Aseptic technique
- Use and disposal of needleless supplies
- How to obtain medications and other supplies
- Medication storage requirements and medication preparation (if applicable)
- How to administer the drug
- Infusion pump operation (if applicable)
- Expectations for medical follow-up, such as physician visit or laboratory sampling
- Adverse drug effects and what should be done if these occur
- The importance of strict compliance with the medication regimen and how to recognize symptoms of a worsening condition
- Care of the IV access site, including problem recognition and troubleshooting techniques

Guidelines for Home Care
IV Medications

Successful home IV medication administration depends on the patient's and caregiver's abilities and competence to safely and accurately administer medications with the availability of a reliable venous access.

- Instruct the patient and caregiver to know drug name, purpose for drug infusion, drug infusion schedule (e.g., every 6 hours, every 12 hours), side effects of the drug, and the importance of reporting immediately to the physician/home care agency symptoms such as shortness of breath, rash, itching, hives, fever, abdominal cramps, or nausea/vomiting.
- Discuss an emergency plan with the patient and caregiver.
- Instruct the patient and caregiver regarding the medication (drug, dose, route, time, and appropriate drug infusion solution and infusion time).
- Demonstrate with return demonstration aseptic technique regarding connecting and disconnecting from the venous access device.
- Demonstrate with return demonstration aseptic technique regarding flushing the infusion line and venous access device with sterile normal saline solution.
- Demonstrate with return demonstration problem-solving techniques for infusion pump alarms, how to start and stop medication infusion, and how to change the pump battery.
- Discuss issues regarding medication preparation, storage, supply, and discarding of supplies used for medication preparation and administration.
- Inform the patient and caregiver that *usually, the initial dose of a new medication is given in the physician's office, clinic, or acute care setting.*
- Instruct the patient and caregiver regarding documentation specifics for drug, dose, time, and any unusual side effects incurred.
- Clearly document all education (to both patient and caregiver) provided.
- Home care agency documentation should include patient history regarding diagnosis, medication (drug, dose, time, route, infusion solution, purpose for medication, monitoring technique—e.g., culture and sensitivity reports, peak and trough levels), scheduled frequency of home care agency visits, and how to contact home care agency staff.

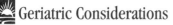

Geriatric Considerations

Both the use of many drugs (polypharmacy) and the physiologic changes that occur with aging place elderly people at high risk for adverse drug reactions. Some factors to consider include the following:

- Reduced lean body mass (an increased percentage of total body fat) alters the number of receptor sites available for drug binding. This phenomenon increases serum drug levels, so toxic levels can be achieved using even usual drug doses.
- Elderly people normally have a decreased cardiac output and decreased total body water. These conditions adversely affect both drug metabolism and drug excretion in older individuals and predispose this population to more adverse drug effects.
- When the elderly patient experiences disease in one part of the body, there is a reduced ability to maintain physiologic homeostasis. Renal function is often compromised in illness, and thus drug excretion is negatively affected.

Resources

Clinical Competency—IV Medication Administration

	Yes	No	NA
Medication Administration			
1. Verifies medication orders with physician orders.			
2. Verifies that the medication matches the patient for whom it is ordered.			
3. Verifies that the patient is not allergic to medication.			
4. Administers medication in			
a. Prescribed dose			
b. Prescribed time			
c. Prescribed route			
5. Documents			
a. Name of medication			
b. Dose			
c. Route			
d. Time			

Clinical Competency—IV Medication Administration—cont'd

	Yes	No	NA
e. Nurse's name or initial, according to policy			
f. Response of the patient to the medication, if indicated			
g. Patient education regarding potential side effects of drugs			
h. Blood return status and frequency			

Routes of Drug Administration

1. IV push medications
   a. Verifies IV site for infiltration and patency.
   b. Administers medication without introducing contaminate.
   c. Administers IV infusion at prescribed rate.
   d. Validates blood return before, during, and at the end of drug administration.
   e. After IV push medication, locks the IV catheter according to agency policy.
2. IV piggyback medications
   a. Verifies IV site for infiltration/patency.
   b. Administers medication without introducing contaminate.
   c. Administers IV infusion at prescribed rate.
   d. Administers IV drug with prescribed dilution.
   e. Flushes IV site in a timely manner after completion of infusion to ensure site patency.
3. Continuous IV infusions
   a. Verifies IV site for infiltration/patency.

Continued

Clinical Competency—IV Medication Administration—cont'd

	Yes	No	NA
b. Administers medication without introducing contaminate.			
c. Administers IV infusion at prescribed rate.			
d. Uses electronic-controlled devices to monitor and assist in administration of drug infusion.			
e. Attaches time-tape label to IV solution bag.			
f. After completion of the IV continuous infusion, locks the IV catheter or discontinues the peripheral IV site.			

Indications for Use of Pumps or Controllers

	Yes	No	NA
1. Correctly selects type of pump appropriate for patient and therapy.			
2. Correctly selects tubing and/or or necessary equipment for pump.			
3. Uses aseptic technique to prime infusion solution before inserting tubing into the pump.			
4. Correctly selects infusion pump controls: infusion volume, rate, and alarms settings.			
5. Follows manufacturer's guidelines for pump alarms and/or pump malfunction.			
6. Promptly reports pump malfunction and selects secondary pump for drug or solution infusion.			
7. Documents infusion pump use and all designated settings according to agency policy.			

Study Questions

1. The half-life of a drug refers to the following:
   a. Half of the loading dose
   b. A value measured after the third dose
   c. Time for plasma levels to fall to half original level
   d. A value that is not measured if a drug is given continuously

2. The following is true of drug peak levels:
   a. The level is measured before a drug dose.
   b. The level is measured within 30 minutes of dose completion.
   c. Levels must be measured daily for the first 2 days
   d. Levels are measured if toxicity is suspected.

3. Which of the following is *false* regarding adverse drug reactions?
   a. They may be a side effect that is documented in the literature.
   b. They are usually a predictable medical emergency.
   c. Hypersensitivity occurs more rapidly with IV drug administration.
   d. Very young and elderly patients are at greatest risk.

4. Which of the following is *false* for drug incompatibility?
   a. Visual inspection will detect particulate formation in an IV solution.
   b. Chemical effects are often not detected with visual inspection of a solution.
   c. Drug incompatibility results in physical, chemical, and therapeutic changes.
   d. Refrigeration improves drug stability.

5. Adverse effects of epidural analgesia include:
   a. Increased respiratory and pulse rate, agitation
   b. Increased respiratory rate, pulse rate, and blood pressure
   c. Decreased respiratory and pulse rate, decreased sedation
   d. Decreased respiratory and pulse rate, increased sedation

6. Conscious sedation preparation, administration, and monitoring requirements include:
   a. Food and fluid restrictions, airway maintenance, patent IV

access, intermittent assessment and documentation: blood pressure, pulse, respirations, oxygen saturation, and responsiveness to commands

b. Fluid restrictions, airway maintenance, patent IV access, intermittent assessment and documentation: blood pressure, pulse, respirations, oxygen saturation, and responsive to commands

c. Food and fluid restrictions, airway maintenance, patent IV access, continuous assessment and documentation: blood pressure, pulse, respirations, oxygen saturation, and responsive to commands

d. Food restrictions, airway maintenance, patent IV access, intermittent assessment and documentation: blood pressure, pulse, respirations, oxygen saturation, and responsive to commands

7. Drug metabolism and drug excretion predispose the elderly population to various major system malfunctions such as:

a. Decreased cardiac output and total body water, increased lean body mass

b. Decreased cardiac output and total body water, increased lean body mass

c. Decreased cardiac output, increased total body water and lean body mass

d. Decreased cardiac output and total body water, reduced lean body mass

8. Safeguards to monitor PCA infusions include:

a. Dose volume, frequency, volume and time lock-out intervals

b. Drug option, incompatibility, maximum volume lock-out intervals

c. Drug option, frequency, incompatibility, time lock-out interval

d. Drug volume, option, incompatibility, time lock-out interval

9. The major side effects of aminoglycosides include:

a. Ototoxicity, nephrotoxicity, cardiac toxicity, balance

b. Ototoxicity, nephrotoxicity, balance, tinnitus

c. Ototoxicity, hepatic toxicity, balance, tinnitus

d. Ototoxicity, bladder infections, balance, nausea

10. Drug categories that have an *increased potential* for adverse side effects include:
    a. Anticoagulants, antiemetics, antimicrobials, antifungals
    b. Anticoagulants, antimicrobials, antifungals, diuretics
    c. Anticoagulants, antimicrobials, antifungals, antineoplastics
    d. Anticoagulants, antifungals, antiemetics, diuretics

Answers   1. c   2. b   3. b   4. a   5. d   6. c
7. d   8. a   9. b   10. c

Blood and Blood Component Administration

7

Objectives

1. List critical verification elements of blood product, donor, and recipient before initiating a blood product transfusion.

2. Discuss the nursing management process for initiating blood product transfusions related to equipment, patient monitoring, and documentation.

3. Recognize potential signs and symptoms for acute hemolytic transfusion reaction.

4. Describe the nursing management process for blood and blood product transfusion reaction.

5. Summarize elements for the informed consent process for blood product administration.

General Principles of Blood Transfusion Therapy

Blood transfusions are a major factor in restoring and maintaining quality of life for patients with cancer, hematologic disorders, obstetric emergencies, solid organ transplantation, and trauma-related injuries and for those who have undergone major surgical procedures. Although blood transfusions are significant for the return to homeostasis, they can be detrimental. Many complications can result from blood component therapy, such as potentially lethal acute hemolytic reactions, transmission of infectious disease (hepatitis, acquired immune deficiency syndrome [AIDS]), and febrile reactions. Most life-threatening transfusion reactions *result from incorrect identification of patients or inaccurate labeling of blood samples or blood components,* leading to the administration of incompatible blood. Monitoring patients receiving blood and blood components and administration of these products are nursing responsibilities. Blood components should be administered by competent, experienced, and skilled personnel following the guidelines of the accrediting organizations and agencies providing blood component therapy.

Blood Group Antigens, Antibodies, Rh Type, and Human Leukocyte Antigen

Blood is composed of several constituents that play a major role in blood transfusion therapy. These components—antigens, antibodies, Rh type, and human leukocyte antigen (HLA)—contribute greatly to the success of any transfusion. An antigen is a substance that elicits a specific immune response when coming in contact with foreign matter. The body's immune system responds by producing antibodies to destroy the invader. This antigen (Ag) and antibody (AB) reaction is demonstrated by agglutination or hemolysis. The antibody in the serum responds to the invading antigen by clumping the red cells together and rendering them ineffective or by completely destroying the red cell. Blood typing systems are based on Ag-AB reactions that determine blood compatibility.

The ABO blood group is important in transfusion therapy. Blood type is determined by detection of both antigens on the red cells and corresponding antibodies in the plasma. The antigens on the red cells that are important in the ABO system are the A antigen and the B antigen. Individuals with type A blood have A antigen present on red blood cells (RBCs), individuals with type B blood have B antigen present, and individuals with type O blood have neither antigen present.

Corresponding antibodies exist in the plasma for each of the antigens (A and B). These antibodies occur naturally in the blood. The antibodies anti-A and anti-B act against the antigen normally present. If the patient's ABO blood type is B, the B antigen is present on the s and the anti-A antibody occurs naturally in the plasma.

After the ABO system, the Rh type is the group of red cell antigens with greatest clinical importance. Unlike anti-A and anti-B, which occur in normal, unimmunized individuals, Rh antibodies do not develop without an immunizing stimulus. Persons whose RBCs possess antibody D are called *Rh positive;* those whose cells lack antibody D are called *Rh negative,* no matter what other Rh antigens are present. The presence of this antibody (anti-D) may cause destruction of the RBC, as in the case of a delayed hemolytic transfusion reaction.

Blood typing identifies the ABO and Rh groupings in the donor blood. Crossmatching then determines the compatibility of donor and recipient cells. ABO and Rh compatibility criteria are essential in blood transfusion therapy.

The HLA system is the next component to consider in transfusion therapy. It is based on antigens present on leukocytes, platelets, and other cells. HLA typing and crossmatching are sometimes necessary before repeated platelet transfusions. Platelets with HLA typing compatible with the patient's have a longer life span when infused. HLA-matched. platelet product (HLA-matched) infusions are avoided in patients who are expected to be candidates for a bone marrow transplant (BMT) to diminish potential graft-versus-host disease (GVHD).

Indications for Transfusion

The primary indications for transfusion are to provide adequate blood volume and prevent hemorrhagic shock, increase the oxygen-carrying capacity of blood, and replace blood platelets or clotting factors to maintain hemostasis. Numerous blood components are available, each with its own potential benefits and adverse effects.

Whole Blood

Transfusing a unit of whole blood (500 ml) over 30 to 60 minutes increases the blood volume by this amount. The seven general rules for transfusion of whole blood are as follows:

1. Transfuse whole blood only for the treatment of acute, massive hemorrhage.
2. Use platelet concentrates and fresh-frozen plasma to correct documented impaired homeostasis when large volumes of whole blood have been transfused.
3. Administration of whole blood should be synonymous with multiple transfusions.
4. Use whole blood to treat patients who have active bleeding and who have lost more than 25% of total blood volume.
5. Whole blood is indicated only for patients with a symptomatic deficit in oxygen-carrying capacity combined with hypovolemia of such a degree to be associated with shock.

6. Whole blood is indicated for patients undergoing cardiopulmonary bypass, intraoperatively and during the first 6 hours postoperatively.
7. Do not give whole blood when the ABO group is unknown.

Red Blood Cells

RBCs are the component of choice to restore or maintain oxygen-carrying capacity. Transfusing RBCs increases the oxygen-carrying capacity with minimal expansion of blood volume and therefore is indicated when chronic anemia and congestive heart failure exist. RBC transfusions may be administered for red cell loss (hemoglobin greater than 8 g/dl) or for losses related to childbirth, surgery, trauma, or treatment-related side effects, such as losses incurred in chemotherapy, radiation therapy, or BMT.

Two major types of RBC products are available. The first is an RBC product with CPDA-1 (citrate-phosphate-dextrose-adenine) anticoagulant with a final hematocrit value of 70% to 80%. This product has a shelf life of 35 days. The second RBC product has 100 ml of additive solution (AS-1) containing RBCs with 90% of the plasma removed and 100 ml of a special solution containing necessary additional preservative to decrease viscosity. This product has a shelf life of 42 days. A unit of packed RBCs should increase the hematocrit 3% to 5% or hemoglobulin level 1 to 1.5 g/dl.

Leukocyte-poor RBCs are given to multiparous women and previously transfused patients who develop antibodies to leukocytes or platelets. These products prevent recurrence of febrile, nonhemolytic transfusion reactions caused by donor white blood cell (WBC) antigens reacting with recipient WBC antibody.

Indications for RBC transfusion include the following:
1. Hemoglobulin level less than 8 g/dl
2. Tachycardia, hypotension with adequate volume replacement
3. Tissue hypoxia
4. Increased risk of adverse consequences (e.g., in patients with sickle cell disease to prevent stroke)

Platelet Types

Two types of platelet products are available: (1) single-donor platelets (obtained by apheresis), whereby a single donor's platelets are harvested while returning red cells, yielding a product of 6 to

10 units of transfusable platelets; and (2) multidonor (random) platelets, which are obtained by centrifuging units of whole blood and expressing off the platelet-rich plasma. One unit of whole blood yields 1 unit of platelets; therefore multiple platelet units must be pooled together to obtain a sufficient quantity for a transfusion.

Indications for platelet transfusion relate to the platelet count, the functional ability of the patient's platelets, and the patient's clinical condition. Individuals with platelet counts of $20,000/mm^3$ or less and who do not have a specific platelet-destroying disease benefit from prophylactic transfusion. Patients who are actively bleeding or who require major surgery require a platelet count of $50,000/mm^3$. Platelets are transfused to control or prevent bleeding associated with deficiencies in the number or function of a patient's platelets. Each unit of platelet concentrate should increase the platelet count 5000 to 10,000 mm^3. It is recommended that 1 unit of random platelets be given for every 10 kg of body weight or one platelet pheresis pack. A platelet count should be obtained at 1 and 24 hours after platelet transfusion.

Indications for platelet transfusion include the following:

1. Thrombocytopenia
2. Decreased production as a result of chemotherapy for malignancy: 20,000/μl
3. Invasive procedures or serious hemorrhage (e.g., disseminated intravascular coagulation [DIC]): less than 50,000/μl

Granulocyte Transfusion

The use of granulocyte transfusions to treat neutropenia has decreased in recent years because of difficulties in collecting a sufficient number of granulocytes. The other significant issue is the availability and varied uses of the hematopoietic growth factors (e.g., granulocyte colony-stimulating factor, granulocyte-macrophage colony-stimulating factor, and interleukin-3). The hematopoietic growth factors provide a stimulus response to the bone marrow stem cells to produce more cells in the peripheral blood.

Massive Transfusion

Massive transfusion is the replacement of the patient's total blood volume(s) within a 24-hour period. A blood volume is estimated to be 75 ml/kg or about 5000 ml (10 or more units of whole blood) in a 70-kg adult.

Potential complications that may result from massive transfusion include circulatory overload, microemboli, hypothermia, citrate toxicity, hypokalemia, hyperkalemia, and coagulation disorders. Patients receiving massive transfusions must be observed closely during the transfusion process. Replacement of blood volume requires rapid infusion (more than 100 ml/min) of warmed blood components or isotonic saline solutions. Frequent laboratory testing is performed during and after the transfusion process to monitor critical values—hemoglobin, hematocrit, prothrombin time, platelet count, sodium, potassium, and calcium levels, and arterial blood gases.

Volume Expanders

Volume expanders such as Hespan, dextran, and Plasmanate provide expansion to the plasma volume and may be used in conjunction with blood product infusions. Volume expanders are recommended for use early in the management of shock or impending shock from burns, hemorrhage, surgery, sepsis, or trauma, as well as for maintenance of cardiac output. A physician's order is required to use the various products. Adverse reactions may include circulatory overload, pulmonary edema, nephrotoxicity, hypotension, and hypersensitivity reactions. Because of the potential serious adverse reactions, prudent monitoring of the patient before, during, and after volume expander infusion is required.

Frequently Transfused Patients

After frequent transfusions, alloimmunization to red cells, platelets, and HLA may occur. This results in crossmatching difficulty and febrile and allergic reactions. The risk of alloimmunization may be decreased by limiting the number of transfusions or donors, using leukocyte-depleted components, and using irradiated blood products. The patient receiving frequent transfusions should be monitored closely throughout the transfusion process. The blood component is usually administered over an increased infusion time.

Irradiated Blood Products

Viable lymphocytes (cells capable of division) present in all cellular transfusion products, including stored RBCs, are thought to be capable of triggering GVHD. This rejection reaction of the graft against seemingly "foreign" host tissues can occur in patients receiving both allogeneic and autologous transplantation. GVHD can occur in HLA-matched siblings and allogeneic BMT recipients and is seen more often with lesser degrees of matches. Using irradiated blood products can avert GVHD produced by blood product transfusion. A measured amount of radiation to blood products renders the donor lymphocytes incapable of replication. The usual radiation dosage recommended is between 1.5 and 3.0 Gy (1500 to 3000 cGy) of gamma radiation. The irradiation of blood products usually takes place at the regional blood center, at the hospital blood bank, or in the hospital radiation therapy department.

Irradiated blood products are used to prevent GVHD in immunocompromised patients who are receiving blood components containing viable WBCs. Irradiation destroys the ability of donor lymphocytes to engraft in the patient. Patients susceptible to transfusion-associated GVHD are those who have Hodgkin's or non-Hodgkin's lymphoma, aplastic anemia, acute leukemia, or congenital immunodeficiency disorder; low-birthweight neonates; and patients undergoing BMT or intrauterine transfusions.

A recent problem with directed donations is transfusion-associated graft-versus-host disease (TA-GVHD). Although exceedingly rare, the mortality rate for TA-GVHD approaches 100%. This high mortality rate is associated with bone marrow failure. TA-GVHD has been associated most frequently with directed donations from first-degree relatives such as parents or siblings. TA-GVHD occurs when the transfusion recipient has two nonidentical HLA haplotypes and the transfusion (lymphocyte) donor is homozygous (identical) for either of the HLA haplotypes of the recipient. The recipient is unable to recognize the donor lymphocytes as "not-self" while the donor (transfused) lymphocytes are able to recognize the recipient as "not-self." The lymphocyte reaction is essentially the same as that seen after allogeneic marrow transplantation. Because of the potential for TA-GVHD after directed donation, it is recommended that all blood components from first-degree relatives be irradiated before transfusion.

TA-GVHD occurs with the following:

- Allogeneic peripheral blood stem cell transplantation and/or BMT
- Directed donations from blood relatives
- Exchange transfusions (neonate)
- Intrauterine transfusions (fetus)
- Hodgkin's disease
- Severe combined immunodeficiency disease
- Wiskott-Aldrich syndrome

Quality Control Measures

Blood Bank Responsibilities

Blood collection facilities have the responsibility of providing safe effective blood products. The American Association of Blood Banks (AABB), American Red Cross (ARC), U.S. Food and Drug Administration (FDA), Centers for Disease Control and Prevention (CDC), and Occupational Safety and Health Administration (OSHA) provide rules, regulations, and standards for operation to which all blood bank centers must comply.

Criteria for collection of donor blood are as follows:

1. Detailed health history, especially related to high-risk activities associated with AIDS and hepatitis (hepatitis B and C, human immunodeficiency virus [HIV]-1 and HIV-2), as well as occupation
2. Screening for diseases such as hepatitis B and C, HIV-1 and HIV-2, human T-cell leukemia virus types I (HTLV-1—T-cell leukemia) and II (HTLV-II—hairy-cell leukemia), syphilis, and cytomegalovirus antigen when the blood product will be given to bone marrow and organ transplant patients
3. Verification of vital signs (blood pressure—systolic no greater than 180 mm Hg, diastolic no greater than 100 mm Hg; temperature—not to exceed 99.5° F or 37.5° C; pulse rate between 50 and 100 beats/min)
4. Minimum age of 17 years
5. Weight not less than 110 pounds
6. Freedom from any skin disease
7. Time since last blood donation at least 56 days
8. Hemoglobin level of at least 12.5 g/dl or higher (or hematocrit value at least 38% or higher) for female patients and 13.5 g/dl for male patients
9. Verification of signed informed consent

Who Can Donate Blood?

Some conditions may warrant temporary deferral from donation, such as colds, flu, and therapy with certain drugs, but the following are *permanently* ineligible as homologous donors:

- Anyone who has AIDS or symptoms of AIDS or who has ever had a positive test for AIDS or for the AIDS virus
- Men who have had sex with another man or women who have had sex with a man who has had sex with another man since 1977—even just one time

- Men and women who have ever taken illegal drugs by needle—even just one time
- Men and women who have had sex with a prostitute in the last 12 months
- Anyone who has had sex with someone who fits in the preceding categories
- Anyone who has ever had hepatitis, malaria, or Chagas' disease
- Anyone who has a history of certain types of cancer (other than minor skin cancer)
- Anyone who has hemophilia or who has received clotting factor concentrates
- Anyone who has received Tegison for psoriasis

Procedure for Blood Collection

To prevent any potential contamination to the blood specimen, a thorough, skilled, sterile procedure is used. The skin is scrubbed with povidone-iodine solution, and the blood is collected into sterile, labeled tubes and bags. Tests performed on the donor's blood include ABO grouping, Rh type (including D), antibody screening, rapid plasma reagin (RPR) syphilis (STS), hepatitis B surface antigen, hepatitis C core antibody, alanine aminotransferase (ALT)—also called *serum glutamic-pyruvic transaminase (SGPT)*—hepatitis C antibody, hepatitis B surface antigen (HBsAg), anti–HIV-1 and -2, anti–hepatitis C virus (HCV), anti–hepatitis B core (HB_c), HIV-1 and HIV-2 antibodies, and HTLV-I and HTLV-II antibodies.

Guidelines have been developed to ensure accuracy in collecting blood samples for recipients of transfusions and for those providing blood donation. Box 7-1 lists guidelines for collecting blood samples. (See Table 14-1 to review blood collection equipment, p. 471.)

Storage Techniques

Red cell products are stored under temperature-controlled refrigeration in the range of 1° to 6° C. Platelets are usually stored at 22° to 24° C (room temperature) and require gentle agitation during storage. Plasma separated from whole blood shortly after collection can be frozen at −18° C or lower temperatures for use as coagulation factor–rich plasma (fresh-frozen plasma).

The blood bank cannot refrigerate and later reissue any blood component meant to be stored at 1° to 6° C if the temperature of

---

Box 7-1   Guidelines for Collecting Blood Samples

1. The intended recipient and the blood sample shall be identified positively at the time of the collection.
2. Blood samples shall be obtained in stoppered tubes, each identified with a firmly attached label bearing at least the recipient's first and last names, identification number, and the date.
3. The completed label shall be attached to the tube before leaving the recipient.
4. There must be a mechanism to identify the person who drew the blood.
5. Before a specimen is used for blood typing or compatibility testing, all identification information on the request form shall be confirmed by a qualified person as being in agreement with that on the specimen label; in case of discrepancy or doubt, another specimen shall be obtained. (See Table 14-1 on p. 471.)

---

the component exceeded 10° C (50° F) at any time. This will happen if the blood component is removed from the blood bank refrigerator for longer than 30 minutes.

CLINICAL ALERT: Refrigeration and freezing of blood products in any patient care area does not ensure accurate temperature regulation or monitoring alarms and is *never acceptable*.

Release of Blood Products

Only qualified blood bank personnel may issue any blood components and only after following all the guidelines for proper identification of the blood unit—ABO grouping, Rh type, antibody screening, and expiration date (Fig. 7-1). The ABO group and Rh type must match on the donor unit and the requested transfusion form. On some occasions, substitutions occur in the blood bank.

Group O packed red cells (not whole blood) may be substituted for any ABO group. Rh (D)-negative red cells may be safely transfused to Rh (D)-positive patients. Rh (D)-positive red cells may not be safely transfused to Rh (D)-negative patients. However, it is acceptable to transfuse Rh (D)-positive *plasma products* to Rh (D)-negative patients because Rh (D) antigens are on the red cells only.

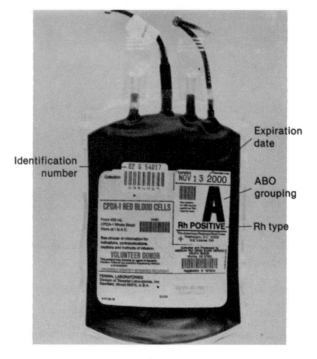

Fig. 7-1
Blood product identification.

Separation Techniques—Apheresis

Apheresis is a process that removes whole blood from the donor and then separates it into component parts by centrifugation, harvesting the desired component. The remainder is returned to the donor, thus allowing collection of large amounts of a single component for an individual recipient. This technique is used for selective collection of platelets to provide matched platelets in sufficient numbers for specific patients.

Currently, apheresis is being used extensively for harvesting peripheral blood stem cells in autologous and allogeneic peripheral stem transplantation. A large-bore double-lumen central catheter is placed to permit the collection of stem cells through apheresis. The patient's blood is circulated through a high-speed cell separator, and the peripheral stem cells are retained and stored. The plasma and erythrocytes are returned to the patient. Approximately 9 to 14 L of blood are processed over 2 to 4 hours. The number of apheresis procedures performed depends on the viability and number of the collected stem cells. Generally, two to four apheresis procedures are performed over 2 to 4 days. Stem cell harvest is usually performed on an outpatient basis.

Autologous Transfusions

Autotransfusion has become an accepted cornerstone in comprehensive blood conservation programs. Autologous transfusion is the collection, filtration, and reinfusion of a patient's own blood by various methods. There are several advantages to autologous transfusions. Because exposure to homologous RBC transfusions is minimized, there is no disease transmission (hepatitis or AIDS) or alloimmunization, and using the patients' own blood is sometimes an acceptable alternative for patients who object to receiving banked blood for religious reasons.

Preoperative autologous blood donation begins 4 to 6 weeks before surgery, with the last donation collected no later than 72 hours before the surgical procedure. The units are collected, properly labeled, and stored using the AABB guidelines. Bacteremia is the only absolute contraindication. A patient must have a hemoglobin level of at least 11 g/dl and a hematocrit level greater than 34% before each donation.

Perioperative blood salvage is performed during surgery (thoracic or cardiovascular surgery, ruptured ectopic pregnancy, liver transplantation, or repair of traumatic injuries). To remove blood from the wound, the surgeon uses a suction wand with a double-lumen catheter. The catheter delivers an anticoagulant (CPDA-1 or heparin) to the tip of the wand. Blood mixes with the anticoagulant and is collected in a sterile plastic container with a flexible lining and filter. The salvaged blood is processed by centrifugation, washing, and filtering and is then reinfused to the patient during or immediately after surgery. Salvaged blood must not be stored because neither filtering nor processing can remove bacteria completely from the blood.

Autotransfusion systems are regulated by the FDA and must meet safety and regulatory guidelines. Some features that are incorporated into the design of the devices include a preset suction control mechanism to regulate the vacuum and allow consistent suction throughout the collection period, a mechanism to protect tissue damage at the wound site and protect RBCs from potential hemolysis, a spill-proof bag and suction port to prevent spillage if the unit is tipped over, and a one-way valve to allow air evacuation while preventing air reentry.

Reinfusion of collected blood must be completed within 6 hours of *initiating* the collection process if the blood is going to be used. Blood salvage is not attempted during procedures that involve spilled intestinal contents, bacterial peritonitis, intraabdominal abscess, osteomyelitis, or cancer resections.

Hemodilution is the process by which the blood is withdrawn from the patient (immediately before surgery in the operative suite) and replaced with an IV infusion of a crystalloid or colloid solution to maintain volume for adequate circulation. The collected blood is reinfused after the bleeding has been controlled.

Reinfusing salvaged blood after surgery is accomplished by collecting the blood through a closed, sterile, plastic drainage system (Fig. 7-2). Collection techniques include carefully regulating suction (not to exceed 100 mm Hg), adding anticoagulant ACD-A per the physician's order, monitoring the fluid level in the sterile container at least every hour, and keeping the system closed and free of air. Because of bacterial growth risks, the blood should not remain in the collection reservoir for more than 6 hours. The blood can be reinfused by gravity drip or infusion pump. The blood must be reinfused within 6 hours of *initiating* the collection process if it is going to be used. Use of microaggregate filter for reinfusion of the blood product is required.

CLINICAL ALERT: Follow all the AABB guidelines for patient identification: Correctly write the patient's name, identification number, date, time collection was initiated, and anticoagulant used on the space provided on the autotransfusion collection device. Consult the manufacturer's guidelines and instructions for setup and use of postoperative autotransfusion systems.

Time of Blood Production Administration

Identification of the patient and the proper blood component are the most important procedures in transfusion safety. The correct blood product must be verified, and all labels must be read carefully. All information on the blood product (donor number, ABO group, Rh type, and expiration date) must be compared and matched with the patient's identification bracelet and the transfusion requisition in

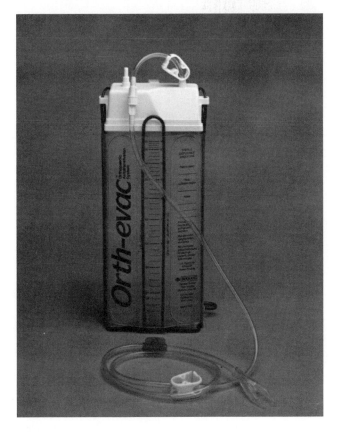

Fig. 7-2
Orthopedic autotransfusion system.
(Courtesy Deknatel Snowden Pencer, Fluid Management Systems, Tucker, Ga.)

the presence of the patient. Discrepancies in spelling, identification numbers, or expiration dates should not exist. All the identification steps must be confirmed by two licensed nursing personnel or blood bank personnel before the transfusion is initiated. Baseline vital signs must be obtained, and the patient must be monitored throughout the transfusion process. On completion of the infusion, the date and time the blood unit was initiated and infusion completed must be documented on the transfusion requisition. Signatures of the personnel confirming all identification information and initiation of the transfusion must also be recorded on the requisition.

Equipment and Supplies Used for Transfusions
Equipment
Blood Warmers

The warming of the blood to the body temperature is necessary during transfusions in certain clinical situations. Research indicates that rapid or massive administration of cold blood has a hypothermic effect on the patient and could have lethal consequences. Patients with cold agglutinin disease (cold-type autoimmune hemolytic anemia in which unexpected antibodies in the patient's serum react at temperatures below 20° C) need to have the blood warmed before transfusion to diminish potential adverse effects. Exchange transfusions in neonates and children receiving rapid or massive transfusions must always be warmed, especially when given through a central line. Hypothermia produced by the rapid infusion of cold blood may lead to arrhythmia and cardiac arrest. For patients requiring extensive operative procedures, a 2° C body temperature loss is not uncommon, reducing the normal body temperature to 35° C. In these situations, blood must be infused at this temperature (35° C) to prevent further heat loss.

An effective blood warmer provides a constant temperature between 32° and 37° C and flows to 150 ml/min. Because warm blood dilates veins, reduced resistance helps offset flow loss that may result when a warmer is attached. Commercial blood warmers may use a warm bath or dry incubator through which blood passes in sterile, disposable plastic coils to warm the blood. Safety mechanisms include thermostats and audible and visual alarm systems for close monitoring of the blood temperature. The manufacturer's prescribed directions for appropriate use and the specific tubings and supplies required must be followed.

CLINICAL ALERT: Heating blood under hot-water faucets, in incubators, or in microwave ovens can cause hemolysis and is *never acceptable*.

Pressure Cuffs

A pressure cuff is the most commonly used device for increasing the flow rate during transfusion. To increase flow rate, the pressure cuff sleeve is secured snugly around the blood bag. The pressure cuff is then filled by a pressure manometer (similar to a blood pressure cuff) that inflates the sleeve with air. As the blood unit empties, the pressure decreases. Agency guidelines for use of pressure cuffs should be followed. Only cuffs specifically designed for blood infusion should be used. When pressure-transfusing components containing RBCs, 300 mm Hg should be not exceeded.

Electronic Infusion Devices

The use of an electronic infusion pump is strongly advised for all pediatric transfusions, although the flow rate is difficult to regulate when small volumes are administered. Gravity flow administration (as used in the adult) is contraindicated because of its potential for allowing too much blood flow over a short time. When electronic infusion devices are used, the nurse should be knowledgeable of the features of the device used—for example, alarm operation and rate consistency, rate and volume of infusion, memory, power supply, and maintenance—and the manufacturer's recommendations for the types of solutions the device is capable of delivering. Not all electronic infusion devices are acceptable for use in transfusing blood products.

Supplies
Filters

Blood and components must always be transfused through a filter designed to retain blood product debris. Standard filters have a pore size of about 170 μm. Proper use of a blood filter requires that the tubings and filter be primed adequately. The filter needs to be completely covered with blood or component, and the drip chamber in the tubing should be approximately half full. Incomplete priming can result in air being trapped in the filter, thus causing an inaccurate drop rate. Damage to blood cells may occur if they fall on the exposed filter. Priming procedures differ slightly from one brand of filter and tubing to another; therefore it is important to follow the manufacturer's instructions included with each set.

Microaggregate filters with a pore size of 20 to 40 μm are designed to remove very small aggregates and fibrin. They may be used for massive transfusions, open-heart surgery, and preparation of leukocyte-poor blood. These filters trap the smaller particles that have potential for causing microemboli. For routine blood transfusions, microaggregate filters are used more often with children than with adults. The manufacturer's guidelines for the correct procedure in priming the filter and (if applicable) for flushing the filter after the transfusion should be followed.

CLINICAL ALERT: Do not use a blood filter set for more than 4 hours. If the flow rate decreases after more than 1 unit has been transfused, you may have to change the filter set.

High-Efficiency Leukocyte Depletion Filters

Considerable data link nonhemolytic febrile transfusion reactions, HLA alloimmunizations, and cytomegalovirus (CMV) transmission of infection to white cells in homologous transfusions. In many high-risk populations, leukocyte filtration is a standard of care and has been demonstrated to be cost-effective. The new information concerning leukocyte-associated viral reactivation and postoperative infections suggests that a wider population of patients would benefit from leukocyte reduction. Patients undergoing surgical procedures such as cardiac procedures, joint replacement, transplants, transurethral resection of the prostate, and vascular surgery are the major consumers of blood and blood products. These patients should be evaluated for leukoreduction blood and blood products.

High-efficiency leukocyte removal devices use a surface modification that is permanently integrated into the microfibrous filter medium (Figs. 7-3 and 7-4). These fibers have an affinity for leukocytes; therefore, as the blood component passes through the filter, more than 99.9% of the leukocytes are removed. When used according to the manufacturer's instructions, these filters provide consistent performance; however, when used improperly, they can cause difficulties during the transfusion. For example, not properly priming a leukocyte depletion filter according to the manufacturer's directions can create an air lock. To prevent misuse and to achieve the manufacturer's stated claims, platelets and RBCs should be given through a leukocyte removal filter designed for that specific transfusion. Filters used for more than the manufacturer's recommended number of units will no longer remove the desired number of leukocytes.

CLINICAL ALERT: High-efficiency leukocyte removal filters for RBCs and platelets are not interchangeable. For example, a leukocyte-depleting RBC filter is not recommended to transfuse platelets or a leukocyte-depleting platelet filter to transfuse RBCs.

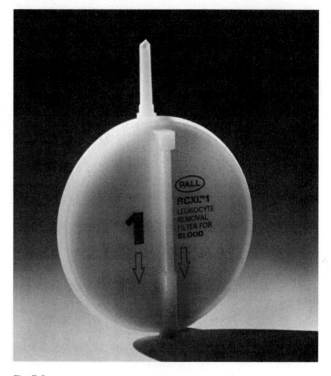

Fig. 7-3
Pall RCXL 1 high-efficiency leukocyte removal filter for red cell transfusion.
(Courtesy Pall Specialty Materials, Port Washington, NY.)

Follow the manufacturer's instructions. Leukocyte depletion filters are not indicated for transfusion of granulocytes.

Tubings

Filtered IV tubings may contain a single line from the blood bag to the patient or a Y-type (dual) line. The Y-type set allows the infusion of normal saline while the blood component bags are being initiated or changed. This dual line offers the availability of normal saline to be used as a diluent for RBCs that are too viscous to flow properly. However, AS-1 RBCs are already diluted with 100 ml of the adenine saline preservative. Therefore additional saline is not

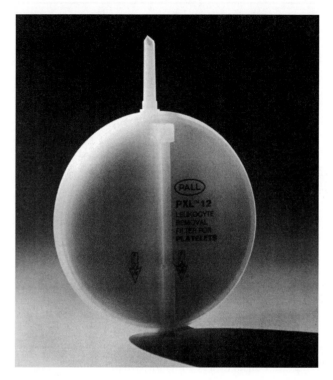

Fig. 7-4
Pall PXL 12 high-efficiency leukocyte removal filter for platelet transfusion.
(Courtesy Pall Specialty Materials, Port Washington, NY.)

needed to increase flow. CPDA-1 RBCs would flow better with the addition of normal saline. If a blood transfusion reaction occurs, the dual line provides an immediate IV access for isotonic solutions (Fig. 7-5).

Only normal saline (0.9% USP) may be administered with blood. Solutions such as 5% dextrose in water or Ringer's lactate can cause in vivo hemolysis or initiate coagulation of the donor blood. Medications should never be added to a unit of blood.

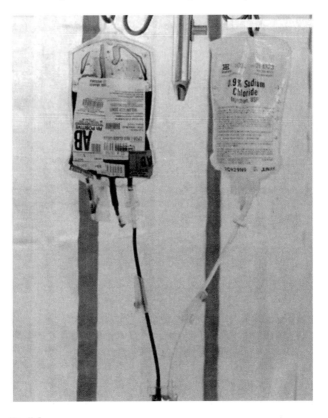

Fig. 7-5
Blood administration with normal saline. Note that the red blood cell infusion is CPDA-1 RBCs.
(From Perry AG, Potter PA: *Clinical nursing skills and techniques,* ed 4, St Louis, 1998, Mosby.)

Blood and Blood Components

Table 7-1 lists blood and many blood components with the approximate volume of each unit, the recommended filter, and the administration rate. The Comment section refers to ABO and Rh compatibility and specific product preparation for infusion. The agency blood bank or blood center should be referred to for blood product information. *Text continued on p. 220*

Table 7-1   Blood and blood components

Product	Infusion Guidelines/Comments
Red Blood Cells *Volume* AS-1 RBC 375-425 ml CPDA-1 RBC 300-350 ml *Filter* Standard 170-μm blood filter or micro-aggregate filter High-efficiency leukocyte depletion filter	Infuse over 1½-2 hr; maximum: 4 hr/unit; if blood loss, transfuse as rapidly as the patient can tolerate; if the patient is in unstable cardiovascular balance (chronic severe anemia, congestive heart failure, very small, or young) and circulatory overload is a concern, rate should be 1 ml/kg/hr; average pediatric dose and rate: 10 ml/kg, 2-4 ml/kg/hr. *Comments* Must be ABO and Rh compatible; occasionally RhO negative will be transfused to an RhO-positive patient, but never RhO positive to an RhO-negative person; group O packed red cells may be given to any blood group, provided the Rh type is appropriate; crossmatch is required.
Washed Red Cells (WRCs) (Leukocyte-Poor) *Volume* 200-280 ml *Filter* Standard 170-μm blood filter	Infuse over 1½-2 hr. *Comments* Same as RBCs; blood bank requires notification to prepare WRCs; expires 24 hr after washing.

Continued

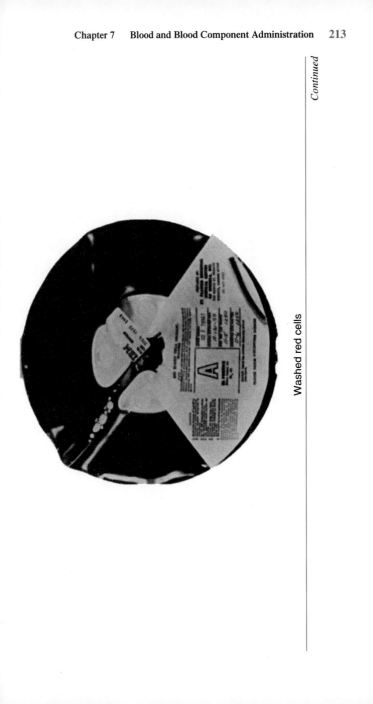

Washed red cells

Table 7-1 Blood and blood components—cont'd

Product	Infusion Guidelines/Comments
Frozen Deglycerolized Red Cells (FDRCs) *Volume* 200-250 ml *Filter* Standard 170-μm blood filter	Infuse over 1½- 2 hr. *Comments* Same as RBCs; blood bank will not deglycerolize until requested; required time to deglycerolize, approximately1 hr, used primarily for transplant patients or patients who have multiple antibodies; expires 24 hr after deglycerolizing; frozen must be thawed and washed before administration to remover glycerol.
Whole Blood *Volume* 450-500 ml *Filter* Standard 170-μm blood filter	Infuse over 2-3 hr; maximum 4 hr/unit; average pediatric dose 20 ml/kg initially followed by volume required for stabilization. *Comments* Must be ABO and Rh exact.
Fresh-Frozen Plasma (FFP) *Volume* 200-250 ml *Filter* Special component filter; standard blood filter may be used	Infuse over 15-20 min when given for bleeding or clotting factor replacement; 1-2 hr when given for other reasons; average pediatric dose and rate: acute hemorrhage, infuse 15-30 ml/kg as indicated; clotting deficiency, 10-15 ml/kg; infuse 1-2 ml/min. *Comments* Must be ABO compatible; RhO antigens not in plasma; no crossmatch required; group AB plasma may be given to any blood group; blood bank does not thaw until required to do so; required time to thaw, 20 min; expires 24 hr after thawing.

Albumin—25% Salt Poor

Volume
12.5 g/50 ml
Filter
Special tubing comes with this product

Infuse within 1 hr at 1 ml/min; average pediatric dose and rate: 1 g/kg, infuse 4 ml/kg.
Comments
Dosage based on bovine serum albumin (BSA) requirements (estimating blood and plasma volume); refer to manufacturer's package insert; very hypertonic.

Albumin—5%

Volume
12.5 g/50 ml
Filter
Special tubing comes with this product

Infuse within 1 hr at 2-4 ml/min; average pediatric dose and rate: 1 g/kg, infuse 10 ml/kg.
Comments
Dosage based on BSA requirements (estimating blood and plasma volume): refer to manufacturer's package insert.

Plasma Protein Fraction (PPF)

Volume
Varies according to scheduled dose
Filter
Special tubing comes with this product

Infuse no more than 1-10 ml/min.
Comments
No typing or crossmatching required; used for volume expansion.

RhO Immune Globulin (RhoGAM)

Volume
1 ml
Filter
None

Give intramuscularly (IM).
Comments
Usually ordered from blood bank; to achieve optimal effect, must be administered within 72 hr to Rh-negative patients who have been exposed to Rh(D) antigens through transfusion or pregnancy.
Usually given prenatally 28-30 wk to protect during delivery exposure after negative Coombs test results.

Table 7-1   Blood and blood components—cont'd

Product	Infusion Guidelines/Comments
Rho (D) Immune Globin (WinRho SDF) *Volume and concentration vary* 600 IU (120 µg) 2.5-ml vial 1500 IU (300 µg) 2.5-ml vial 5000 IU (1000 µg) 8.5-ml vial *Filter* None	Used for treatment of chronic or acute immune thrombocytopenia purpura in adults and children; drug is administered IV; muse be diluted with 0.9% normal saline; dose is adjusted according to hemoglobin level for initial dose and then subsequent dosing is based on platelet level and hemoglobin. Dose is administered IU/kg body weight.
Immune Serum Globulin (ISG) Gamimune (Miles Inc.) Gammagard (Baxter) Gammar (Armour) Gamastan Iveegam (Immuno-US Inc.) Sandoglobulin (Sandoz) Venoglobulin (Alpha Therapeutic Corp.) *Volume* Diluent provided by manufacturer Each bottle of IVIG for single use and should not be stored beyond manufacturer's recommended date *Filter* Manufacturer product specific supplied with product	*To ensure the safety of IVIG products, all donors are meticulously screened, and all plasma donations are now tested for hepatitis B surface antigen, antibodies to HIV, and hepatitis C.* Each IVIG product/brand different and *should not be substituted for another product or brand.* May be given IV or IM. Recommended IV infusion rates: infusion initially is slow (0.01-0.02 ml/kg/min) and then increased incrementally every 15 to 30 min until the maximum infusion rate is achieved; most infusion times 2-4 hr; Appropriate rate depends on IVIG brand, dosage, patient's weight and diagnosis; previously received IVIG, how well dose tolerated, and health/illness state. *Comments* IVIG should not be mixed with other medications or infusion solutions. Product is usually ordered from pharmacy. Supplies IgG antibodies, note patient allergy status.

Purified Factor VIII Concentrate (Hemofil, Hyland)

Volume

10-30 ml freeze-dried

Reconstitute with diluent provided

Filter

Filter needle or IV drip using component recipient set provided with product

Administered intravenously as fast as tolerated by patient to a maximum of 6 ml/min; monitor pulse rate while infusing.

Dose is calculated according to body weight and designated level of factor activity.

Comments

Use for hemophilia A patient (classical hemophilia or factor VIII deficiency); usually ordered from pharmacy; preheat diluent to 37° C before reconstituting and use within 3 hr.

Purified Factor IX Concentrate (Complex, Hyland)

Volume

20-30 ml freeze-dried

Reconstitute with diluent provided

Filter

Filter needle provided with product

Same as Purified Factor VIII

Comments

Use for hemophilia B patient (Christmas factor IX deficiency); usually ordered from pharmacy; preheat diluent to 37° C before reconstituting and use within 3 hr.

Fibrinogen

Use cryoprecipitate

Comments

Each unit of cryoprecipitate contains approximately 250 mg fibrinogen/15 ml plasma; average pediatric dose: 1 unit/7-10 kg.

Continued

Table 7-1   Blood and blood components—cont'd

Product	Infusion Guidelines/Comments
Platelets (Random)	Administer intravenously as rapidly as patient can tolerate; recommend 150-200 ml/hr; may be given more usual order of 6-10 units slowly if danger of circulatory overload exists; maximum transfusion time 4 hr.
Volume	
60-70 ml/unit; minimum order for adult: 1 unit/10 kg body weight, usual order: 6-10 units	*Comments*
Filter	ABO and Rh compatible preferred but not necessary; no crossmatch required; request blood bank to pool (combine units); required cooling time: 20 min; blood bank will not pool until ready to infuse product.
Special component filter use of micro-aggregate filter may be controversial. High-efficiency leukocyte depletion filter	
Platelets (Apheresis)	Same as Platelets (Random).
Volume	*Comments*
200-400 ml	Arrangements must be made with blood center apheresis department before need; must be ABO and Rh compatible; crossmatch required unless red cell-free product is provided.
Filter	
Same as Platelets (Random); dose: 1 platelet pheresis pack	

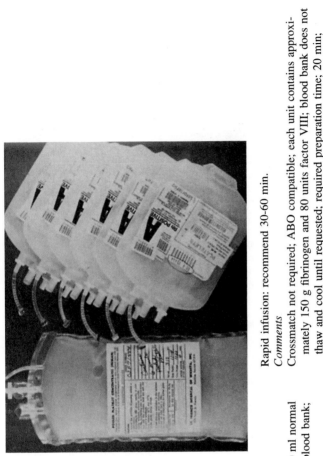

Cryoprecipitate

Volume

10-20 ml/unit; total of 10 ml normal saline is added in the blood bank; usual order 8-10 units

Filter

Special component filter

Rapid infusion: recommend 30-60 min.

Comments

Crossmatch not required; ABO compatible; each unit contains approximately 150 g fibrinogen and 80 units factor VIII; blood bank does not thaw and cool until requested; required preparation time; 20 min; expires 6 hr after pooling.

Protocol for Blood and Blood Component Administration

Pretransfusion

1. Verify prescribed physician's order for specific blood or blood component with the appropriate date of transfusion administration.
2. Verify patient's informed consent (see guidelines for obtaining informed consent in Box 7-2).
3. Obtain the patient's transfusion history, and report any incidence of previous adverse reaction during or after previous blood transfusion.

 Box 7-2   Guidelines for Obtaining Informed Consent

---

1. What do you convey?
   a. The reason for the transfusion
   b. The benefits and risks of the transfusion
   c. What to expect during and after the transfusion
   d. The transfusion options available to the patient
   e. The message that we do not have a completely risk-free blood supply
   f. The assurance that every step is being taken to make the blood supply as safe as possible
   g. Risk information that can be put into reasonable perspective (numbers and percentages are not always useful by themselves); comparisons to other risks in life the patient may have taken
2. How do you obtain consent?
   a. When possible, get the consent several days before the transfusion.
   b. Evaluate comprehension by asking the patients to tell you what they heard you say and what they understand from the written consent. Try to arrange more than one opportunity for discussion.
   c. Provide reading material.
   d. Give the patient a copy of the consent form.
   e. Respect the patient's religious and cultural beliefs about transfusion, especially any that preclude the receipt of blood.

---

4. Follow agency-prescribed procedure for type and crossmatching for blood and blood component therapy.

5. Establish patent peripheral or central line site. To ensure safety of blood product administration for patients with multilumen catheters, reserve one lumen of the catheter for blood and blood component infusions. This technique minimizes the potential of infection for patients with these catheters.

6. Select appropriate tubing. All blood and components must be administered through a filter designed to retain blood clots and other debris. Follow agency policy for use of the appropriate filter.

7. Blood bank personnel issuing the blood unit and nursing personnel administering the transfusion must identify the blood product, the identification number on the transfusion request, and the identical information on the recipient's medical record.

   a. The identification number and name on the patient's wrist band must be identical with the name and number on the transfusion unit and on the compatibility label.

   b. Donor's ABO group and Rh type must be present on the donor unit and transfusion request.

   c. Patient's (recipient) ABO group and Rh type must be present on the transfusion request. Verify ABO and Rh compatibility between the patient (recipient) and donor.

   d. Verify the expiration date on the blood bag.

   e. Inspect the blood product for any abnormalities.

   f. Ask patients to identify themselves by giving their complete name. If a patient is unable to state name, follow appropriate agency procedure in validating patient identification.

   g. Never administer blood to a patient without a correct, appropriate identifying bracelet or tag.

   h. Explain the procedure to the patient. Verify the written consent form.

   i. Inform the patient of potential adverse effects of blood transfusion (Table 7-2) and instruct the patient to report symptoms experienced promptly to the nurse or physician.

   j. Encourage the patient to ask questions about the procedure and potential adverse effects.

   k. On completion of the identification process, the person starting the transfusion and the other licensed person verifying the correct product must record date, time, and their signatures on the transfusion requisition.

Text continued on p. 226

Table 7-2   Adverse effects of blood transfusion

Reactions	Symptoms
Air Embolism Cause: Improper maintenance of a closed administration system	Shortness of breath, chest pain, cough, hypotension, cyanosis, dyspnea, shock
Anaphylaxis Cause: Previous sensitization by IgA-deficient patients who develop anti-IgA antibodies	Shock, respiratory distress (wheezing, cyanosis), nausea, hypotension, abdominal cramps; absence of fever; occurs quickly after only a few milliliters of blood or plasma
Circulatory Overload Cause: Excessive or rapid volume of blood or blood component	Dyspnea, tightness in chest, dry cough, restlessness, severe headache, increased pulse, respiration, and blood pressure
Citrate Toxicity Cause: Citrate anticoagulant accumulates; toxic effects of ionized calcium in the blood, e.g., hypocalcemia	Tingling in fingers, hypotension, nausea and vomiting, cardiac arrhythmias, muscle cramping, seizures
Febrile Nonhemolysis Cause: Recipient anti-HLA antibodies react to transfused leukocyte or platelet antigens	Fever, flushing, chills, absent RBC hemolysis, lumbar pain, malaise, headache, palpitation, cough, increased pulse, chills

Hemolysis

Immediate cause: Antibodies in recipient's plasma react to donor's antigens on red cells

Delayed cause: Recipient becomes sensitized to foreign RBC antigens not in the ABO system

Anxiety, increased pulse, respiration, and temperature, decreased blood pressure, dyspnea, nausea and vomiting, chills, fever, hemoglobinemia, hemoglobinuria, abnormal bleeding, oliguria, back pain, shock; reactions may occur when as little as 10-15 ml of incompatible blood have been infused; occurs ≥2 days after transfusion; continued anemia, hemoglobinuria, fever, lumbar pain, and mild jaundice

Hyperkalemia

Cause: Prolonged storage of blood; releases potassium into the cell plasma

Onset within few minutes; electrocardiogram (ECG) changes, peaked T wave and widening of QRS, weakness of extremities, abdominal pain

Hypokalemia

Cause: Associated with citrate-induced metabolic alkalosis but may be affected by respiratory or tissue alkalosis

Onset gradual; ECG changes, flattened T wave, depressed ST segment, polyuria, muscle weakness, decreased bowel sounds

Hypothermia

Cause: Rapid administration of cold blood components or when cold blood is administered through a central venous catheter

Shaking chills, hypothermia, cardiac arrhythmias, cardiac arrest, hypotension

---

IgA, Immunoglobulin A; *HLA*, human leukocyte antigen; *RBC*, red blood cell; *HIV*, human immunodeficiency virus; *DIC*, disseminated intravascular coagulation.
Continued

Table 7-2   Adverse effects of blood transfusion—cont'd

Reactions	Symptoms
Urticaria Cause: Allergy to soluble product in the donor plasma	Local erythema, hives, and itching, total body rash, usually without fever
Infections Transmitted by Transfusions	
Acquired Immunodeficiency Syndrome (AIDS) Cause: Donor blood HIV seropositive	Can be asymptomatic for up to several years or develop flulike symptoms within 2-4 wk; later signs and symptoms include fever, night sweats, fatigue, weight loss, adenopathy, and skin lesions; seropositive for HIV virus
Bacterial Contamination Cause: Contamination at time of donation or preparation; gram-negative bacteria release endotoxins	Onset within 2 hr of transfusion; chills, fever, abdominal pain. shock, marked hypertension, hemoglobinuria, bacteria release endotoxins renal failure, DIC
Cytomegalovirus (CMV) CMV can exist in any healthy adult	Immunosuppressed patients are at high risk (bone marrow transplant, open-heart surgery, newborn, positive heterophil); fatigue, weakness, adenopathy, low-grade fever

Graft-versus-Host Disease (GVHD)
Cause: Immunocompetent donor; lymphocytes engraft and multiply in immunodeficient recipient; GVHD may occur in recipients of transfusions from first-degree family members (parents, children, siblings) due to shared specificities at the major histocompatibility complex; irradiation of cellular blood components before administration is useful in reducing the risk of GVHD

Bone marrow-suppressed patients at risk; fever, skin rash, diarrhea, presence of infection, jaundice

Hepatitis
Hepatitis B, hepatitis A extremely rare; chronic liver disease more common with hepatitis C than hepatitis B

Occurs in a few weeks to months after transfusion; nausea and vomiting, fever, dark orange urine, jaundice, weakness, fatigue, anorexia, elevated liver enzyme levels (serum glutamic-oxaloacetic transaminase [SGOT], SGPT)

Malaria

Spiking fever after receiving transfusion containing red cells, platelets, or fresh-frozen plasma; malaria organism isolated in the blood

Syphilis

Rare; blood test positive for syphilis

Thrombocytopenia Purpura

Occurs most often in women; decreased platelet count; generalized purplish rash

Initiating the Transfusion

After the protocol to obtain the blood product from the blood bank has been completed, the blood product should be administered within 30 minutes, because blood can deteriorate and become rapidly contaminated at room temperature. (A blood product cannot be returned to the blood bank if administration of the product is not initiated in appropriate time.)

The transfusion should be initiated slowly and then maintained at an administration rate appropriate for the patient's condition. All blood components should be infused within 4 hours; the nurse must time the transfusion accurately.

During the first 15 minutes of initial transfusion, the nurse should remain and observe the patient for adverse reactions. Any adverse or unusual symptoms should be noted. The earlier these symptoms are detected, the more promptly the infusion can be discontinued and treatment instituted. (See Table 7-2 for effects and symptoms of adverse reactions to blood transfusion.) The patient should be assessed on an ongoing basis. The nurse should take baseline vital signs (temperature, pulse, respirations, and blood pressure) before the transfusion and throughout the transfusion process.

Only compatible IV fluids should be used. No drug should ever be injected into a blood bag; only normal saline solution may be added to or run simultaneously with blood or components before or during transfusion.

Damage to the blood cells must be prevented. For the infusion of most blood components, an 18-gauge catheter is appropriate. For patients with small veins (small children and elderly patients), a thin-walled, 23-gauge "scalp vein" needle may be used. Also, a blood warmer may be considered for massive transfusions and transfusions in the neonate, child, or immunosuppressed patient.

Transfusion Pitfalls to Avoid

- Do not store component in the nursing unit or another unmonitored refrigerator.
- Do not keep blood out of a monitored refrigerator for more than 30 minutes before beginning the transfusion.
- Do not warm blood in an unmonitored water bath or sink or in a microwave oven.

- Do not administer blood component without a blood filter.
- Do not use the same blood filter for more than 4 hours.
- Do not transfuse a unit of blood for more than 4 hours.
- Do not add any medications, including those intended for intravenous use, to blood or components or infuse through the same administration set as the blood component.
- Do not allow any solution other than 0.9% normal saline to come in contact with the blood component or the administration set.

Troubleshooting Tips

Sluggish IV lines and clogged filters that decrease the flow rate may be encountered during transfusion. Investigative questions to ask include the following:

- Is there a kink in the administration set?
- Is the correct gauge of needle or catheter being used?
- Has flushing the tubing with normal saline been attempted?
- Has the filter been used for more than 2 units?
- Has the blood bag been rotated to distribute contents evenly?
- Is the blood bag 36 to 48 inches above the venous access or venipuncture site?
- Does the roller clamp need to be adjusted?

If all the preceding points are negative or problems have been corrected, use of a pressure cuff and infusion pump should be considered (according to your agency's guidelines).

Posttransfusion

1. Complete posttransfusion documentation.
2. Return the completed transfusion form to the blood bank.
3. Continue to observe the patient, and monitor vital signs according to agency policy.
4. Dispose of used supplies in a puncture-proof, leakproof container. NOTE: If a transfusion reaction occurs, return the discontinued bag of blood and blood components with all attached solutions to the blood bank.
5. Follow up with prescribed, scheduled posttransfusion laboratory tests, such as complete blood count, hemoglobin, hematocrit, platelet count, prothrombin time, or factor VIII level.

CLINICAL ALERT: Wear gloves while initiating and discontinuing a blood transfusion to protect against blood-borne infections (hepatitis or AIDS). Immediately and thoroughly wash hands and other skin surfaces contaminated with blood, body fluids containing visible blood, or other body fluids to which universal precautions apply.

Adverse Effects of Blood Transfusion

Of the adverse reactions listed in Table 7-2, hemolytic (immediate and delayed) reactions, febrile nonhemolytic reactions, and allergic reactions occur most frequently. To provide immediate intervention for a transfusion reaction, the most common symptoms of a transfusion reaction and the appropriate interventions need to be studied. The greatest risk of exposure to infectious disease from blood transfusions is a 1% to 2% incidence of posttransfusion hepatitis. If the patient is suspected of having posttransfusion hepatitis, the blood bank service should be notified so that the donor can be investigated.

The avoidance of concurrent infusions of blood components and amphotericin B should be considered. Similar adverse reactions to these products may include fever, chills, nausea, vomiting, hypotension, decreased urine output, dyspnea, and anaphylaxis. It may be difficult to determine the source (blood component or amphotericin B) of the reactions. In addition, there is the potential deleterious effects of amphotericin B on blood cell survival after transfusion. Further studies are needed to clearly evaluate the differences between adverse reactions and the effects of amphotericin B on the blood components.

Management of Transfusion Reactions

The time between suspicion of a transfusion reaction and the initiation of appropriate therapy should be as short as possible. The nurse administering blood component therapy is responsible for obtaining baseline vital signs and monitoring the patient for any changes that may develop during and after a transfusion. An accurate assessment of clinical symptoms and reporting of this information is crucial in life-threatening reactions. Nursing staff should be skilled in blood component therapy, and policies and procedures for management of transfusion reactions should be readily available.

Guidelines established by the AABB for reactions to blood transfusions include the following:

1. Stop the transfusion to limit the amount of blood infused.
2. Notify the physician.

3. Keep the IV line open with an infusion of normal saline.
4. Check all labels, forms, and patient identification to determine whether the patient received the correct blood or component.
5. Report the suspected transfusion reaction to blood bank personnel immediately.
6. Send required blood samples, carefully drawn to avoid mechanical hemolysis, to the blood bank as soon as possible, together with the discontinued bag of blood, the administration set, attached IV solutions, and all the related forms and labels.
7. Send other samples—for example, urine for evaluation of acute hemolysis—as directed by the blood bank director or patient's physician.
8. Complete the agency report or "Suspected Transfusion Reaction" form (if appropriate).
9. Medication and supplies to have readily available include the following:
   a. Injectable: aminophylline, diphenhydramine hydrochloride (Benadryl), dopamine, epinephrine, heparin, hydrocortisone, furosemide (Lasix)
   b. Oral: acetaminophen, aspirin
   c. Oxygen setup, tubing, cannula and/or mask, and airway device
   d. Foley catheterization kit
   e. Blood culture bottles
   f. IV fluids (isotonic solution) with compatible IV tubings

CLINICAL ALERT: The nurse must become familiar with all the equipment used in the employing agency so that intervention for a transfusion reaction can be administered promptly and safely.

Documentation Recommendations

- Location of patent peripheral or central venous access IV site
- Baseline vital signs before transfusion
- Time transfusion was started
- Type of product and identification number
- Signature of person initiating the transfusion and signature of second licensed person verifying correct product
- Total number of units infused and their identification numbers
- Total volume of blood component, saline infused, and filters used
- Time transfusion was completed

- Premedication or postmedication supplies (tubings) used for blood component therapy
- Patient's response to transfusion, especially any symptoms of an adverse reaction (chills, fever, urticaria, sweating, nausea, blood in urine, shortness of breath, dyspnea, hypotension, or anxiety)
- All nursing interventions initiated and performed in response to an adverse reaction

Nursing Diagnoses

- Fluid volume excess, potential, related to infusion of the product or volume of the infusion
- Infection, risk for, related to contamination of supplies or blood product
- Fluid volume deficit, actual or risk for, related to loss of blood volume
- Cardiac output, decreased
- Body temperature, altered: hypothermia/hyperthermia
- Knowledge deficit related to side effects of transfusion reaction
- Injury, risk for, related to allergy, air embolism, hemolytic transfusion reaction related to blood products

Patient/Family Teaching for Self-Management

- Describe the purpose, schedule, and procedure for blood component administration.
- Explain the potential blood transfusion reactions (fever, chills, urticaria, back pain, pain at infusion site, chest pain, dyspnea, and nausea) and the importance of reporting the reactions promptly to the nurse or physician.
- Instruct the patient or caregiver regarding potential delayed reactions to transfusions, which may occur several hours, days, or a week after transfusion; examples are jaundice and generalized purplish rash (purpura); advise to notify the physician promptly.
- If blood component therapy is to be administered in the home setting, assess availability of the caregiver to be present in the home during administration of the blood product.

Guidelines for Home Care
Blood Transfusion Therapy

- The patient must be *homebound* (unable to drive self or leave home without assistance).

- The patient should be alert, cooperative, and able to respond appropriately to body symptoms.
- The patient must have been previously transfused without difficulty.
- A responsible adult must be present in the home to participate in the identification process and to summons assistance (physician or paramedic) if necessary.
- A usable telephone must be available during the transfusion.
- Whole blood must not be administered in the home.
- The blood specimen for type and crossmatch should be obtained 24 to 48 hours before blood product administration.
- Registered nurse and blood band personnel before administration must verify each unit of blood component therapy.
- The registered nurse must work under the direction of a physician in accordance with federal, state, and local regulations and the standards of the American Association of Blood Banks.
- The registered nurse should be knowledgeable and skilled in the procedure of blood product administration.
- The nurse must remain in attendance throughout the blood transfusion process and for at least 30 minutes after the transfusion.
- Blood should be transported in insulated containers with ice packets that maintain the temperature between 1° and 10° C for 24 hours.
- The container, empty bags, and tubing should be returned to the blood bank on completion of the transfusion.
- Posttransfusion instructions must be given in writing, and the patient or caregiver must be provided with the names and phone numbers of individuals available at all times to be called in the event of a delayed problem.
- The nurse should arrange for prescribed posttransfusion laboratory tests to be completed; examples are RBCs (hemoglobin, hematocrit), within 24 hours; platelets, 18 hours after the transfusion(s).

CLINICAL ALERT: Home care nursing personnel should be alert and prepared for possible transfusion reactions. The drugs and supplies necessary to manage these potential reactions must be readily available for use. Protocols for management of transfusion reactions should be clearly defined and easily accessible to home care infusion-nursing staff.

Geriatric Considerations

- Previous history of homebound status may include anemia with bone marrow failure, anemia associated with malignancy, chronic gastrointestinal bleeding, or chronic renal failure.
- There is a potential for compromise of cardiac, renal, and respiratory systems: Adjust the flow rate if the patient cannot tolerate the prescribed flow rate. Flow rate should be 1 ml/kg/hr in the patient at risk for circulatory overload.
- Sensory deficits may occur.
- Consult medical records or family members for previous blood transfusion reactions.
- The patient may require assistance with elimination needs before the blood product transfusion.
- Premedications may cause drowsiness; encourage the patient to use transportation resources (family, public, American Cancer Society, American Red Cross) if receiving blood transfusions on an outpatient basis.
- Venous integrity may be compromised; ensure catheter or needle patency before transfusion.
- Consult with community resources if the homebound situation becomes compromised.

Resources

Patient and Professional Information Booklets

The American Red Cross and the U.S. Public Health Service have made available the following publications regarding the blood supply and AIDS:

- AIDS and the Blood Supply
- AIDS and the Health Care Workers
- AIDS and Your Job
- Caring for the AIDS Patient at Home
- AIDS and Your Children
- If Your Antibody Test Is Positive
- AIDS, Sex and You

Clinical Competency—Blood and Blood Component Administration

	Yes	No	NA
1. Verify the physician's order for specific product to be given on a stated date.			
2. Verify appropriate laboratory data; allergy status and informed consent.			
3. Review transfusion history of the patient.			
4. Select correct tubing and filter for the blood and blood product.			
5. Explain the procedure to the patient.			
6. Obtain baseline vital signs (blood pressure, temperature, pulse, respirations).			
7. Identify the patient by name and by written ID number on the patient bracelet.			
8. Confirm blood unit number, ABO group, Rh type, expiration date of product on donor unit, patient transfusion request form, and patient identification number on patient bracelet with another licensed professional.			
9. Prime blood tubing and filter, taking care to cover the entire filter.			
10. Initiate the transfusion slowly (5 ml/min for initial 15 minutes).			
11. Readjust the transfusion rate after 15 minutes to the desired infusion rate.			
12. Use only normal saline for flushing of IV line.			
13. Obtain the patient's vital signs throughout the transfusion according to agency policy.			

Continued

Clinical Competency—Blood and Blood Component Administration—cont'd

	Yes	No	NA
14. Document the procedure according to agency policy.			
15. Return completed posttransfusion request to blood bank.			

Study Questions

1. The primary cause of bacterial contamination of blood products is:
   a. Gram-positive bacteria, contamination at time of donation or preparation
   b. Gram-negative bacteria, contamination at time of donation or preparation
   c. Gram-positive bacteria, contamination at time of administration or preparation
   d. Gram-negative bacteria, contamination at time of administration or preparation

2. Chills, fever, headache, low back pain, hypotension, tachycardia are clinical features for:
   a. Acute hemolytic reaction
   b. Circulatory overload
   c. Delayed transfusion reaction
   d. Hyperkalemia

3. The intravenous solution most compatible with blood or blood products is:
   a. 0.33% saline
   b. 0.45% saline
   c. 0.9% normal saline
   d. Ringer's lactate

4. The initial infusion rate and total infusion time, respectively, for blood products are:
   a. 2-5 ml/min over 1 hour
   b. 5-10 ml/min over 1 hour
   c. 10-15 ml/min over 2-4 hours
   d. 2-5 ml/min over 2-4 hours

5. Nursing interventions for blood transfusion reaction include:
   a. Notifying the physician; stopping the infusion for 30 minutes then resuming infusion; reporting the incident to the blood bank immediately
   b. Notifying the physician; stopping the transfusion; reporting the incident to the blood bank within 24 hours
   c. Notifying the physician; stopping the transfusion; reporting the incident to the blood bank immediately
   d. Notifying the physician; stopping the transfusion for 15 minutes then resuming the infusion; notifying the blood bank immediately

6. Patients that are at risk for TA-GVHD include:
   a. Bone marrow transplant recipients, exchange transfusion neonates, those with Hodgkin's disease, those who directed blood donation to self
   b. Bone marrow transplant recipients, exchange transfusion neonates, those with Hodgkin's disease, those who directed donation from blood relatives
   c. Bone marrow transplant recipients, those who received platelet transfusions, individuals with breast cancer, those who directed donation from blood relatives
   d. Bone marrow transplant recipients, those who received platelet transfusions, individuals with breast cancer, those who directed blood donation to self

7. A unit of RBCs should elevate the hematocrit and hemoglobin by:
   a. Hematocrit between 1% and 3% and hemoglobin by 1-1.5 g/dl
   b. Hematocrit between 1% and 3% and hemoglobin by 1.5-2 g/dl
   c. Hematocrit between 3% and 5% and hemoglobin by 2-3.5 g/dl
   d. Hematocrit between 3% and 5% and hemoglobin by 1-1.5 g/dl

8. Critical elements of verifying blood product before administration include:
   a. Blood product, blood bank product form, physician's order, patient blood armband

b. Blood product, blood bank donor form, physician's order, patient blood armband

c. Blood product, blood bank product form, donor informed consent, patient blood armband

d. Blood product, blood bank donor form, donor informed consent, patient blood armband

9. Agencies that regulate blood and blood product collection, storage, and administration include:
   a. AABB, ARC, CDC, FDA, JCAHO
   b. AABB, ACS, ARC, CDC, FDA
   c. AABB, ARC, CDC, FDA, OSHA
   d. AABB, ARC, CDC, FDA, FBI

10. Compatibilities for ABO and Rh for donor and recipient is required for which blood products:
    a. RBCs, whole blood, fresh-frozen plasma, platelets
    b. RBCs, cryoprecipitate, fresh-frozen plasma, platelets
    c. RBCs, washed red cells, cryoprecipitate, platelets
    d. RBCs, plasma protein fraction, whole blood, platelets

Answers   1. b   2. a   3. c   4. d   5. c   6. b
7. d   8. a   9. c   10. a

Chemotherapy Administration

Objectives

1. Identify the goals of chemotherapy and the patient factors that influence drug selection.

2. Define *nadir* as it relates to chemotherapy drug side effects.

3. List the sequential steps for chemotherapy drug safe handling and extravasation management.

4. Discuss the use of test dosing and premedication sequence for chemotherapy drug-related anaphylaxis.

5. Describe the major system toxicities associated with chemotherapy drugs.

Chemotherapy is the use of cytotoxic drugs in the treatment of cancer. These drugs have been available since the early 1940s. Chemotherapy is recognized as one of the major treatment modalities (e.g., surgery, radiation therapy, biotherapy, and/or bone marrow/stem cell transplantation) that provide a cure, control, or palliation as a cancer treatment goal. Chemotherapy may be used separately or in conjunction with these other modalities.

Nursing has major responsibilities in caring for patients who receive chemotherapeutic agents. It is important that nurses know the cancer treatment goal, drug classification with modes of action, principles of tumor growth and cell kill, and the drug administration protocol. Chemotherapeutic agents should be administered by nurses who are knowledgeable and clinically competent in the various procedures. The patient and family/caregivers require

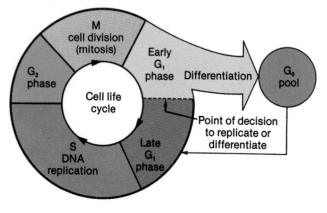

Fig. 8-1
Cell generation cycle.
(Courtesy Adria Laboratories, Columbus, Ohio.)

information on the many aspects of chemotherapy (e.g., drug administration procedure, potential side effects/toxicities, and self-care intervention strategies). The patient and family/caregivers should be encouraged to participate and become an integral part of the treatment planning and implementation. Competent nursing assessment and intervention are essential throughout the patient's disease and treatment process. These many responsibilities offer unique opportunities and challenges for the nurse administering and monitoring chemotherapy drugs.

Principles of Chemotherapy
Cell Generation Cycle
Normal cells and cancer cells go through the same cell cycle division, which is characterized by a sequential series of phases or steps (Fig. 8-1). The time it takes for a cell to complete the phase or cycle varies. This time is called *generation time*. Chemotherapeutic drugs are most active against frequently dividing cells. Normal cells with rapid growth changes most commonly affected by chemotherapeutic agents include bone marrow (platelets and red and white blood cells), hair follicles, mucosal lining of the gastrointestinal tract, skin, and germ cells (sperm and ova).

CLINICAL ALERT: Chemotherapy is given according to scheduled sequences or cycles that are planned to allow recovery of the normal cells. *Nadir* is defined as the time when the patients' blood counts are at their lowest level, related to the specific chemotherapy drugs and/or dosing principles.

The nurse must anticipate changes such as low red and white blood cell counts that may increase a patient's risk for anemia and infection and incorporate protective measures into the patient's plan of care.

Drug Classification

Chemotherapeutic agents are classified according to their pharmacologic action and their interference with cellular reproduction. The basic groups are cell cycle phase specific and cell cycle phase nonspecific. Their potential actions are the following.

Cell Cycle Phase–Specific Drugs

Cell cycle phase–specific drugs act on cells undergoing division in the cell cycle. These drugs have the greatest tumor cell kill when administered in divided doses or as a continuous infusion over short intermittent cycle times (e.g., drug volume is infused over 2 hours at scheduled increments of every 12 hours).

G_1 Phase	G_2 Phase
Asparaginase	Bleomycin (Blenoxane)
Capecitabine (Xeloda)	Docetaxel (Taxotere)
Prednisone	Etoposide (VP-16)
Vincristine (Oncovin)	Paclitaxel (Taxol)
	Vinorelbine (Navelbine)

S Phase	M Phase
Cytarabine (ara-C)	Docetaxel (Taxotere)
Floxuridine (FUDR)	Paclitaxel (Taxol)
Fludarabine (Fludara)	Vindesine (Eldisine)
5-Fluorouracil	Gemcitabine (Gemzar)
Hydroxyurea (Hydrea)	

Idarubicin (Idamycin)

Irinotecan (Camptosar)

6-Mercaptopurine

Methotrexate (Mexate)

Pentostatin (2'-deoxycoformycin)

Teniposide (VM-26, Vumon)

6-Thioguanine

Topotecan (Hycamtin)

Vinblastine (Velban)

Vincristine (Oncovin)

Cell Cycle Phase–Nonspecific Drugs

Cell cycle phase–nonspecific drugs act on cells in all phases of the cell cycle, including the resting phase. The cell-kill effect is proportional to the administered drug dose. Drugs of this nature are often given as single bolus injections and/or infusions.

Alkylating Agents	Nitrosoureas
Busulfan (Busulfex)	Carmustine (BCNU)
Carboplatin (Paraplatin)	Lomustine (CeeNu)
Chlorambucil (Leukeran)	Semustine (MeCCNU)
Cisplatin (Platinol)	Streptozocin (Zanosar)
Cyclophosphamide (Cytoxan)	
Ifosfamide (IFEX)	
Mechlorethamine hydrochloride (Mustargen)	
Melphalan (Alkeran)	
Thioplex (Thiotepa)	

Antitumor Antibiotics	Miscellaneous
Bleomycin (Blenoxane)	Cladribine (Leustatin) (2-CdA)
Dactinomycin (actinomycin, Cosmegen)	Dacarbazine (DTIC-Dome)
Daunorubicin (daunomycin, Cerubidine)	Hexamethylmelamine
Doxorubicin (Adriamycin)	Hydroxyurea (Hydrea)
Idarubicin (Idamycin)	L-Asparaginase (Elspar)
Mithramycin, mitomycin-C (Mutamycin)	Pegaspargase (Oncaspar)
Mitoxantrone (Novantrone)	Procarbazine (Matulane)
Plicamycin (Mithracin)	

Hormone and Steroid Drugs

The remaining group of drugs that affect tumor cell growth by altering the intracellular environment is hormone and steroid drugs. The mechanism of action for each drug is different. Steroidal drugs provide an antiinflammatory effect on the body tissues. These drugs all recruit malignant cells out of G_0 phase, making them vulnerable to damage, caused by cell cycle phase–specific agents. Hormones are cell cycle phase nonspecific. These chemicals, secreted by the endocrine glands, alter the environment of the cell by affecting the cell membrane permeability. By manipulating hormone levels, they can suppress tumor growth. Antihormonal agents derive their antineoplastic effect from their ability to neutralize the effect of or inhibit the production of natural hormones used by hormone-dependent tumors.

Hormones	Corticosteroids
Androgens	Dexamethasone (Decadron)
Androgens	Dexamethasone
Fluoxymesterone (Halotestin)	Hydrocortisone sodium succinate (Solu-Cortef)
Testosterone	Prednisone (Deltasone)
	Prednisolone (Prelone)

Progestins	Estrogens
Medroxyprogesterone acetate (Depo-Provera intramuscular; Provera oral)	Chlorotrianisene (TACE)
Megestrol acetate (Megace)	Conjugated estrogens (Premarin)
	Diethylstilbestrol (DES)

Antihormonal Agents

Finasteride (Proscar)

Flutamide (Eulexin)

Letrozole (Femara)

Leuprolide (Lupron)

Mitotane (Lysodren)

Tamoxifen (Nolvadex)

Goserelin (Zoladex)

CLINICAL ALERT: Chemotherapy drugs have multiple side effects related to the dose, route, schedule frequency, and specific body system toxicity. Become familiar with all the potential side effects and toxicities associated with chemotherapeutic drugs in all the drug categories.

Tumor Growth

The regulatory mechanism controlling the growth of cancer cells differs from that of normal cells. Unlike normal cells, cancer cells grow via a pyramid effect; however, they grow at the same rate as the tissue from which they originated. The time required for a tumor mass to reach a certain size is called *doubling time*. Between the 7th and 10th doubling time, the possibility arises for the tumor to shed cells, a process called *micrometastasis*. During the early stages of tumor growth, doubling time is more rapid than in later stages. This pattern of growth is called the *Gompertzian growth curve* (Fig. 8-2).

CLINICAL ALERT: Chemotherapy is used as an effective treatment modality in the treatment approach for the micrometastasis process. Tumor cells are more sensitive to chemotherapeutic agents that are toxic to rapidly dividing cells. Treatment protocols for patients with leukemia and lymphoma may include interven-

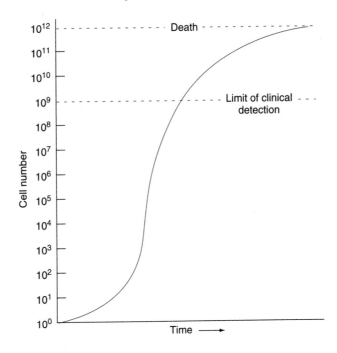

Fig. 8-2
The Gompertzian growth curve.
(From *The American Cancer Society textbook of clinical oncology,*
Atlanta, 1995, American Cancer Society.)

tions for rapid cell destruction. This protocol may include extensive
fluid hydration with administration of allopurinol to minimize renal
toxicity 24 to 48 hours before the initial chemotherapeutic drug
dose is given.

Cell Kill Hypothesis

A single cancer cell is capable of multiplying and eventually killing
the host. The last tumor cell needs to be killed to achieve a cure in
the treatment of cancer. With each course of the drug therapy, a
given dose of chemotherapeutic drug kills only a fraction or
percentage of all of the cancer cells present. Repeated courses of

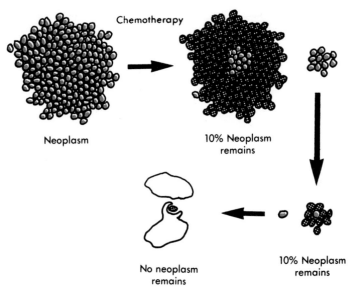

Fig. 8-3
Cell kill hypothesis.
(From Goodman MS: *Cancer chemotherapy and care,* part 1, Evansville, Ind, 1995, Bristol Laboratories, Division of Bristol-Myers Co.)

chemotherapy must then be used to reduce the total cancer cell number (Fig. 8-3).

CLINICAL ALERT: Anticipation of potential drug cumulative side effects is required for sequential scheduled courses of chemotherapy drugs. Infusion of multiple drugs at varied dose intensity and/or schedule sequence intensifies the cumulative side effects. Assess major system toxicities, side effects, and laboratory values that will be affected by these treatment regimens.

Factors Considered in Drug Selection

1. Patient's eligibility for chemotherapy (confirmed diagnosis; age; bone marrow, nutritional, cardiac, hepatic, renal, and respiratory status; expectation of longevity; previous history of chemotherapy and radiation therapy)
2. Cancer cell type (e.g., squamous cell, adenocarcinoma)

3. Rate of drug absorption (e.g., treatment interval and routes—oral, intravenous, intraarterial)
4. Tumor location (e.g., many drugs do not cross the blood-brain barrier)
5. Tumor burden (e.g., larger tumors are generally less responsive to chemotherapy)
6. Tumor resistance to chemotherapy (e.g., tumor cells can mutate and produce variant cells distinct from the tumor stem cell of origin)

Combination Chemotherapy

Chemotherapeutic drugs are most commonly given in combination. This process enhances the effect of the drugs on the tumor cell kill. Consideration for drugs used in combination include effectiveness as a single agent, increased tumor cell kill, increased patient survival, prevention or delay in the development of disease/drug resistance, presence of a synergistic action, varied toxicities, different mechanisms of action, and administration in repeated courses to minimize the immunosuppressive effects that might otherwise occur. Table 8-1 lists combination chemotherapy regimens.

Combination chemotherapy provides additional benefits not possible with single drug treatment. These benefits include maximal cell kill within the range of toxicity tolerated by the patient for each drug, a broader range of coverage of resistant cell lines in a heterogeneous tumor population, and prevention or slowing of the development of new resistant cell lines. By the time a tumor that has metastasized is detected, numerous cellular variants exist within the tumor; therapy for the metastatic disease is often directed toward characteristics of the secondary tumor rather than the primary tumor. Combination chemotherapy rather than single sequential therapy maximizes therapeutic response by addressing the diversity of cellular response.

Additional drugs that maybe used in combination chemotherapy regimens are monoclonal antibodies (trastuzumab [Herceptin] and rituximab [Rituxan]). These drugs have disease specificity (e.g., breast cancer and B-cell lymphoma). Monoclonal antibodies exert their cancer treatment effects by altering cell regulation process (e.g., turn off cell production). Manufacturer and agency guidelines should be followed for preparation, administration, and patient monitoring.

Table 8-1   Combination chemotherapy regimens

Breast

CMF: cyclophosphamide, methotrexate, 5-fluorouracil

CMFVP: cyclophosphamide, methotrexate, 5-fluorouracil, vincristine, prednisone

FUVAC: 5-fluorouracil, vinblastine, adriamycin, cyclophosphamide

Hodgkin's Disease

ABVD: adriamycin, bleomycin, vinblastine, dacarbazine

MOPP: nitrogen mustard, Oncovin, prednisone, procarbazine

Lung

CAV: cisplatin, adriamycin, vinblastine

CAMP: cyclophosphamide, adriamycin, methotrexate, procarbazine

Lymphoma

CHOP-BLEO: cyclophosphamide, adriamycin, Oncovin, prednisone, bleomycin

PROMACE-Cyta-BOM: prednisone, oncovin, methotrexate, adriamycin, cyclophosphamide, etoposide, cytarabine, bleomycin, leucovorin, dexamethasone, trimethoprim-sulfamethoxazole

Chemotherapy Administration
Drug Dosage Calculation

Drug dosage for cancer chemotherapy is based on body surface area (BSA) for both adults and children. BSA is determined by a correlation of body weight and height via a designated nomogram. The nurse must ensure that accurate patient height and weight measurements are obtained on a scheduled frequency. Fluctuations in weight may occur as result of chemotherapy drug-related side effects (e.g., nausea and vomiting or anorexia). All drug calculations should be verified by a second person to ensure dose accuracy. The dosage range of one drug may vary with different routes and/or protocols. Multiple, cost-effective calculation tools are available for nurses (e.g., programmable BSA calculators) to facilitate accurate drug dose calculation. (See Chapter 13 for specific details of drug calculations.)

Drug Reconstitution

The nurse should prepare and reconstitute drugs using aseptic technique in accordance with the manufacturer's current recommendations. To ensure safe and accurate drug administration, all syringes of reconstituted drugs should be labeled immediately with the name and dose of the drug. Many of the chemotherapeutic agents are colorless and cannot be distinguished from one another after reconstitution or from normal saline that is used to flush the venous access device. (See "Safe Handling of Chemotherapeutic Agents" on page 265.) Guidelines for route of administration are outlined in Table 8-2.

CLINICAL ALERT: Validate blood return before, during, and after *bolus or continuous* infusion of all chemotherapeutic drugs. Follow the agency guidelines for frequency of monitoring continuous chemotherapeutic infusions. For continuous infusion of vesicant drugs, suggestions include validating blood return every 2 hours; for continuous infusion of nonvesicant drugs, validate blood return every 4 hours.

Vein Selection and Venipuncture

Many chemotherapeutic agents can be irritating to veins and surrounding tissues. Peripheral sites should be changed daily before administration of vesicant drugs. (See "Extravasation Management" on page 270.) The number of available veins may be limited as a result of previous therapy. (See Chapter 2, pages 28-30.)

Procedure for Chemotherapeutic Drug Administration

1. Verify patient identification, drug, dose, route, and time of administration with the physician's order.
2. Review drug allergy history with the patient.
3. Review appropriate laboratory data and other tests.
4. Verify informed consent for treatment.
5. Select the appropriate equipment and supplies.
6. Calculate the dose (verify calculation with second nurse) and reconstitute the drug using aseptic technique (follow safe handling guidelines).
7. Explain the procedure to patient and family. (See "Patient/ Family Teaching for Self-Management" on page 278.)
8. Administer prescribed antiemetics or other medications.
9. Initiate the peripheral IV site or prepare a central venous access site.

10. Validate blood return status.
11. Administer chemotherapeutic agents.
12. Monitor the patient at scheduled frequencies throughout the course of drug administration.
13. Anticipate and plan interventions for potential side effects or major system toxicity. (See Tables 8-3 and 8-4.)
14. Dispose of all used supplies and unused drugs into approved punctureproof, leakproof containers, with closeable lid, outside of the patient area.
15. Document the procedure according to agency policy and procedure. (See "Documentation Recommendations" on page 278.) *Text continued on p. 265*

 Table 8-2   Guidelines—route of administration

1. *Oral:* Emphasize importance of patient compliance with prescribed dose schedule.
2. *Subcutaneous and intramuscular:* May require demonstration with return demonstration to teach patient/caregiver medication administration techniques. Encourage site rotation and keeping log of drug dosing schedule.
3. *Topical:* Cover surface area with thin film of medication; instruct patient to wear loose-fitting, cotton clothing. Wear gloves and be sure to wash hands thoroughly after procedure. Caution patient not to touch area of topical ointment application.
4. *Intraarterial:* Requires temporary catheter placement in artery near tumor site. The drug is usually administered in heparinized solution via infusion pump to overcome arterial pressure resistance. Monitor vital signs, color and temperature of extremity, catheter placement, and potential for bleeding at insertion site during infusion process. Instruct patient and family on care components for catheter insertion procedure and restrictions during drug infusion. Specialized education and skills are required for nurse if chemotherapy is administered via implantable infusion pump.
5. *Intraperitoneal:* Warm infusate solution (with dry heat) to body temperature of 38° C before administration. Administer drug solution into abdominal cavity through implantable port or external suprapubic catheter (Fig. 8-4). Monitor patient for abdominal pressure, pain, fever, and electrolyte status. Measure and record abdominal girth for 48 hr.

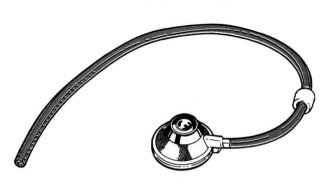

Fig. 8-4
Implantable intraperitoneal port.
(Courtesy CR Bard, Inc, Cranston, RI.)

Table 8-2   Guidelines—route of administration—cont'd

6. *Intrapleural:* Drug is administered through chest tube into pleural cavity. Administer prescribed premedication drugs (analgesia) for comfort measures. After drug instillation, clamp chest tubes and reposition (e.g., side to back to side) every 15 min for 2 hr or per protocol. Monitor vital signs, pain, and chest tube status on scheduled frequency.

7. *Intrathecal:* Reconstitute all intrathecal medications with preservative-free, sterile normal saline or sterile water. Infusion of medication may be given through an Ommaya reservoir and/or lumbar puncture procedure. Usual volume of medication instilled is 15 ml or less (Fig. 8-5). Medication should be injected slowly. If ara-C or methotrexate is given in large dose, monitor patient closely for potential neurotoxicity. Usually *physicians* administer intrathecal drugs.

8. *Intravesicular:* Maintain sterile technique when inserting Foley catheter. Instill solution, *clamp and unclamp* catheter to drain according to protocol.

9. *IV:* May be given through central venous catheters or peripheral venous access. Methods of IV administration include the following:

   - *Push* (bolus): Medication is administered through syringe by direct IV method.
   - *Piggyback* (secondary setup): Drug is administered using secondary bag (bottle) and tubing; primary infusion is concurrently maintained throughout drug administration.
   - *Side arm:* Drug is administered through syringe into side port of running (free-flowing) IV infusion.
   - *Infusion:* Drug is added to prescribed volume of fluid IV bag (bottle); continuous or intermittent flow.

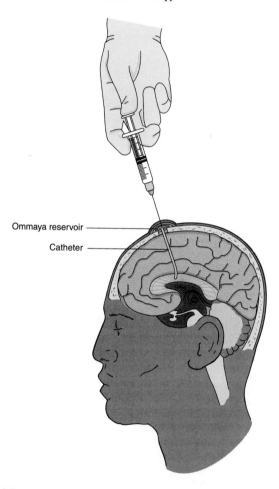

Fig. 8-5

The Ommaya reservoir. The reservoir is a mushroom-shaped device with an attached catheter that is implanted into the lateral ventricle through a burr hole. A silicone injection dome rests over the burr hole under the scalp. Drugs can be injected directly into the reservoir with a syringe.

(From Phipps WJ, Sands JK, Marek JF: *Medical-surgical nursing: concepts & clinical practice*, St Louis, 1999, Mosby.)

Table 8-3   Patient teaching for self-management of most common side effects from chemotherapeutic drugs

Side Effects	Points to Cover
Aches and Pains	Pain medication should be taken on a regular and duration of pain schedule.
Nursing intervention	Side effects of pain medicine are constipation, dry mouth, and
Assess location, intensity, and quality.	drowsiness.
	Rest and relaxation strategies include music, progressive relaxation exercise, distraction, and positive imaging.
Alopecia	Hair loss occurs 10-21 days after drug administration.
Hair loss	Hair loss is temporary, and hair will regrow when drug is
Drugs causing: bleomycin, cyclophosphamide, dacarbazine, dactinomycin, daunorubicin, doxorubicin idarubicin, ifosfamide, irinotecan mechlorethamine, mitomycin, paclitaxel, teniposide, topotecan, vinblastine, and vinorelbine.	stopped. Hair loss may occur suddenly and in large amounts; select wig, cap, scarf, or turban before hair loss occurs. Avoid use of hair dryers, curling irons, and harsh shampoos and frequent shampooing.
Hair thinning	Keep head covered in summer to prevent severe sunburn and in
Drugs causing: bleomycin, etoposide, 5-fluorouracil, floxuridine, and vincristine.	winter to prevent heat loss.

Continued

Table 8-3   Patient teaching for self-management of most common side effects from chemotherapeutic drugs—cont'd

Side Effects	Points to Cover
Anorexia	Eating is a social event; eat with others in a pleasant area with soft music and attractive settings.
Nursing intervention	Freshen up before meals (e.g., with mouth care and exercise).
Assess dietary history; monitor serum transferrin levels and weight loss.	Eat small, frequent meals (5-6 meals daily); avoid drinking fluids with meals to prevent feeling of fullness.
	Concentrate on eating foods high in protein, such as eggs, milk products, peanut butter, tuna, beans, and peas.
	Breakfast may be the most tolerable meal of the day; try to include one third of daily calories at this time.
	Monitor and record weight weekly; report weight loss.
Constipation	Increase intake of high-fiber foods, such as whole grain products, bran, fresh fruit, raw vegetables, and popcorn.
Drugs associated with potential for: vinblastine, vincristine, vindesine, vinorelbine, and opioids.	Increase fluid intake to 2-3 quarts of liquids daily; encourage fresh fruit juices, prunes, and hot liquids on waking.
Nursing intervention	Follow prescribed schedule for use of stool softener; follow prescribed physician's orders if no bowel movement for ≥3 days.
Determine normal bowel habits; advise patient not to strain with bowel evacuation, and to respond immediately to urge to defecate.	

Cystitis

Drug associated with potential for: cyclophosphamide and ifosfamide.

Nursing intervention

Observe urine for color and amount, and assess frequency of voiding; advise patient to take oral cyclophosphamide early in the day.

Increase fluid intake to 3 quarts daily.

Empty bladder at least every 4 hr, especially at bedtime and at least once during the night.

Report increasing symptoms and frequency of bleeding, burning, pain, fever, and chills promptly to physician.

Depression

Nursing intervention

Assess for changes in mood or affect.

Set small goals that are achievable daily.

Participate in enjoyable and diversionary activities, such as music, reading, and outings.

Share feelings and concerns with someone.

Diarrhea

Drugs associated with potential for: 5-fluorouracil, irinotecan, and methotrexate.

Nursing intervention

Monitor serum fluid and electrolytes and number, color, frequency, and consistency of diarrhea stools.

Avoid eating high-roughage, greasy, and spicy foods and beverages.

Avoid using milk products or use boiled skim milk.

Avoid caffeine and alcoholic products.

Eat a bland diet.

Increase fluid intake to 3 quarts of liquids daily (weak, tepid tea, bouillon, grape juice).

Record number and consistency of daily bowel movements; report information to physician.

Follow prescribed medication schedule if problem persists beyond 1 day.

Cleanse rectal area after each bowel movement.

Continued

Table 8-3 Patient teaching for self-management of most common side effects from chemotherapeutic drugs—cont'd

Side Effects	Points to Cover
Fatigue	Conserve energy; rest when tired; plan rest periods.
Nursing intervention	Plan for gradual accommodation of activities into lifestyle.
Assess for possible causes (anemia, chronic pain, stress, depression, and insufficient rest, or nutritional intake).	Monitor dietary and fluid intake daily.
Hematopoietic Changes	
Leukopenia	Avoid sources of infection, such as people with bacterial infections, colds, sore throats, flu, chickenpox, measles, or cold sores or people recently vaccinated with live vaccines such as measles-mumps-rubella (MMR) or diphtheria-pertussis-tetanus (DPT).
Most myelosuppressive agents produce white blood cell (WBC) nadir 7-14 days after drug administration; myelosuppression will be severe and prolonged with increased dosages: for example, with cytarabine 3-6 g; busulfan 2-6 g; cyclophosphamide 2-3 g, methotrexate 6-8 g, or etoposide 2-3 g.	Avoid having fresh fruit, live plants, and flowers at or near bedside.
	Avoid eating raw vegetables, fruits, and eggs.
	Avoid cleaning animal litter boxes since feces contain high levels of bacteria and fungi.
Nursing intervention	Maintain good personal hygiene, e.g., bathe daily, wash hands before eating and preparing food, clean carefully after bowel movements, and keep nails clean and clipped short and straight across.
Monitor WBC count and differential; change equipment as indicated—e.g., O₂ set up, denture cups, and IV supplies; teach sexual hygiene.	

Maintain adequate fluid intake.

Conserve energy; get adequate rest and exercise.

Prevent trauma to the skin and mucous membranes.

Avoid elective dental work or surgery. Avoid enemas, rectal suppositories, use of rectal thermometers, and catheterizations.

Use toothettes or nonabrasive dental cleaning devices.

Report signs and symptoms of infection immediately to the physician; for example, report fever of 38° C or greater, cough, sore throat, a shaking chill, painful or frequent urination, or vaginal discharge.

Avoid use of straight-edge razor or power tools; avoid physical activity that could cause injury.

Avoid use of drugs containing aspirin.

Humidify air; use lotion and lubricants on skin and lips; use soft bristle toothbrush.

Avoid invasive procedures: no intramuscular injections, rectal or vaginal examinations, enemas, suppositories, or use of rectal thermometers.

Discourage bare feet when ambulatory.

Use sanitary pads instead of tampons.

Report these signs and symptoms immediately to physician: bleeding gums, increased bruising, petechiae, purpura, hypermenorrhea, tarry-colored stools, blood in urine, or coffee-ground emesis.

Check with physician before any dental work.

Continued

Thrombocytopenia

Drugs associated with a delayed cumulative effect: mitomycin and all nitrosureas.

Nursing intervention

Monitor platelet counts; observe bleeding precautions; apply firm pressure to venipuncture site for 3-5 min; monitor pad count for menstruating females; monitor environment for sharp objects.

Table 8-3 Patient teaching for self-management of most common side effects from chemotherapeutic drugs—cont'd

Side Effects	Points to Cover
Anemia *Nursing intervention* Monitor hematocrit and hemoglobin, especially during drug nadir.	Adjust physical activity to accommodate periods of rest. Report these signs and symptoms promptly to physician: fatigue, dizziness, shortness of breath, and palpitations.
Mucositis, Rectal Symptoms occur 3-5 days after chemotherapy. *Nursing intervention* Monitor for electrolyte imbalance and granulocyte count; monitor number, consistency, and amount of bowel movements and urine output; assess for rectal bleeding.	Report weight loss to physician. Eat low-residue and easily digestible foods. Increase intake of liquids to replace fluid loss. Follow prescribed medication schedule, such as antidiarrheal and pain control drugs. Wash rectal area with soap and water after each bowel movement; pat or air dry.
Mucositis, Vaginal Symptoms occur 3-5 days after chemotherapy and subside in 7-10 days after therapy.	Report pain, ulceration, or bleeding of mucous membranes lining the perineum and vagina to physician. Sitz bath with warm salt water may provide relief of vaginal itching and odor.

Use hydrogen peroxide (one-quarter strength) with warm water after voiding to rinse perineal area.

Avoid commercial douches, tampons, and vaginal pads or liners containing deodorants.

Nausea and Vomiting

Drugs with high emetic potential: asparaginase, carmustine, cisplatin, dacarbazine dactinomycin, daunorubicin, doxorubicin, idarubicin, ifosfamide, mechlorethamine, methotrexate, mitoxantrone, procarbazine, streptozocin teniposide, and high-dose cytarabine, cyclophosphamide, and methotrexate.

Nursing intervention

Premedicate with antiemetic before nausea begins, for example, ½ hr before meals; patient may require routine antiemetics for 3-5 days after some chemotherapy protocols; monitor fluid and electrolyte status.

Eat frequent, small meals.

Avoid greasy or fatty foods and very sweet foods or candies.

Avoid unpleasant sights, odors, and tastes.

Cold foods, salty foods, dry crackers, and dry toast may be more tolerable.

If vomiting is severe, restrict diet to clear liquids and notify physician.

Consider diversionary activities, such as music therapy and relaxation techniques.

Recall strategies that were successful during pregnancy, illness, or other times of stress, for example, sipping on a flat cola drink.

Continued

Table 8-3   Patient teaching for self-management of most common side effects from chemotherapeutic drugs—cont'd

Side Effects	Points to Cover
Pharyngitis and Esophagitis Symptoms are often first noted by difficult or painful swallowing.	Eat a soft pureed or liquid diet. Follow prescribed scheduled medication to relieve discomfort. Report to physician symptoms that persist more than 3 days.
Skin Changes	Maintain good personal hygiene. Use topical preparations to minimize itching, such as creams or lotions containing vitamins A, D, or E. Avoid use of perfume and perfumed lotion, wearing fabrics such as wool or corduroy, and wearing tight-fitting clothes such as jeans or pantyhose.

Stomatitis (Oral)

Symptoms occur 5-7 days after chemotherapy and persist up to 10 days.

Continue brushing regularly; use soft toothbrush.

Use nonirritant mouthwash, such as salt, soda, and water solution (¼ tsp salt, pinch of soda, 8 oz water) at least 4 times daily.

Avoid irritants to the mouth, such as tobacco, alcoholic beverages, spices, and commercial mouthwashes.

Avoid wearing dentures until mouth soreness heals.

Maintain good nutritional intake; eat soft or liquid foods high in protein; add sauces or gravies to make food soupier.

Follow prescribed medication schedule, such as scheduled drugs for oral candidiasis.

Report persistent symptoms promptly to physician, and report if white patches occur on tongue, back of throat, or gums.

Table 8-4   Major system toxicity or dysfunction and nursing management

Toxicity/Dysfunction	Nursing Management
Cardiac Toxicity	
Drugs associated with potential for: chlorambucil, cyclophosphamide, dactinomycin, daunorubicin, doxorubicin, mitoxantrone, and high-dose ifosfamide, and paclitaxel	Verify baseline cardiac studies (e.g., electrocardiogram, ejection fraction, cardiac enzymes) before drug administration.
	Monitor cardiac status and report symptoms of tachycardia, shortness of breath, distended neck veins, gallop heart rhythm, and ankle edema.
	Monitor and record total cumulative dose of drug in patient's medical record; approximate maximum lifetime dose is 500 mg/m^2.
Hematopoietic Toxicity (see Table 8-3)	
Hepatic Toxicity	
Drugs associated with potential for: asparaginase, busulfan, carmustine, chlorambucil, cytarabine, doxorubicin, 5-fluorouricil, lomustine, mercaptopurine, methotrexate, mitoxantrone, mithramycin, mitomycin, paclitaxel, and streptozocin	Monitor liver function studies, such as lactic dehydrogenase, bilirubin, prothrombin time, and liver function tests (SGOT, SGPT).
	Report to physician signs of jaundice, tenderness over liver, and urine and stool color changes.

Hypersensitivity Reaction

Drugs associated with potential for: asparaginase, bleomycin, docetaxel, doxorubicin (local erythema), etoposide, paclitaxel, and teniposide

Review patient's allergy history.

Monitor for symptoms of hypersensitivity and anaphylaxis, such as agitation, urticaria, rash, chills, cyanosis, bronchospasm, abdominal cramping, and hypotension; onset may be rapid or delayed; advise patient to report subjective symptoms promptly.

Ensure that proper medical equipment is nearby and in good working condition. Emergency drugs for intervention should be readily available.

When administering a drug with potential for a reaction, give test dose, monitor vital signs, and observe for allergic response.

If allergic response occurs, stop drug administration and notify physician immediately.

Metabolic Alterations

Hypercalcemia

Monitor serum level; observe for anorexia, constipation, nausea, vomiting, polyuria, and mental status change.

Hyperglycemia

Monitor serum and urine levels; observe for symptoms of thirst, hunger, glucosuria, and weight loss.

Hyperkalemia

Monitor serum level: observe for symptoms of confusion, complaints of numbness or tingling, weakness, and cardiac arrhythmias.

Continued

Table 8-4 Major system toxicity or dysfunction and nursing management—cont'd

Toxicity/Dysfunction	Nursing Management
Metabolic Alterations—cont'd	
Hypernatremia	Monitor serum level and weight loss; observe for symptoms of thirst, dry mucous membranes, poor skin turgor, rapid thready pulse, restlessness, lethargy.
Hyperuricemia Potential with treatment of highly proliferative tumors, such as leukemia and lymphoma (e.g., allopurinol)	Monitor serum and urine levels; daily intake and output. Initiate prescribed drug therapy to inhibit the formation of uric acid before administration of chemotherapy drug. Provide vigorous hydration, such as oral and IV fluid intake (2000-3000 ml), beginning 12-24 hr after initiation of chemotherapy. Alkalize urine to pH ≥7.0 by administration of IV $NaHCO_3$ (sodium bicarbonate). Report symptoms of pain, chills, fever, and diminished urinary output.
Hypocalcemia	Monitor serum level; observe for symptoms of muscle cramping, tingling of extremities, depression, and tetany.
Hypomagnesemia	Monitor serum level; observe for symptoms of personality changes, anorexia, nausea, vomiting, lethargy, weakness, and tetany.
Hyponatremia	Monitor serum level; observe for symptoms of rales, shortness of breath, distended neck vein, weight gain, edema of sacrum or lower extremity, increasing mental status changes.

Neurotoxicity

Drugs associated with potential for: ifosfamide, vinblastine, vincristine, high peak plasma levels of etoposide, 5-fluorouracil; high-dose intrathecal administration of cytarabine, carboplatin, cisplatin, and methotrexate

Monitor and report symptoms of weakness, numbness, and tingling sensation of hands, arms, and feet; also monitor and report symptoms of hoarseness, jaw pain, hallucinations, mental depression, and/or decreased or absent deep tendon reflexes, slapping gait or foot drop, severe constipation, and paralytic ileus.

Ototoxicity

Drug associated with potential for: cisplatin

Verify baseline audiogram.

Monitor and report symptoms of tinnitus, hearing loss, and vertigo.

Pulmonary Toxicity

Drugs associated with potential for: bleomycin, busulfan, and carmustine

Verify baseline respiratory function.

Individuals older than age 70 years have increased risk.

Monitor respiratory status and report symptoms of dyspnea, dry cough, rales, tachypnea, and fever.

Renal System Toxicity

Drugs associated with potential for: carmustine, cisplatin, cyclophosphamide, ifosfamide, methotrexate, mitomycin-C, streptozocin, and thiotepa

Assess 24-hr urine creatinine clearance before treatment, 2-3 L for 24 hr before and after therapy.

Verify baseline renal function.

Encourage adequate fluid intake, such as 2-3 L for 24 hr before and after therapy.

Monitor intake and output and weight changes.

Report diminished output to physician (e.g., <500 ml in 24 hr).

Administer drug mesna concomitant with ifosfamide, high-dose cyclophosphamide, and thiotepa.

Continued

Table 8-4   Major system toxicity or dysfunction and nursing management—cont'd

Toxicity/Dysfunction	Nursing Management
Reproductive System Dysfunction	Assess for nature and frequency of sexual dysfunction.
Drugs associated with potential for: busulfan, chlorambucil, cyclophosphamide, mechlorethamine, melphalan, nitrogen mustard, thiotepa, vinblastine, and vincristine	Counsel patients regarding avoidance of pregnancy and sperm banking before chemotherapy administration; provide information on contraceptives.
Antihormonal agents: finasteride, flutamide, leuprolide, tamoxifen, goserelin, and goserelin	Birth control practices are recommended by most practitioners for 2 yr after chemotherapy to provide for evaluation of disease response, avoidance of possible teratogenic drug effects, and in male patients, recovery of spermatogenesis.
	Inform the patients of potential for temporary or permanent infertility and loss of libido.
	Women may experience symptoms including amenorrhea, "hot flashes," insomnia, dyspareunia, and vaginal dryness; estrogen therapy may be helpful in management of these symptoms.

Chemotherapeutic Toxicities

Chemotherapeutic drugs have the potential for causing adverse side effects and major system toxicity and dysfunction in the patients receiving these agents. Each side effect or toxic effect varies in severity according to the patient's individual response to the drug therapy. Nursing responsibilities include evaluating individual patient response to the drugs, teaching the patient or caregiver management interventions, and monitoring various laboratory data and symptoms observed or reported by the patient.

The information listed in Tables 8-3 and 8-4 may be referred to in developing the plan of care for the patient receiving chemotherapeutic drugs.

Safe Handling of Chemotherapeutic Agents

The number and use of chemotherapeutic agents have increased considerably in recent years. A concern among health care workers has emerged regarding the potential occupational hazard associated with the handling of these drugs. Clinical studies have indicated that many agents are carcinogenic, mutagenic, and/or teratogenic. Exposure to these chemotherapeutic agents can occur from inhalation, absorption, and/or ingestion. Recommended safe handling practice guidelines should be referred to when establishing policies and procedures within each agency that prepares, administers, stores, or disposes of supplies for unused chemotherapeutic agents.*

Safe handling practice guidelines include the following:

- Drug preparation
- Drug administration
- Disposal of supplies and unused drugs
- Management of chemotherapy spill
- Caring for patients receiving chemotherapy, such as handling of linen contamination or patient excreta
- Staff education
- Employment practice regarding reproductive issues

---

*Recommendations for safe handling of chemotherapeutic drugs are available from OSHA, National Cytotoxic Study Commission, and American Society of Hospital Pharmacists.

Drug Preparation

To ensure safe handling, all chemotherapeutic drugs should be prepared according to the package insert in a class II biologic safety cabinet (BSC). Venting to the outside is preferable where feasible. Personal protective equipment includes disposable surgical latex or latex-free gloves and a gown made of lint-free, low-permeability fabric with a closed front, long sleeves, and elastic or knit cuffs. Eye-protective splash goggles or a face shield should be worn when preparing drugs if not using a BSC.

Suggestions to minimize exposure include the following:

- Wash hands before and after drug handling.
- Limit access to the drug preparation area.
- Keep a labeled drug spill kit near preparation area.
- Apply gloves before drug handling.
- Prepare drugs using aseptic technique.
- Avoid eating, drinking, chewing gum, applying cosmetics, or storing food in or near the drug preparation area.
- Place an absorbent pad on the work surface.
- Use Luer-Lok equipment.
- Open drug vials or ampules away from the body.
- Vent vials with a hydrophobic filter needle or pin to prevent spray of the drug.
- Wrap an alcohol wipe around the neck of the ampule before opening it.
- Prime tubing containing drugs inside BSC in sealable bag.
- Cover the tip of the needle with an alcohol wipe when expelling air from the syringe.
- Label all chemotherapeutic drugs with a chemotherapy hazard label.
- Clean up any spills immediately.
- Transport drugs to the delivery area in a leak-proof container.

 CLINICAL ALERT: A variety of surgical latex, powdered latex, and/or latex-free gloves are available from many product supply companies. Change gloves between drug preparation and administration and at least every 30 minutes during drug preparation or administration to ensure maximum protection.

Drug Administration

1. Wear protective equipment (gloves, gown, and eye-wear) as mentioned in "Drug Preparation" above.

2. Inform the patient that chemotherapeutic drugs are harmful to normal cells and that protective measures used by personnel minimize their exposure to these drugs throughout their workday.
3. Administer drugs in a safe and unhurried environment.
4. Place a plastic-backed absorbent pad under the tubing during administration of the drug to catch any drug or solution spillage.
5. Do not dispose of any supplies or unused drugs in patient care areas. (See "Disposal of Supplies and Unused Drugs" below.)
6. Avoid hand-to-eye or hand-to-mouth contact when handling chemotherapeutic drugs.

CLINICAL ALERT: Drugs such as docetaxel, paclitaxel, and high-dose etoposide require glass bottles with nonpolyvinyl tubing for accurate and safe drug preparation and administration. These drugs have a cremophor component and/or a pH alteration that causes melting of products (e.g., polyvinyl products such as IV tubings and IV bags).

Disposal of Supplies and Unused Drugs

1. Avoid clipping or recapping needles and breaking syringes.
2. Place all supplies used intact in a closable, leakproof, puncture-proof, appropriately labeled container.
3. Place all unused drugs in containers into a leakproof, puncture-proof, appropriately labeled container; position these containers in every area where drugs are prepared or administered so that waste materials need not be moved from one area to another.
4. Dispose of containers filled with chemotherapeutic supplies and unused drugs in accordance with regulations regarding hazardous wastes, including use of a licensed sanitary landfill or incineration at 1000° C.

Management of Chemotherapy Spills

Chemotherapy spills should be cleaned up immediately by properly protected personnel trained in the appropriate procedures. A spill should be identified with a warning sign so that other persons in the area will not be contaminated. Recommended supplies and procedures to manage a chemotherapy spill on hard surfaces, linens, personnel, or patients include the following.

Supplies

1. Chemotherapy spill kit
   a. Respirator mask for airborne powder spills
   b. Plastic safety glasses or goggles
   c. Heavy-duty rubber gloves
   d. Absorbent pads to contain liquid spills
   e. Absorbent towels for cleanup after spill
   f. Small scoop to collect glass fragments
   g. Two large waste disposal bags
2. Protective disposable gown (See "Drug Preparation" on page 266.)
3. Containers of detergent solution and clear tap water for postspill cleanup
4. Approved chemotherapy waste disposal closeable lid, puncture-proof, and leakproof container
5. Approved, specially labeled, impervious laundry bag
6. Eye wash faucet adapters or fountain available in or near work area

Procedure for a Spill on a Hard Surface

1. Restrict the area of the spill.
2. Obtain a drug spill kit.
3. Put on protective gown, gloves, and goggles (respirator mask if powder spill).
4. Open waste disposal bags (double bag).
5. Place absorbent pads gently on the spill; be careful not to touch the spill.
6. Place saturated absorbent pads into the waste bag.
7. Cleanse the surface with absorbent towels using detergent solution; wipe clean with clean tap water.
8. Place all contaminated materials (e.g., gown, gloves, saturated absorbent pads, and towels) into double-bagged waste disposal bags.
9. Discard the waste bag with contents into an approved waste disposal container.
10. Wash hands thoroughly with soap and water.

Procedure for a Spill on Linen

1. Restrict the area of the spill.
2. Obtain a drug spill kit.

3. Obtain a specially marked, approved laundry bag, and a labeled, impervious bag.
4. Put on protective gown, gloves, and goggles.
5. Remove soiled, contaminated linen from the patient's bedside.
6. Place linen in an approved, specially marked, impervious laundry bag.
7. Contaminated linen should be washed two times in the laundry; laundry personnel should wear surgical latex gloves and gown when handling this material.
8. Clean the contaminated area with absorbent towels and a detergent solution.
9. Place all contaminated supplies used for management of the spill into a waste disposal bag and discard it in an approved waste disposal container.
10. Wash hands thoroughly with soap and water.

Procedure for a Spill on Personnel or a Patient

1. Restrict the area of spill.
2. Obtain a drug spill kit.
3. Immediately remove the contaminated protective garments or linen.
4. Wash the affected skin area with soap and water.
5. For eye exposure, immediately flood the affected eye with water for at least 5 minutes; obtain medical attention promptly.
6. Properly care for contaminated linen. (See "Procedure for a Spill on Linen" on page 268.)
7. Notify the physician if the drug spills on the patient.
8. Follow agency guidelines for employee health interventions and monitoring.

Documentation

1. Document in the patient's medical record management of the drug spill and notification of the patient's physician.
2. Document on the agency's approved forms management of any spill occurring on a hard surface, linen, or personnel.

Caring for Patients Receiving Chemotherapeutic Drugs

Personnel handling blood, vomitus, or excreta from patients who have received chemotherapy during and within the previous 48 hours should wear disposable surgical latex gloves and gowns to be discarded after use. (See "Disposal of Supplies and Unused Drugs" on page 267.) Linen contaminated with chemotherapeutic drugs, blood, vomitus, or excreta from a patient who has received these drugs up to 48 hours before should be placed in a specially marked, impervious laundry bag. (See "Procedure for a Spill on Linen" on page 268.)

Staff Education

All personnel involved in any aspect of the handling of chemo-therapeutic agents should receive an orientation to chemotherapy drugs, including their known risks, relevant techniques and procedures for handling, proper use of protective equipment and materials, spill procedures, and medical policies; this personnel category includes those who are pregnant or actively trying to conceive children (per OSHA requirements). Evaluation of staff compliance may be achieved by quality monitoring on a regular basis. When possible, a peer-review system should be used. Peer pressure often induces improved compliance.

Employment Practices Regarding Reproductive Issues

The handling of chemotherapeutic agents by women who are either pregnant or actively trying to conceive and by those who are breast-feeding remains a sensitive issue. Suggestions have been made to offer these personnel the opportunity to transfer to areas that do not involve chemotherapeutic agents. All safe handling guidelines should be practiced with utmost care by all pregnant personnel. Refer to the OSHA guidelines (chemotherapy bibliography) for detailed information on the topic or to obtain copy of the document.

Extravasation Management
Definition

Extravasation is the accidental infiltration of vesicant or irritant chemotherapeutic drugs from the vein into surrounding tissues at the IV site. A *vesicant* is an agent that can produce a blister, tissue destruction, or both. An *irritant* is an agent capable of producing venous pain at the site of and along the vein with or without an inflammatory reaction. Injuries that may occur as the result of extravasation include sloughing of tissue, infection, pain, and loss of mobility of an extremity. The degree of tissue damage is related

Table 8-5   Chemotherapeutic drugs, nonvesicants

Generic Name	Trade Name
Asparaginase	Elspar
Bleomycin	Blenoxane
Busulfan	Bulsufex
Carboplatin	Paraplatin
Cisplatin	Platinol
Cladribine	Leustatin (2-CdA)
Cyclophosphamide	Cytoxan
Cytarabine (ara-C)	Cytosar-U
Docetaxel	Taxotere
Floxuridine	FUDR
Fludarabine	Fludara
Fluorouracil	Efudex
Gemcitabine	Gemzar
Irinotecan	Camptosar
Methotrexate	Methotrexate
Mitoxantrone	Novantrone
Pentostatin	Deoxycoformycin
Thioplex	Thiotepa
Topotecan	Hycamtin

to several factors such as drug concentration, the quantity of drug extravasated, individual tissue responses, and anatomic location (e.g., dorsum of hand, wrist, or antecubital fossa). (See Tables 8-5 to 8-7 for lists of nonvesicant drugs and drugs with irritant and vesicant potential.) An additional factor that influences the potential injury from extravasation is what action or intervention was implemented to minimize harm (e.g., type and volume of drug infiltrated and immediate intervention by the nurse, following a protocol directed by the physician prescribing the chemotherapy drug).

Clinical Studies

Because of the harmful effect of vesicants on tissues, studies using patients as subjects are ethically and morally prohibitive. As a result, controlled clinical trials demonstrating effectiveness of treatment have been difficult to attain. Most extravasation interventions have been based on preclinical studies using animal model systems, including mice, pigs, rabbits, and dogs. Treatment

Table 8-6   Chemotherapeutic drugs with irritant potential

Generic Name	Trade Name
Carmustine (BCNU)	BiCNU
Dacarbazine	DTIC-Dome
Etoposide (VP-16)	VePesid
Ifosfamide	Ifex
Mitoguazone	Methyl-GAG, MGBG
Streptozocin	Zanosar
Teniposide (VM-26)	Vumon VM-26

Table 8-7   Chemotherapeutic drugs with vesicant potential

Generic Name	Trade Name
Dactinomycin	Actinomycin D, Cosmegen
Daunorubicin	Cerubidine, Daunomycin
Doxorubicin	Adriamycin
Epirubicin HCl	Ellence (Pharmorubicin)
Esorubicin	4-Deoxydrorubicin
Idarubicin	Idamycin
Mechlorethamine (Nitrogen mustard)	Mustargen
Mitomycin-C	Mutamycin
Menogaril	Tomasar
Paclitaxel	Taxol
Piroxantrone	Oxantrazole
Plicamycin	Mithracin
Vinblastine	Velban
Vincristine	Oncovin
Vindesine	Eldisine
Vinorelbine	Navelbine

strategies for extravasation management include the use of specific antidotes based on their mechanism of action and guidelines for immediate intervention to minimize the tissue damage. Prevention of extravasation and prompt intervention are the key elements for successful extravasation management.

Controversial Issues*

The management of extravasation of chemotherapeutic drugs involves some controversial issues. These issues include the following.

Use of Antecubital Fossa for Drug Administration

1. Favoring antecubital fossa access
   a. Larger veins permit more rapid infusion of drug.
   b. Larger veins permit potentially irritating drugs to reach the general circulation sooner, with less irritation.
2. Opposing antecubital fossa access
   a. Arm mobility is restricted.
   b. Infiltration could cause extensive reconstructive efforts.
   c. Early infiltration may be difficult to assess.
   d. There is a potential for venous fibrosis; blood drawing from antecubital fossa may be more difficult.

Methods of drug sequencing

1. Favoring the administration of vesicants first
   a. Vascular integrity decreases over time.
   b. Initial assessment of vein patency is most accurate.
   c. There is a potential for diminishing patient awareness of symptoms related to drug infiltration.
2. Favoring the administration of vesicants last
   a. Vesicants are irritating and may increase vein fragility.
   b. Venous spasm may occur at onset of drug administration and alter assessment of venous access.

Needle or Catheter Size

1. Favoring the use of larger gauge, such as 18 or 19 gauge
   a. Potentially irritating chemotherapeutic agents can reach circulation sooner, with less irritating effect on the peripheral veins (see Table 8-6).
2. Favoring the use of smaller gauge, such as 20 or 23 gauge
   a. Smaller-gauge devices are less likely to puncture the wall of a small vein.

---

*Adapted from Oncology Nursing Society Task Force: *Cancer chemotherapy guidelines and recommendations for nursing education and practice, 1999 guidelines,* Pittsburgh, 1999, The Society.

b. Increased blood flow around a smaller-gauge device increases dilution of chemotherapeutic agents.

c. Phlebitis may be minimized with a smaller-gauge device.

Prevention of Extravasation

Nursing staff responsibilities for the prevention of extravasation include the following:

- Knowledge of drugs with vesicant potential (see Table 8-7)
- Skill in drug administration
- Identification of risk factors, such as multiple vein punctures or previous treatment
- Anticipation of extravasation and knowledge of approved management protocol
- Establishment of a new venipuncture site daily if peripheral access is used
- Consideration of central venous access for difficult peripheral access
- Administration of drug in a quiet, unhurried environment
- Testing of vein patency without using chemotherapeutic agents
- Adequate drug dilution, such as side port infusion via free-flowing IV infusion
- Careful observation (visualization of access site and extremity) throughout the procedure
- Validation of blood return from IV site before, during, and after vesicant drug infusion
- Education of patients regarding symptoms of drug infiltration, such as pain, burning, and stinging sensations at the IV site

Protocol for Extravasation Management (Peripheral Site)

Agency policy and procedure guidelines for management of extravasation with the responsible physician's prescription should be easily accessible to the staff. The approved antidote should be readily available, and the following procedure should be initiated with a physician's prescription as soon as extravasation of a vesicant or irritant agent is suspected or occurs.

1. Stop the administration of the chemotherapeutic drug.
2. Leave the needle or catheter in place.
3. Aspirate any residual drug and blood in the IV tubing, needle or catheter, and suspected infiltration site.
4. Instill the IV antidote (Table 8-8).

Table 8-8   Chemotherapeutic vesicant drugs with recommended antidotes

Drug	Antidote
Alkylating Agent Mechlorethamine (Mustargen, nitrogen mustard)	Isotonic Sodium thiosulfate ⅙ M (4.4 g/10 ml) Dilute 1.6 ml of sodium thiosulfate 25% with 8.4 ml sterile water for injection; apply cold compresses
Antibiotics Daunorubicin (daunomycin, Cerubidine), doxorubicin (Adriamycin), mitomycin-C (Mutamycin)	Apply *ice cold* compresses immediately for 30-60 min Alternative protocol: topical dimethyl sulfoxide (DMSO) 1-2 ml of 1 mM DMSO 50%-100%; apply topically one time at the site; apply *cold* compresses
Vinca Alkaloids Teniposide, vinblastine, vincristine, vindesine, vinorelbine	Apply warm compresses; *do not* inject corticosteroids

The following drugs have no known specific antidotes: dactinomycin, epirubicin, esorubicin, idarubicin, menogaril, mitoxantrone, paclitaxel piroxantrone

5. Remove the needle.
6. If unable to aspirate the residual drug from the IV tubing, remove the needle or catheter.
7. Inject the antidote subcutaneously clockwise into the infiltrated site using a 25-gauge needle; change the needle with each new injection.
8. Avoid applying pressure to the suspected infiltration site.
9. Photograph the suspected area of extravasation according to the agency's policy and procedure for documentation and follow-up.
10. Apply topical ointment if ordered.
11. Cover lightly with an occlusive sterile dressing.
12. Apply cold or warm compresses as indicated (see Table 8-8).
13. Elevate the extremity.
14. Observe regularly for pain, erythema, induration, and necrosis.
15. Document the following elements of extravasation management:
    a. Date
    b. Time
    c. Needle or catheter size and type
    d. Insertion site, location, and description
    e. Number and location of previous venipuncture attempts; any difficulty in venipuncture or venous access device
    f. Drug sequence
    g. Approximate amount of drug extravasated
    h. Nursing management of extravasation
    i. Photo documentation
    j. Patient complaints and statements
    k. Appearance of site
    l. Physician notification and/or additional physician consultation
    m. Follow-up interventions
    n. Nurse's signature

CLINICAL ALERT: The process of tissue destruction resulting from drug extravasation may be subtle and progressive. Initial symptoms may include pain or burning at IV site, progressing to erythema, edema, and superficial skin loss. Tissue necrosis may not develop until 1 to 4 weeks after the drug extravasation.

Anaphylaxis

Nursing personnel administering chemotherapy should be alert and prepared for the possible complications of anaphylaxis. The drugs and supplies necessary to manage these complications must be readily available. Emergency medications and supplies for management of anaphylaxis include the following:

- Injectable aminophylline, diphenhydramine hydrochloride (Benadryl), dopamine, epinephrine, heparin, hydrocortisone (Solu-Cortef), methylprednisolone (Solu-Medrol)
- Oxygen setup, tubing cannula or mask, and airway device
- IV fluids (isotonic solutions)
- IV tubings and supplies for venous access

All or some of these symptoms may be present: anxiety, hypotension, tachycardia, urticaria, cyanosis, respiratory distress, wheezing, abdominal cramping, flushed appearance, facial edema, tightness in chest, and/or chills. The calm and reassuring presence of the nurse will facilitate in the management of these symptoms. Management proceeds as follows.

1. Immediately stop the drug infusion.
2. Maintain an IV line with isotonic saline.
3. Position the patient for comfort and to promote perfusion of the vital organs.
4. Notify the physician, nursing agency, and emergency medical services.
5. Maintain the airway and anticipate the need for cardiopulmonary resuscitation.
6. Monitor the vital signs according to agency policy.
7. Administer the appropriate medications with the approved physician's order.
8. Follow the nursing agency's protocol for follow-up care (e.g., evaluation of the patient by the physician).
9. Document the incident in the patient's medical record.

CLINICAL ALERT: *Always* review the patient's allergy history before chemotherapy drug administration. Administer premedications (e.g., corticosteroids, antihistamines, or antipyretics) as ordered. Ensure the emergency equipment and medications are readily available. Follow guidelines for drug *test-dose procedures*. Prompt and effective nursing interventions for anaphylaxis decrease complications. The nurse must be alert to the signs and symptoms of an anaphylactic response and provide an immediate intervention for a chemotherapeutic drug hypersensitivity or anaphylaxis event.

Table 8-9 lists potentials of chemotherapy drugs for anaphylaxis.

Documentation Recommendations

- Site assessment before and after infusion or injection of chemotherapeutic drug
- Establishment of blood return before, during, and after IV and intraarterial infusion of chemotherapy
- Needle or catheter size and type
- Establishment of catheter or device patency before, during, and after infusion of chemotherapy—for example, intraperitoneal or intrathecal
- Drug sequence and administration technique
- Patient/family education regarding chemotherapy protocol— potential side effects and toxicities, self-management of side effects, and schedule of follow-up blood counts, tests, and procedures
- Chemotherapeutic drug, dose, route, time, and date
- Premedications, test-dose procedure drugs, or postmedications, flushing solutions, other infusions, and supplies used for chemotherapy drug regimen
- Any patient complaints of discomfort and symptoms experienced before, during, and after chemotherapeutic infusion

Nursing Diagnoses

- Knowledge deficit, related to chemotherapeutic side effects
- Oral mucous membrane, altered, related to side effects of drugs
- Injury, risk for, related to alteration in immune system
- Injury, risk for, related to alteration in clotting factors
- Sexual dysfunction, related to effects of chemotherapeutic drugs (alkylating agents)
- Nutrition, altered: less than body requirements, related to nausea and vomiting

Patient/Family Teaching for Self-Management

- Assess the patient's ability and willingness to learn, availability of caregiver, environment at home, ability to assume self-care, and compliance with treatment regimen.

Table 8-9   Potential for anaphylaxis of chemotherapy drugs

Drugs	Signs and Symptoms	Nursing Interventions
Asparaginase (Elspar)	Respiratory distress, increased pulse, respirations, hypotension, facial edema, anxiety, flushed appearance, hives, itching; risk for anaphylaxis increases with each dose	Test dose before initial IV/IM dosing; monitor 30 min IM or 60 min after drug administration; keep vein open with IV normal saline (NS) before, during and 30/60 min after IV administration of asparaginase. Initiate drug infusion slowly (mg/m^2/titrate infusion). Crash cart, O$_2$, suction, drugs for anaphylaxis at or near patient's bedside.

Test-Dose Procedure
Prepare 10,000 IU asparaginase with 5 ml N/S; inject 0.1 ml of this solution (200 IU) into 9.9 ml NS; inject intradermally 0.1 ml of this concentration (2 IU) to make a wheal in inner aspect of arm; observe wheal for 60 min for erythema, swelling, itching before doing infusion.

Continued

Table 8-9 Potential for anaphylaxis of chemotherapy drugs—cont'd

Drugs	Signs and Symptoms	Nursing Interventions
Bleomycin	Dyspnea, hypotension, rash increased pulse, and respiration	Test dose before initial IV dosing. Initiate drug infusion slowly (10-20 ml/15 min). Monitor vital signs and auscultate breath sounds q4h during and for 24 hr postinfusion and/or on scheduled basis in outpatient setting.
Test-Dose Procedure Inject 2 units of bleomycin intradermal to make a wheal in inner aspect of arm; observe for erythema or edema itching before first 2 doses of bleomycin infusion		
Etoposide (VP-16)	Hypotension, bronchospasm, chest pain, increased pulse, respirations, facial flush, fever, chills, diaphoresis	Initiate drug infusion slowly (10-20 ml/15 min). Infuse total volume over at least 60 min. Monitor vital signs q15min × 4, q30min × 2, and q4h, during and 24 hr after infusion.

| Teniposide (VM-26) | Severe hypotension, anxiety, increased pulse, respirations, fever | Initiate drug infusion slowly (10-20 ml/30 min) for total infusion time of 60-120 min.
Monitor vital signs q15min × 4 and q30min × 2, during and after infusion; then monitor q4h × 24 hr. |
| Paclitaxel (Taxol) (Fig. 8-6), docetaxel (Taxotere) | Increased or decreased blood pressure; increased temperature and pulse; restlessness, dyspnea, bronchospasm, facial flushing, hives
If any of these symptoms occur, stop the drug infusion and notify the physician immediately. | Premedicate with the following before Taxol or Taxotere infusion: dexamethasone 10-20 mg PO/IV 12 and 6 hr; diphenhydramine 50 mg IV push 30-60 min; cimetidine 300 mg IV over 30 min; infuse Taxol/Taxotere in a glass bottle immediately with non-PVC tubing and a 0.22-μ filter.
Obtain baseline vital signs; then monitor q15min × 4, qh × 4, q4h × 4 during the infusion. Ensure emergency medications: Benadryl 50 mg; hydrocortisone 100 mg; adrenalin (epinephrine) 1:1000—all IV bolus; oxygen and suction, equipment assembled and ready for use. |

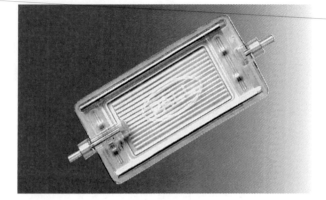

Fig. 8-6
Posidyne ELD Intravenous Filter Set. Air-eliminating filter set with 96-hour bacteria and endotoxin retention.
(Courtesy PALL Medical, Ann Arbor, Mich.)

- Describe purpose, schedule, and procedure of chemotherapeutic regimen.
- Explain to the patient the potential side effects from chemotherapeutic drugs (nausea and vomiting, anorexia, stomatitis, constipation, diarrhea, alopecia, and skin and hemopoietic changes).
- Instruct the patient or the caregiver on self-management interventions specific to each of the side effects.
- Review symptoms such as temperature elevation over 38° C, severe constipation or diarrhea, persistent bleeding from any site, sudden weight gain or loss, shortness of breath, pain not relieved by prescribed medications, and severe nausea and vomiting more than 24 hours after treatment, and reporting of these symptoms promptly to the physician.
- Instruct the patient or the caregiver regarding management of infusion devices for a patient receiving chemotherapy in the home.
- Validate the aseptic technique and skills of the patient or the caregiver for prescribed self-administration and discontinuation of chemotherapeutic drugs.
- Explain safe handling precautions for administration and disposal of chemotherapy drugs and supplies.

- Provide information and a list of resources for obtaining, storing, and disposing of drugs and supplies, and schedule of follow-up tests and care.
- Discuss requirements for scheduled physician and diagnostic appointments.
- Provide patient teaching materials from the National Cancer Institute and American Cancer Society (titles such as *Chemotherapy and You, What Are Clinical Trials All About?*, and *When Someone in Your Family Has Cancer*).
- Consider culture-sensitive materials and interventions.

Guidelines for Home Care
Chemotherapy Administration

- Store drugs in a safe recommended environment, such as refrigeration, away from sunlight.
- Follow procedures for preparation and administration of chemotherapy as in agency or hospital.
- Record the drug, dose, route, and time given in the home and provide this information to the agency responsible for care management.
- Discard all unused drugs and used supplies into a recommended closable, punctureproof, leakproof container, and return this container to the appropriate agency for disposal.
- Provide prompt linen and clothing change with meticulous skin care for the patient with incontinence.
- Use plastic sheeting to protect the bedding or furniture if incontinence is possible.
- Carefully handle linen contaminated from chemotherapeutic drugs and excreta, and wash two times separately from all other linen.
- The patient should receive the first dose of the drug(s) in an acute care setting or in an outpatient setting.

Geriatric Considerations

- The potential for increased toxic effects of drugs exists, as do related compromised cardiac, respiratory, and renal systems; compromised endocrine and liver functions; and neuromuscular deficits.
- Anticipate potential sedative effects related to antiemetic therapy and analgesics.

- Monitor serum electrolyte values closely: The potential exists for alterations related to concomitant diseases such as arthritis, diabetes, and hypertension.
- Query the patient or caregiver about other current medications (prescribed and over-the-counter) that may interfere with or increase toxic effects of the chemotherapy drugs.
- Age-related neuromuscular sensory deficits may include but are not limited to visual, hearing, fine motor skills, and mobility status deficits and changes to patterns of bowel and bladder elimination. Assess the potential for changes and deficits and plan for appropriate intervention.
- Follow these basic guidelines:

    Introduce yourself and face the patient while speaking.

    Provide simple, step-by-step instructions for tasks.

    Include the caregiver in the instructions.

    Monitor bowel and bladder function; for example, increased fluid intake may require limits because of bladder toxicity.

    Provide for rest or naps; reduce mental activity late in the day.

    Assess and monitor skin integrity; for example, plan and provide body position changes on a scheduled frequency for the activity-compromised patient.

- Consult with community resources for patient health mainte-nance management. For example, consult social services (finan-cial, housing, and companion care), home health care agencies (physical care), Meals on Wheels programs (nutrition), and senior citizen programs (recreation and socialization).
- Consider and plan developmental age-related interventions for sexuality issues such as dry vaginal mucous membrane and impotence related to side effects of chemotherapy drugs.

Resources

Clinical Competency—Chemotherapy Administration

	Yes	No	NA
1. Verifies allergy and laboratory data; verifies informed consent if investigational protocol before administration of chemotherapy.			
2. Verifies physician's written order for specific dosage, route, and mode of administration.			
3. Calculates drug dosage based on patient's height and weight; verifies information with a second nurse.			
4. Uses protective coverings and follows precautions in drug preparation and handling.			
5. Maintains aseptic technique during preparation and administration.			
6. Reconstitutes drugs under sterile conditions according to the package insert.			
7. Discards unused portion of drug in proper container.			
8. Follows safe handling guidelines in the event of drug spillage.			
9. Follows safe handling in the event of drug spray or contact with skin or mucous membranes.			
10. Correctly labels drug with patient's name, drug: name, dose, concentration/volume, route and rate of administration, date and time prepared; note if vesicant.			
11. Verifies drug dosage a second time, at the patient's bedside.			
12. Correctly states immediate and delayed side effects of the drugs.			
13. Verifies patient identification.			

Continued

Clinical Competency—Chemotherapy Administration—cont'd

	Yes	No	NA
14. Introduces self to patient.			
15. Follows prescribed premedication(s) administration.			
16. Explains procedure and drug side effects to patient/family/caregiver and answers questions appropriately.			
17. Assesses patient's response to previous therapy.			
18. Instructs patient/family/caregiver to report any adverse reactions immediately.			
19. Assembles equipment before validating venous access.			
20. Washes hands.			
21. Selects appropriate supplies for venous access.			
22. Prepares venous access site and device (subclavian catheter; tunneled catheter; implantable port; peripherally inserted central catheter).			
23. Validates blood return check from above mentioned venous access devices.			
24. Flushes venous access device with >5 ml normal saline.			
25. Securely connects chemotherapy infusion bag tubing/chemotherapy drug syringe.			
26. Reconfirms vein patency periodically by validating blood return status.			
27. Flushes tubing upon completion of one drug before administering another drug.			
28. Infuses drugs at the appropriate rate to minimize untoward sensations/complications.			

Clinical Competency—Chemotherapy Administration—cont'd

	Yes	No	NA
29. Follows extravasation protocol should infiltration of a drug occur.			
30. Observes for allergic or hypersensitivity reactions to the drugs; follows anaphylaxis or hypersensitivity protocol.			
31. Flushes IV tubing with a sufficient amount of saline to clear the line before removing the chemotherapy drug/infusion.			
32. Instructs the patient on posttreatment care and precautions.			
33. Disposes of all used supplies and/or drugs in proper container according to agency guidelines.			
34. Documents procedure in the medical record according to agency guidelines.			

Study Questions

1. Chemotherapy drugs that have potential for cardiac toxicity include:
   a. Dactinomycin, daunorubicin, doxorubicin, deoxycoformycin
   b. Dactinomycin, daunorubicin, docetaxel, dexamethasone
   c. Chlorambucil, cyclophosphamide, daunorubicin, doxorubicin
   d. Carmustine, cisplatin, dactinomycin, daunorubicin

2. Chemotherapy vesicant drugs with extravasation potential include:
   a. Antitumor antibiotics, alkylating agents, antiestrogens
   b. Antitumor antibiotics, alkylating agents, vinca alkaloids
   c. Antitumor antibiotics, antimetabolites, vinca alkaloids
   d. Antitumor antibiotics, alkylating agents, antihormonal agents

3. Clinical features that may occur during a hypersensitivity or anaphylaxis event include:
   a. Anxiety, cyanosis, dyspnea, urticaria
   b. Anxiety, chills, fever, hives
   c. Anxiety, facial edema, hoarseness, weakness
   d. Cyanosis, dyspnea, hives, vertigo

4. Chemotherapy drugs that cause neurotoxicity symptoms, such as numbness, jaw pain, absent deep tendon reflexes, and/or severe constipation include:
   a. Alkeran, busulfan, cisplatin, dactinomycin
   b. Bleomycin, carboplatin, cytarabine, doxorubicin
   c. Cisplatin, dactinomycin, etoposide, fludarabine
   d. Etoposide, ifosfamide, vinblastine, vincristine

5. Factors considered in chemotherapy drug selection for cancer treatment include:
   a. Patient's age, diagnosis, pain status, tumor burden
   b. Cancer cell type, bone marrow status, tumor burden, tumor resistance
   c. Rate of drug absorption, nausea potential, renal status, tumor burden
   d. Cardiac, hepatic, renal, sexuality status

6. Interventions for nausea and vomiting associated with chemotherapy drugs include:
   a. Offering antiemetics at least every 12 hours, avoiding greasy or cold foods, eating large meals
   b. Offering antiemetics at least every 24 hours, avoiding fatty foods, eating small meals and dry toast
   c. Offering antiemetics before chemotherapy, avoiding greasy or fatty foods, eating small meals
   d. Offering antiemetics after chemotherapy, eating cold or salty foods, dry crackers, or toast

7. Nursing interventions for chemotherapy drug extravasation include:
   a. Knowing drugs with vesicant potential, testing the vein with normal saline, carefully observing drug administration, validating blood return before, during, and after
   b. Knowing drugs with irritant potential, testing the vein with distilled water, carefully observing drug administration, validating blood return before, during, and after

    c. Knowing drugs with nonvesicant potential, testing the vein with normal saline, carefully observing drug administration, validating blood return before and after

    d. Knowing drugs with vesicant potential, testing the vein with normal saline, carefully observing drug administration, validating blood return during and after

8. The following treatments that are considered major treatment modalities for cancer include:
    a. Antiemetic therapy, biotherapy, bone marrow transplantation, chemotherapy
    b. Bone marrow transplantation, chemotherapy, surgery, pain management
    c. Chemotherapy, radiation therapy, surgery, therapeutic touch
    d. Biotherapy, chemotherapy, radiation therapy, surgery

9. Recommendations for safe handling of chemotherapy drugs include:
    a. Wear protective covering during preparation, administration, and disposal; dispose of used products in trash container; use chemotherapy spill kit for drug spill
    b. Wear protective covering during preparation, administration, and disposal; dispose of used products in chemotherapy disposal box; use chemotherapy spill kit for drug spill
    c. Wear protective covering during administration and disposal; dispose of used products in chemotherapy disposal box; use chemotherapy spill kit for drug spill
    d. Wear protective clothing during preparation and disposal; dispose of used products in chemotherapy disposal box; use chemotherapy spill kit for drug spill

10. Critical elements of chemotherapy documentation include:
    a. Drug dose, route, site assessment, pharmacy preparation of drug
    b. Drug dose, route, IV access, pharmacy preparation of drug
    c. Drug dose, route, IV access, blood return status
    d. Drug dose, route, IV access, safe handling preparation

Answers   1. c   2. b   3. a   4. d   5. b   6. c
7. a   8. d   9. b   10. c

Parenteral Nutrition

9

Objectives

1. Describe the indications and contraindications of total parenteral nutrition (TPN).

2. Discuss the components of a nutritional assessment.

3. Describe the nurse's role in providing TPN for the critically ill patient or patient with acute or chronic disease.

4. Recognize the common diagnostic laboratory values used to monitor TPN.

5. Identify the potential complications of TPN.

Providing nutritional and metabolic support via a central intravenous (IV) route is termed *parenteral nutrition* or *total parenteral nutrition* (TPN). The term *TPN* is used throughout this chapter when referring to nutritional support via central venous access. The decision to use the IV route for nutritional support is made when the gastrointestinal (GI) tract cannot be used. Common disease- or treatment-related conditions that require TPN include bowel obstruction, peritonitis, intractable vomiting, acute pancreatitis, short bowel syndrome, and ileus.

Components of TPN

The components of TPN are dextrose, amino acids, fats or lipids, fluids and electrolytes, vitamins, and trace elements. Medications may be added if they are compatible with the solution (e.g., heparin, insulin, and/or histamine antagonists [H_2 blockers]) (Fig. 9-1). TPN

```
                  Department of Pharmacy
                                           7019-01
11/19/99    Location:7 SW        Volume:2000ml  IV#:    8
                  ADULT TPN ORDERS
Aminosyn II 10% 1000.000  ML     K Acetate ......  20.000  mEq
Dextrose 70% ...  160.000  ML     Ca Gluconate    9.000  mEq
Liposyn III 20% .  250.000  ml    MgSO4 ..........  10.000  mEq
Na Chloride ......   70.000 mEq   M.V.I. Conc ....  10.000    ml
Na Phosphate ...   20.000  mM    M.T.E.-4 ........    1.000    ml
KCl ....................   50.000 mEq   Selenium ....... 100.000  mcg
```

(barcode)

```
Flow rate:  83.0 ml/hr   (24.0 hours) Cont.    serial #011274
Date due: 11/19/99   at 18:00              Entered by: DLN
Mixed by:      Checked by:      Discard after:        11/21/99

Patient wt.  =  0.000 kg      Soln Osmolarity  =  930 mOsm/L
                  This unit contains:
CHO kcal Fat kcal   Total kcal  Gm pro.  Gm N    kcal/ml
  380.0    500.0      1280.8      100.0    15.3     0.640
        In 24 hours this therapy delivers 1992 ml and:
   Total kcal/day    kcal/kg/day    Gm Pro/day   kcal/gm N
      1275.7            0.0            99.6          83.7
```

Fig. 9-1

Label for bag of total parenteral nutrition solution.
(Courtesy Via Christi Regional Medical Center, Wichita, Kans.)

provides dextrose and fat for energy, whereas amino acids meet the protein needs. Fats and lipids provide a source of caloric intake and are essential for enzyme reactions at a cellular level. Fluids, electrolytes, vitamins, trace elements, and medications support cellular and metabolic demands and enhance wound healing.

Peripheral parenteral nutrition (PPN) is a method of giving diluted solutions of protein and calories in a peripheral IV site. PPN is nutritionally incomplete. The amino acid products must be diluted with 2.5%, 5%, or 10% dextrose for use in peripheral veins. Osmolarity of the solution should be less than 600 mOsm/L. The maximum osmolar concentration should not exceed 900 mOsm/L. Prophylaxis to prevent thrombophlebitis may include heparin, hydrocortisone, or topical nonsteroidal antiinflammatory creams and gels. Use of PPN is usually short term, 5 to 14 days, after GI surgery for a patient who was well nourished preoperatively or for a patient with poor intake who refuses an enteral feeding tube. If use of the IV route is projected to be long term, a central venous access should be obtained because of the potential for phlebitis in the peripheral site. Research has not demonstrated improved outcomes using PPN over 5% crystalloid solutions.

Identification of the patient who requires TPN for nutritional support should be an interdisciplinary effort and addressed along the care continuum. This interdisciplinary team includes dietitians, nurses, pharmacists, and physicians. Depending on agency policy, orders for TPN may be written by the clinical dietitian, a member of a nutritional support team following protocols, or the physician. In an acute or critical care setting, laboratory values may be evaluated daily and adjustments made in the components of the TPN solution. In extended care or home care settings, adjustments are made less frequently by the nurse via consultation with the physician.

Indications for TPN

The basic rule of nutrition is when the gut works, use it. Research supports the use of early enteral feeding when oral intake is not possible. The IV route for nutrition is indicated for the following conditions (Guidelines for TPN Administration from the American Association of Parenteral and Enteral Nutrition [ASPEN]):

- Cancer if treatment is expected to cause GI toxicity that will preclude oral intake for more than 7 days
- Preoperatively for 7 to 10 days for severely malnourished patients
- After surgery when the GI tract cannot be used for an extended period of time; TPN may be initiated by the third postoperative day
- Inflammatory bowel disease such as Crohn's disease
- Renal failure secondary to acute tubular necrosis to maintain calorie intake
- Hepatic dysfunction secondary to cirrhosis
- Pancreatitis when abdominal pain, serum amylase level, or pancreatic fistula drainage is increased by enteral feeding
- Critical illness such as burns, trauma, or sepsis in patients whose hypermetabolism is expected to last more than 4 to 5 days and enteral nutrition is not possible
- Acquired immunodeficiency syndrome (AIDS) when other methods of nutritional support have failed

- Short bowel syndrome when oral or enteral nutrients cannot be absorbed because of mesenteric vascular thrombosis, internal herniation with infarction, massive abdominal trauma, multiple bowel resections, malignancy, or radiation enteritis; if less than 60 cm of bowel remains, TPN is administered indefinitely
- Eating disorders with the presence of severe malnutrition (65% of ideal body weight [IBW] or more than 30% recent weight loss)

Clinical research has shown improved outcomes after the administration of TPN for patients with the following conditions: GI cutaneous fistulas, renal failure (acute tubular necrosis), short bowel syndrome, acute burns, hepatic failure (acute decompensation, superimposed on cirrhosis), acute radiation enteritis, acute chemotherapy toxicity, prolonged ileus, and weight loss before major surgery.

General Contraindications for TPN

- Treatment anticipated for less than 5 days in patients without severe malnutrition and a functioning GI tract
- Inability to obtain central venous access placement
- Irreversible terminal illness or a vegetative state with no reasonable hope to return to a cognitive state

Nutritional Assessment

Nutritional assessment is an interdisciplinary process. A nutritional assessment consists of three components: screening for nutrition support, patient nutritional assessment, and nutrition support decisions.

Screening for Nutrition Support

A nutritional assessment begins with the patient's admission to care status that includes a history and physical examination and a comprehensive nursing assessment. The initial part of a nutritional assessment is to identify patients with alterations in nutritional status and those with the potential to develop malnutrition because of inadequate intake. During the assessment process, information is obtained about recent weight loss/gain, previous medical conditions, and medications. The nursing physical examination assesses for signs and symptoms of malnutrition and/or nutrition deficiencies. Agency screening criteria prompt further nutrition assessment and referral to the clinical dietitian.

Components of Screening for Nutritional Status

ASPEN has identified the following criteria as components for screening nutritional status. Verify agency screening criteria that call for nutritional assessment by the clinical dietitian.

- Identification of patients at increased risk for malnutrition through physical examination and a focused nutritional assessment
- Patients with stress or hypermetabolism from trauma, burns, surgery, or sepsis who may develop malnutrition without adequate nutrition intake
- Patients at increased nutritional risk: weight loss of more than 10% of ideal body weight or low body mass index (less than 22)
- Decreased visceral protein as indicated by albumin level of less than 3.5 g/dl
- Identification of well-nourished patients without excessive metabolic stress who may tolerate little or no nutritional intake for up to 7 days

Patient Nutritional Assessment

Assessing a patient's nutritional status is important when deciding whether parenteral nutrition is necessary and also when monitoring therapy. The first component of this assessment is an evaluation of the effect of the patient's underlying medical condition on nutritional status. The following tools and indicators are key nutritional assessment components: subjective global assessment (SGA), degree of weight loss, estimation of lean body mass, anthropometric measurements, degree of catabolism, status of immune response, and serum laboratory values of albumin, prealbumin, or transferrin. Each method currently used to assess the extent of malnutrition experienced by a patient has limitations. Currently, there is no single, best test for evaluating nutritional status because many factors influence an individual's nutritional condition.

Nutritional Status Indicators	Comments
Diet history	Includes 24-hour recall, special diets, food allergies or intolerance, appetite, chewing and swallowing difficulties, changes in food intake, and diarrhea associated with eating.
Height and weight	Compared against standard height and weight tables. Actual body weight is calculated as percentage of ideal weight.
SGA	Tool components include history about weight change, changes in dietary intake, GI symptoms, patient's functional capacity, and disease nutritional requirements. SGA ratings are well nourished, moderately malnourished, or severely malnourished.
Weight loss	Determine the degree of weight loss. Weight loss of 10% or more is an indicator of malnutrition if it occurred within 6 months.
Basal energy expenditure (BEE)	Estimate of energy requirements at rest (Harris-Benedict equation) (see "Resources").
Anthropometric measurements	Measurements of the midarm circumference, skinfold thickness, and arm muscle are compared against standard values as a way of inferring patient body mass. Fluid shifts and changes in hydration status affect measurements.

Creatinine/height index (CHI) — Indicates the status of muscle stores in patients with normal renal function. Creatinine is released from muscle at a constant rate in proportion to muscle mass; the patient's index is compared with standards to determine the degree of depletion: ≥80%—zero to mild depletion; 60%-80%—moderate depletion; <60% severe depletion (see "Resources").

Bioelectrical impedance analysis (BIA) — Analysis technique used to determine body fat stores, based on the principle of higher electrical conductivity in lean tissue and a lower impedance related to water and electrolyte content. This tool does not have widespread clinical use.

Albumin levels — Indirect measures of visceral protein mass; low values are associated with reduced dietary protein or excessive losses. It does not reflect immediate changes—20-day half-life; normal range 3.5-5 g/dl. Not a good indicator in acute or critically ill patients because of dehydration and long half-life. Refer to agency guidelines for albumin level criteria as a screening mechanism for nutrition consultation.

Prealbumin — Short half-life; provides an analysis of protein changes during previous 2 days; 10-40 mg/dl is normal. This is the most commonly used tool for ongoing monitoring.

Serum transferrin — Short half-life; indicates a combination of protein depletion and iron deficiency; 200-400 mg/dl is normal. Transferrin transports iron in plasma and is sensitive to iron levels.

Retinol-binding protein — Highly sensitive to nutritional status. Shows change over 12 hours and is affected by renal insufficiency.

CLINICAL ALERT: The preceding serum proteins are manufactured in the liver. Hepatic insufficiency will affect the values.

Total lymphocyte count (TLC)	Used to identify malnutrition-related immunosuppression. TLC of <1500 mm^3 is an indication of malnutrition.
Delayed hypersensitivity reactivity (DHR)	Skin antigen tests include purified protein derivative (PPD), *Candida,* and dinitrochlorobenzene (DNCB); DHR is not nutritionally specific and is not a useful tool in the hospitalized patient.
CD8 cell counts	Measure cellular and humoral immune function; normal CD4:CD8 ratio is 2.
Nitrogen balance	Determines the degree of catabolism. Nitrogen is an essential element of protein required for tissue building; measured as the total nitrogen excreted in urine, plus a correction factor for unmeasured losses minus the total nitrogen consumed in the form of protein. Positive nitrogen balance exists when nitrogen intake is greater than nitrogen loss. Negative nitrogen balance is found in persons who are inadequately fed relative to protein needs; protein is broken down to meet their metabolic needs, and thus these persons excrete more nitrogen than they take in. Goal is 0 for maintenance or +2 to +4 for repletion (see "Resources").

Nutrition Support Decisions

A consultation by the clinical dietitian is initiated when the nursing assessment and agency triggers indicate malnutrition or the potential exists for malnutrition caused by inadequate nutrition. For example, the nursing assessment would have noted a weight loss or gain, nothing by mouth (NPO) status and decreased oral intake, or a decreased albumin level. Upon referral, the dietitian will expand the assessment using the aforementioned indicators to calculate specific information related to nutritional status. Recommendations for oral, enteral, and IV nutritional are made. If it is determined that the patient's nutritional needs are best met by TPN, calculation of the energy, protein, and calorie needs is necessary.

Determining Nutritional Needs

A member of the health care team will calculate the energy, protein, and calorie needs of the patient. All persons, in health and in illness, require both energy and nutrient sources. Without adequate nonprotein calories, the body uses its own protein from muscles, visceral stores, and the amino acids provided in the parenteral nutrition solution. An objective of parenteral nutrition is to meet energy needs through nonprotein calorie sources so that the infused amino acids can be directed toward protein synthesis. Protein breakdown for energy is a catabolic process. Protein synthesis is an anabolic process.

Nutritional Requirements

Parenteral nutrition solutions contain energy sources in the forms of dextrose and lipids, as well as nitrogen sources in the form of amino acids, vitamins, and trace elements. Research in the area of parenteral nutrition is focusing on the pharmacologic role of individual nutrients. In the future, it is hoped that precise nutrient prescriptions may be used to treat specific diseases. The amounts of the various components of parenteral nutrition vary according to the patient's condition; however, combinations of components tend to be standard. Each of the basic components of parenteral nutrition is discussed in the following sections.

Energy

The source of energy in TPN is the carbohydrates and lipids.

Energy required by the body for metabolic processes, heat production, and physical activity can be provided by carbohydrates, protein, or fat. Energy needs are met in parenteral nutrition through dextrose (carbohydrate) and lipid (fat) administration. The greater the intake of carbohydrates and fat, the less protein needed to achieve nitrogen balance. Even though basal levels of glucose and fat are required for normal body processes, there is not a fixed recommendation for the ratio of glucose to fat that should be provided. The energy expenditure of healthy individuals depends mostly on the basal metabolic rate and the level of physical activity. When a person has an illness, a greater amount of energy is often required because the individual's metabolic rate is increased. For example, prolonged fever increases energy requirement by 7% per Fahrenheit degree and 13% per Centigrade degree. A widely used method for calculating resting energy expenditure is the Harris-Benedict equation (see "Resources"). During illness, caloric (energy) needs vary according to age, sex, height, weight, activity, and the presence of catabolic states such as sepsis, severe injuries, and burns.

Carbohydrates

The carbohydrate source in TPN is glucose (dextrose). When glucose is available, amino acid breakdown is prevented. The action is protein sparing. Glucose is essential at a tissue and cellular level, particularly the brain. The central nervous system (CNS) requires about 150 g of glucose per day. Dextrose is the least expensive source of glucose and is available in concentrations of 5% to 70% dextrose in water. Concentrated dextrose is the primary calorie source in TPN. Glycerol, a naturally occurring sugar alcohol, may be used as an alternative caloric source in TPN. A widely used method for calculating resting energy expenditure is the Harris-Benedict equation (see "Resources," p. 319).

Fat Emulsion

Fat emulsion provides essential fatty acids and is the other major energy source in TPN. Lipid solutions are made from soybean oil and water and emulsified with phospholipids. Fat is the chief storage source of energy in the body. Fat emulsions are available in 10%, 20%, and 30% concentrations. In addition, lipids are a source of essential fatty acids and thus can prevent or correct fatty acid deficiencies. Because use of fatty acids can provide fuel for most tissues, glucose can then be made available for use by the CNS and protein for anabolic processes.

Protein

The goal is to keep the patient in a state of positive nitrogen balance. When a negative nitrogen balance occurs, there is wasting of the patient's tissue protein. Protein is provided in parenteral nutrition in the form of crystalline amino acids, either standard or modified. Optimal amino acid levels have not been established. Standard preparations containing varying amounts of essential and nonessential amino acids are available in concentrations of 3.5% to 15%. Modified amino acid solutions contain amino acids for age-specific or disease-specific requirements. A healthy adult requires 0.82 g/kg of protein, and a stressed, critically ill patient requires 1.5 to 2.0 g/kg body weight. The nitrogen from protein metabolization is excreted principally through urine, so nitrogen loss is measured through urine sampling. Because a small amount of nitrogen is lost through the hair, skin, saliva, and stool, a correction factor for these losses is added to the Harris-Benedict equation (see "Resources"). Research on substrates such as glutamine, arginine, omega-3 fatty acids, and nucleotides have not demonstrated improved outcomes over standard formulas. A marker for determining protein needs is a nitrogen balance study called a *24-hour urine urea nitrogen* (UUN) (see "Resources").

Patients who have renal or liver disease or who are critically ill may require an adjustment in the amount of protein in the TPN. The site of plasma protein synthesis in the body is the liver. If there is hepatic insufficiency or failure, amino acid concentrations in the TPN may need to be adjusted. To achieve a positive nitrogen balance in the presence of impaired renal function, adjustments should be made in the amino acids in TPN.

A patient experiences greater improvement in weight gain and wound healing with the use of IV amino acids than with the use of IV dextrose. Although protein can provide energy, the continued breakdown of protein for energy adversely affects body functioning, growth, and tissue repair. Enough protein must be administered to replace essential amino acids; otherwise, the body will convert its own protein to glucose to meet energy requirements. If body protein is converted to glucose, the patient experiences a persistent loss of protein primarily from muscle tissue, causing a negative nitrogen balance. Because excess protein is metabolized and not stored in the body, maintenance of adequate protein stores is a major objective of nutritional support.

Vitamins

The fat-soluble vitamins are A, D, E, and K. Water-soluble vitamins are vitamin C, folate, and the B-complex vitamins: thiamine, riboflavin, niacin, pantothenic acid, pyridoxine, and biotin. Vitamin

K is unstable in TPN and is not included in most commercially prepared IV vitamin solutions because of possible adverse effects in patients taking oral anticoagulants. A weekly dose of vitamin K intramuscularly or subcutaneously is recommended during the administration of TPN. Vitamins function as essential cofactors in a number of enzymatic processes and cannot be manufactured within the body. Although actual IV vitamin requirements are unknown, IV requirements are considered greater than oral requirements because of increased renal excretion and absorption of vitamins to IV bags and tubing. Vitamins are added per the American Medical Association Nutrition Advisory Group's (AMA-NAG) recommendations.

Trace Elements

Trace elements are essential for normal metabolism. The amount required is small; however, deficiencies can develop rapidly in an acute or critically ill patient. Trace elements must be provided in long-term parenteral therapy for normal metabolism to take place. All trace elements participate in enzymatic reactions and act as cofactors for other metabolic processes. Trace elements thought to be essential are iron, iodine, cobalt, zinc, copper, chromium, molybdenum, selenium, zinc, and manganese. Commercially prepared trace element combinations are available. The AMA-NAG recommendations should be followed for trace elements for TPN.

Vitamin and Trace Element	Function	Deficiency
Vitamin A	Retinal function Prevents night blindness Bone metabolism	Night blindness Reproductive failure
Vitamin C	Wound healing	Scurvy
Vitamin D	Calcium absorption	Rickets
Vitamin E	Protects cellular membrane Prevents oxidation of vitamins A and C	May contribute to hemolytic anemia and liver necrosis
Vitamin K	Prothrombin formation	Prolonged clotting time and bleeding

Iron	Oxygen transport	Anemia
Zinc	Cofactor of many enzymes	Poor wound healing Growth retardation Diminished taste/smell Gonadal dysfunction
Copper	Hemoglobin synthesis	Associated with neutropenia
Calcium	Bone metabolism Neuromuscular function	Neuromuscular irritability
Phosphate	Found in bone Serum levels regulated by kidney reabsorption	Skeletal and cardiac muscle dysfunction
Potassium	Principal cation in intracellular fluid (ICF)	Critical cardiac arrhythmias
Sodium	Principal cation in extracellular fluid (ECF) Regulates acid-base balance Neuromuscular function	Alteration in balance of ICF and ECF
Sulfate	Protein synthesis	Wasting
Iodine	Thyroid function	Hypothyroidism

Fluids and Electrolytes

Electrolytes are essential to physiologic processes. Alterations in electrolyte balance can have critical consequences such as heart arrhythmias. Because they are determined by the patient's condition, fluid and electrolyte needs vary widely. Fluid needs vary when a condition causing fluid loss, fever, or renal or cardiac impairment is present. The amount of water provided in parenteral fluids depends on the patient's fluid needs. Water needs are determined by closely monitoring the patient's weight and intake and output. Sterile water is added to adjust the 24-hour fluid volume based on the patient's 24-hour needs. The physician may adjust electrolytes daily in the acute or critically ill patient, according to serum levels. In long-term therapy, adjustments are made less frequently.

Other Additives

Other agents are sometimes added to parenteral nutrition fluids. The physician may prescribe medications such as regular insulin, heparin, and H_2 blockers when a patient need exists.

CLINICAL ALERT: All additives must be mixed in a pharmacy under a laminar flow hood to reduce the risk of infection.

Administration of Parenteral Nutrition
Total Parenteral Nutrition

TPN orders (Fig. 9-2) are adjusted as the patient's condition warrants. The nurse should review agency preprinted TPN orders. Note guidelines for determining calorie, protein, and fluid needs (Fig. 9-3). TPN orders are written per agency guidelines. The basic guidelines are as follows: Estimate calorie needs (dextrose and fat emulsion/intralipid). The Harris-Benedict equation is most commonly used to determine BEE (see "Resources").

In a critically ill patient, indirect calorimetry is the reference standard for determining energy expenditure. This method measures oxygen consumption and carbon dioxide production to calculate resting energy expenditure and the respiratory quotient (RQ). *RQ* is the ratio of carbon dioxide expired/amount of oxygen inspired. RQ = carbon dioxide production/oxygen consumption. The normal RQ range is 0.7 to 1.0. The overfeeding RQ range is greater than 1.0.

- Adjust for stress, injury, or disease and activity level of the patient.
- Estimate protein needs (amino acids).
- Estimate fluid needs (sterile H_2O).
- Review laboratory values for electrolyte needs.
- Assess for other additives such as multivitamins, trace elements, heparin, insulin, and H_2 blockers. Orders are sent to the pharmacy in advance to allow for preparation of the next bag of solution before infusion of the current bag is complete.

Total Nutritional Admixture, or 3-in-1 Admixture

Total nutritional admixtures (TNAs) combine a 24-hour supply of TPN in a 3-L container. Clinical research on the chemical stability of TPN solutions, growth of microorganisms, and compounding

Text continued on p. 308

DATE	TIME	PHYSICIAN ORDER SET NOTE: specify route of administration on Medication Orders
		Generic or therapeutic substitutions (as deemed appropriate by the Pharmacy and Therapeutics Committee) may be made unless the physician writes "NO SUBSTITUTION" on EACH medication order.

PARENTERAL NUTRITION ORDERS

Orders must be written daily on this form. Additional days supply may be ordered for patients who are stable. Orders received in the pharmacy **by 1200** will begin at the standard start time of approximately **1800** hours. Order Amino Acid, Dextrose, Electrolytes, & Fat Emulsion for 3-in-1 TPN. Pharmacy will calculate rate based on total volume divided by infusion hours. (24 hour default unless otherwise specified.) A pharmacist will assist with orders per request.

STEP 1: Parenteral Nutrition is to be given via (circle one):

Central line   PICC Line   Peripheral line

STEP 2: BASE SOLUTION.   Bag #(s): _____

Infuse over _____ **hours.**

☐ Dietitian to estimate requirements & write order for base solution.

If checked, specify total volume _____ **and skip to Step 3.**

Amino Acid 10%	_____ mL
Dextrose 70%	_____ mL
Fat Emulsion 20%	_____ mL
Sterile H2O	_____ mL
TOTAL VOLUME	_____ mL

Amino Acid _____ %	_____ mL **or**	_____ gms
Renal Amino Acids 5.2%	_____ mL **or**	_____ gms
Hepatic Amino Acids 8%	_____ mL **or**	_____ gms
Dextrose _____ %	_____ mL **or**	_____ gms
TOTAL VOLUME	_____ mL	

STEP 4: MONITORING

LABORATORY (see back side for contents of lab panels)

Date/time lab to be drawn: _____ @ _____

☐ Comprehensive Metabolic Panel

☐ Phosphorous   ☐ Basic Metabolic Panel
☐ Prealbumin   ☐ Magnesium
☐ Triglyceride   ☐ Nitrogen Balance—Order: *Urine Urea Nitrogen and *24° Calorie Count

OTHER MONITORING

☐ Indirect Calorimetry

Bedside Blood Glucose monitoring before TPN begins-call physician if > _____ (200 mg/dL if not specified)
Bedside blood glucose monitoring q 6 hrs. for 72 hrs., then:

• continue q 6 hrs. if diabetic

• q day if not diabetic and glucose is stable and WNL.

I & O q shift

Height: _____   Today's weight: _____

PIGGYBACK FAT EMULSION (if ordering separately)		CENTRAL MAXIMUM AMOUNTS:
Fat Emulsion 20% _____ ml. at _____ ml/hr over _____ hrs.		Dextrose 7.2 gm/kg/day
		Fat: 1 gm/kg/day (1 ml 20% Intralipid = 0.2 gm fat.)
		Peripheral maximum final concentration:
STEP 3: ADDITIVES		Since electrolytes affect osmolarity, a pharmacist will contact the physician if osmolarity is ≥ 940 mOsm/L.
Sodium Chloride	mEq	**ADDITIVE GUIDELINES:**
		Recommended Daily Allowance:
Sodium Phosphate	mM	
Sodium Acetate	mEq	
Potassium Chloride	mEq	Magnesium 10-30 mEq/day Chloride 80-100 mEq/day
Potassium Phosphate	mM	Potassium 80-100 mEq/day Calcium 10-15 mEq/day
Potassium Acetate	mEq	Phosphate 10-50 mMol/day Sodium 80-100 mEq/day
Calcium Gluconate	mEq	Acetate (Order to balance cations or specify amount. May be used in place of part of chloride to prevent metabolic acidosis).
Magnesium Sulfate	mEq	
Multivitamin (1 amp. contains RDA)	Amp	
Trace Elements (Cu, Zn, Mn, Cr.)	Amp	_____ _____
Regular Human Insulin	Units	Date Physician's Signature
Heparin	Units	
		_____ _____
		Date Dietitian's Signature
		VC -234 CHG 11/98

DRUG ALLERGIES	UNIT	ROOM #	PATIENT IDENTIFICATION

PATIENT NAME - HAND WRITTEN

Original - Retain on Chart   Copy- To Pharmacy
VIA CHRISTI REGIONAL MEDICAL CENTER, WICHITA, KS.
PHYSICIAN ORDER SET

Fig. 9-2
Parenteral nutrition orders and physician order set.
(Courtesy Via Christi Regional Medical Center, Wichita, Kans.)

PARENTERAL NUTRITION INFORMATION

Recommendations:

1. Radiographic verification of central catheter placement should be obtained before the initial bottle is hung.
2. TPN may be started at a low rate: 40 ml/hr, if tolerated (ie. glucose, fluid status, electrolytes), then may wish to advance rate increments of 20-40 ml/hr until goal infusion rate is achieved.

ESTIMATING CALORIE NEEDS:

Harris Benedict Equation

Step 1. (Weight in pounds*, Height in inches)

BEE: Male = 66 + (6.3 x wt) + (12.7 x ht) - (6.8 x age)

Female = 655 + (4.3 x wt) + (4.7 x ht) - (4.7 x age)

***Adjustment formula for obesity** (>125% of IBW):

[(ABW - IBW) x 0.25) + IBW] = weight for BEE

ABW = actual body weight

IBW = ideal body weight

Step 2. Multiply BEE and activity / stress factor:

1.2 - Bedrest

1.3 - Ambulatory

1.5 - Anabolic

Calorie needs may be estimated at 20-30 cal/kg (less accurate if patient is overweight).

Indirect calorimetry may aid in estimation of calorie needs when multiple stress factors are present.

ESTIMATING PROTEIN NEEDS:

0.8 - 1.0 gms protein / kg IBW for normal maintenance level

1.2 - 2.0 gms protein / kg IBW for increased protein demands

INFORMATION:

	VOLUME	PROTEIN	CALORIES
10% Amino Acid	500 ml	50 gm	200
8.5% Amino Acid	500 ml	43 gm	170
Aminosyn RF 5.2%	500 ml	26 gm	104
Aminosyn HF 8%	500 ml	40 gm	160
		CHO	
70% Dextrose	500 ml	350 gm	1190
50% Dextrose	500 ml	250 gm	850
20% Dextrose	500 ml	100 gm	340
10% Dextrose	500 ml	50 gm	171
		Fat	
20% Fat Emulsion	500 ml	100 gm	1000

Multivitamin	Trace Element
	Zinc
Ascorbic Acid	Copper
Vitamin A	Manganese
Vitamin D	Chromium
Thiamin	Selenium
Riboflavin	
Pyridoxine	
Niacinamide	
Pantothenic Acid	
Vitamin E	
Biotin	
Folic Acid	
Cyanocobalamin (B12)	

ESTIMATING FLUID NEEDS:
1500 mL for the first 20 kg of body weight
20 mL/ kg for each additional kg of body weight

SAMPLE METHOD TO CALCULATE TPN ORDERS:

Est. calorie needs (from above) **MINUS**

_____ Fat cal. (Est. cal. needs _____ x .30) **MINUS**

_____ Protein cal. (Est. pro. needs _____ gm x 4) **EQUALS**

_____ CHO cal.

10% amino acids: _____ gm pro. x 10 = _____ ml

20% Intralipid: _____ fat cal ÷2 = _____ ml

70% Dextrose:

_____ CHO cal ÷ 3.4 = _____ gm dextrose

_____ gm dextrose ÷ % dextrose (ie. 0.70) = _____ ml

VOLUME (amino acids, lipid, dextrose) = _____ ml

Water: (Est. fluid needs - VOLUME) = _____ ml

Electrolyte Content

	Phosphorus	Sodium	Potassium
Sodium Phosphate / ml	3 mM	4 mEq	---
Potassium Phosphate / ml	3 mM	---	4.4 mEq

LABORATORY MONITORING:
Initial lab: Comprehensive Metabolic Panel, Prealbumin
Subsequent lab:
Electrolytes: first 3 days, then 2-3x/week
BUN and Creatinine: first 3 days, then 2x/week
Magnesium, Calcium, and Phosphorus: 1-2x/ week
Albumin: weekly
Prealbumin: 2x/week until ≥ 18
Triglycerides: daily while lipid infusion is increasing, then weekly.

Laboratory Panels:

COMPREHENSIVE METABOLIC PANEL	Albumin, Total Bilirubin, Total Calcium, Chloride, Creatinine, Glucose, Alkaline Phosphatase, Potassium, Total Protein, Sodium, AST (SGOT), BUN
BASIC METABOLIC PANEL	CO2, Chloride, Creatinine, Glucose, Potassium, Sodium, BUN
PREALBUMIN	not included in standard lab panels
TRIGLYCERIDE	"
MAGNESIUM	"
PHOSPHOROUS	"

PAGE 2 OF PARENTERAL NUTRITION ORDERS

Fig. 9-3
Parenteral nutrition information.
(Courtesy Via Christi Regional Medical Center, Wichita, Kans.)

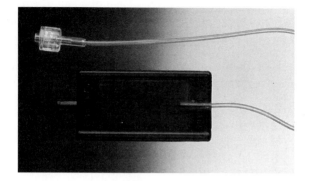

Fig. 9-4
The Lipipor™ TNA Filter Set is an air-eliminating filter for use with any nutritional intravenous administration containing lipids.
(Courtesy PALL Medical, Ann Arbor, Mich.)

techniques has led to procedures that make TNAs safe and convenient. Lipids are mixed with the dextrose and amino acid solution in the pharmacy. TNA solutions are solid white and have a nonreflecting surface, making precipitates difficult to observe. This form of TPN is usually reserved for patients in a stable state because the components are adjusted only once daily.

CLINICAL ALERT: Examine TNA admixtures before hanging for evidence of an unstable solution. Unstable solutions have small, clear, or slightly yellow pools of oil floating on the surface.

If the TPN solution is provided by a contracting agency, the nurse must verify that the TPN solution has been prepared by a pharmacist under a laminar flow hood. He or she should not initiate or infuse TPN solutions if they have been altered after preparation because of the potential for bacteremia.

Central Venous Administration

The type and placement of the access device is related to the need for the therapy to be short or long term. In addition, there are specifically designed filters to be used for administration of TPN-containing lipid products (Fig. 9-4).

TPN may be given in tunneled central venous catheters (Groshong or Hickman), implanted vascular ports (PasPort), percutaneous central venous catheters (basilic, antecubital, or jugular), or single-lumen or multilumen central venous catheters placed in the jugular or subclavian veins. The use of a femoral site for TPN administration is discouraged because of the increased risk of infection.

CLINICAL ALERT: Always obtain a chest x-ray film to confirm placement of the central venous access before use. The tip of the central venous catheter rests in the superior vena cava. The high blood flow rate in the superior vena cava allows rapid dilution of the hypertonic TPN solution.

Initiating and Maintaining Therapy

To ensure glucose tolerance, TPN infusions are initially increased at a rate that allows endogenous insulin production to handle the extra glucose load. Until the patient is in a stable state, daily weight, intake and output, blood glucose tests, electrolyte levels, and all other laboratory reports require close monitoring.

If the infusion falls behind schedule, the nurse should not attempt to catch up. The rate should be readjusted to the prescribed infusion rate. If the rate is too rapid, hyperglycemia will result. If the rate is too slow, hypoglycemia may result. The patient will not receive adequate calories or nitrogen. If the TPN must be interrupted, the nurse should infuse 10% dextrose at a prescribed rate until the TPN is restarted to prevent the development of hypoglycemia.

Equipment Considerations

TPN is always administered via an infusion pump. The nurse must set the rate and the volume to be infused. TNA solutions cannot be filtered with standard IV tubing filters. A 1.2-μ filter should be used to administer TPN (see Fig. 9-4). If the solution does not contain lipids, a 0.22-μ filter can be used.

Cycled TPN

Cycled TPN may be used to improve the patient's tolerance to glucose and to stimulate the patient's appetite. Cycled TPN is usually administered at night to allow patient mobility in the daytime hours.

Considerations When Administering Fat Emulsions

1. Give as prepared by the manufacturer.
2. Use unfiltered tubing because the fat molecules are too large to pass through a filter smaller than 1.2 μ.

3. When administering lipids by the piggyback method, use the Y-tube injection site closest to the catheter hub.
4. Do not use the solution if the oil has separated.
5. Fat emulsions can be administered via a peripheral vein because the solution is isotonic.
6. Monitor blood lipid levels and liver function tests.

Discontinuing Therapy

There are many methods recommended for discontinuing parenteral nutrition. Tapering of the infusion rate over 24 to 48 hours is usually recommended to prevent severe hypoglycemia.

Considerations When Administering Parenteral Nutrition

For safe administration of TPN, the following DO and DO NOT lists should be reviewed:

DO:

- Use five rights of medication: right patient, right drug, right route, right amount, and right time.
- Verify 24-hour infusion versus cycled.
- Verify rate per hour.
- Always monitor rate and volume on a scheduled interval.
- Administer via an infusion pump.
- Use a dedicated lumen of the central venous access.
- Discard any TPN and tubing more than 24 hours old.
- Store TPN in the refrigerator until time for administration. Allow the solution to warm to room temperature 1 hour before administration.
- Follow strict aseptic technique at all times when handling the catheter, dressing, tubing, or solution.
- Monitor bedside blood glucose levels every 6 hours or as prescribed. Patients who are critically ill may have hyperglycemia, and the addition of TPN may further elevate blood glucose. An insulin infusion may be required. Adjustment of the insulin in the next bag of TPN solution may be necessary.

CLINICAL ALERT: Frequent mouth care such as brushing teeth and using mouthwash and lip gloss is often helpful for the patient who is not eating. If the patient is allowed to eat but is experiencing anorexia, encourage small, frequent meals with others present.

DO NOT:

- Interrupt the TPN line (general rule). Turning the TPN off and on creates fluctuations in blood glucose. The pancreas will secrete insulin to alter the changes in blood glucose.

- Attach stopcocks or extension tubing on the TPN line.
- Use the TPN line for piggybacking medications.
- Use the TPN line for central venous pressure monitoring.
- Use the TPN line for blood sampling.

CLINICAL ALERT: Blood samples should never be drawn via the TPN infusion line because of the increased risk of bacteremia and the potential for incorrect laboratory values. Turn TPN and other IV solutions off for at least 5 minutes before drawing blood samples via the central venous access. Blood discard should be up to 10 ml. Verify agency policy for time interval and discard volumes.

Report the following information to the physician:

1. Hyperglycemia—blood glucose levels greater than 200 mg/dl
2. Hypoglycemia—blood glucose levels less than 60 mg/dl
3. Abnormal electrolyte results
4. Signs and symptoms of fluid overload
5. Temperature elevation
6. Weight gains or losses—the goal for most patients is 1 pound/wk
7. Alteration in TPN infusion:
   a. Inability to infuse TPN related to vascular access
   b. Volume infused too fast or too slow
8. Redness, swelling, drainage from the IV catheter site

TPN Continuous Monitoring

Nursing physical assessment during TPN includes the following:

1. Monitor vital signs: blood pressure, heart rate, respiratory rate, and temperature.
2. Observe for a trend in the elevation of the temperature to monitor for infection.
3. Observe for clinical signs of excess fluid balance: increased pedal or sacral edema, increased heart rate, and increased blood pressure.
4. Observe for clinical signs of fluid volume deficit or dehydration: skin turgor, thirst, and decreased urine output.
5. Review daily laboratory results. Laboratory monitoring tests during TPN suggested by ASPEN (Table 9-1) provide clinicians with information necessary to make adjustments based on the patient's energy and protein needs.
6. Monitor the patient's comprehensive metabolic profile: serum triglycerides, complete blood count (CBC) with

Table 9-1 Suggested monitoring for parenteral nutrition

Parameter	Baseline	Critically Ill Patients	Stable Patients
Chemistry screen (Ca, Mg, LFTs, P)	Yes	2-3 × week	Weekly
Electrolytes, BUN, creatinine	Yes	Daily	1-2 × week
Serum triglycerides	Yes	Weekly	Weekly
CBC with differential	Yes	Weekly	Weekly
PT, PTT	Yes	Weekly	Weekly
Capillary glucose	3 × day	3 × day (until consistently <200 mg/dl)	3 × day (until consistently <200 mg/dl)
Weight	If possible	Daily	2-3 × weekly
Intake and output	Daily	Daily	Daily unless fluid status is assessed by physical exam
Nitrogen balance	As needed	As needed	As needed
Indirect calorimetry	As needed	As needed	As needed

From Skipper A, Millikan KW: *Parenteral nutrition implementation and management*, Silver Spring, MD, 1998, A.S.P.E.N.
BUN, Blood urea nitrogen; *CBC*, complete blood cell count; *LFT*, liver function test; *PT*, prothrombin time; *PTT*, partial thromboplastin time.

differential, prothrombin time (PT) and partial thromboplastin time (PTT), albumin, prealbumin magnesium, and phosphorus.

7. Validate agency test requirements and scheduled frequency for the tests.

8. Adjust fluid and electrolytes in the acute and critical care setting daily as needed.

Complications of Parenteral Nutrition

Many serious complications may occur during parenteral nutrition. The most common complications are catheter related or metabolic. Catheter technical problems at the time of insertion include pneumothorax, hemothorax, air embolism, intrathoracic hemorrhage, cardiac compromise, arterial injury, neurologic injury, and catheter dysfunction or misplacement. Over time, potential complications from the vascular access device (VAD) are thrombus formation, dislodgment, fibrin clot formation, vessel problems, and catheter tear (see Chapter 3).

Contamination of the infusion system is a major concern. A break in sterile technique at any point during manufacture, compounding, or infusion may cause contamination. Avoidance of contamination requires strict observance of sterile technique. See Table 9-2 for an overview of potential complications and the associated event.

Septic complications (bacterial or fungal) may be related to contamination of the vascular access area. Maintaining meticulous care during dressing changes and administering TPN is the best preventive measure (Fig. 9-5).

CLINICAL ALERT: In the acute and critical care setting, the recommendation is to keep the TPN line dedicated without interruption to decrease the potential for infection.

Psychosocial Needs of Patients and Caregivers

Initiation of TPN disrupts normal eating patterns. Food and eating are associated with many positive feelings, such as security, acceptance, and belonging. Disruption of normal eating patterns, particularly over long periods, removes a major source of pleasure for the patients. Dependence on TPN leads to feelings of loss of control of normal daily life and often leads to periods of depression.

Table 9-2   Potential complications of parenteral nutrition

Complication	Clinical Event
Infusion equipment	Tubing junctions separate; infusion pump malfunctions.
Metabolic glucose, fat, amino acids, and other blood chemistry abnormalities; vitamin and mineral imbalances (see pp. 301 and 302)	Metabolic alterations secondary to administration of TPN and patient's underlying disease process necessitate frequent monitoring to assess for potential complications. Refeeding syndrome may occur within the first 24-48 hr of TPN initiation in severely malnourished patients. Initially, syndrome is evidenced by alterations in potassium, phosphorus, magnesium, fluid (edema), and basal metabolic rate. If symptoms worsen, there is vitamin flux (water soluble) causing complications such as congestive heart failure, pulmonary edema, glucose intolerance, lethargy, confusion, coma, and death.
Liver failure	Prolonged administration of TPN may result in altered liver function tests and complications that lead to liver failure. Continue to monitor liver function tests. Continued administration of parenteral nutrition without lipids results in accumulation of hepatic fat, which can lead to liver failure.
Acquired coagulopathy	Vitamin K deficiency occurs with administration of TPN unless vitamin K is administered. If patient is also receiving antibiotic therapy, enteric sources of vitamin K are eliminated. The patient is at risk for acquired coagulopathies.
Disuse syndrome of the gastrointestinal tract	This is a long-term complication. Intestinal mucosa provides an effective barrier, but with disuse, translocation of bacteria may occur, leading to potential septic complications. Move to enteral or oral nutrition as soon as the underlying condition improves.

TPN, Total parenteral nutrition.

NOTE: Complications can be varied and complex. Follow the monitoring guidelines of the agency and use meticulous care when handling the TPN line and vascular access device.

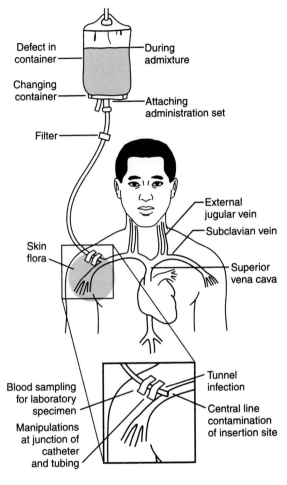

Fig. 9-5
Sites for contamination of parenteral nutrition.

Documentation Recommendations

- Components of parenteral nutrition solution
- Infusion rate and any equipment used for regulation
- Site assessment before and during the infusion
- Observation of catheter or device patency before, during, and after infusion
- All supplies used; date and time of tubing changes per agency policy
- Any complaints of discomfort and symptoms experienced before, during, or after infusion; action taken to correct problems
- Daily weight
- An accurate intake and output record
- All patient and caregiver education
- Discharge teaching when appropriate for long-term TPN therapy; patient's and caregiver's ability to perform all procedures and their understanding of troubleshooting measures, potential complications, and appropriate interventions

Nursing Diagnoses

- Knowledge deficit, regarding the VAD and the reason for TPN; if applicable, home care management of nutrition and VAD
- Nutrition, altered: less than body requirements, related to inadequate intake or absorption of foods
- Infection, risk for, related to high dextrose content of parenteral solution, break in sterile technique when managing catheter, or contamination of supplies
- Self-esteem disturbance, related to body image, placement of VAD

Patient/Family Education for Self-Management

Patient/family education is an important aspect of nursing care. Providing information about the underlying disease process, procedures, and the reason for TPN will decrease patient/family anxiety. Education should include the following:

- Reason for the therapy
- Signs and symptoms to report, such as chills, itching, shortness of breath, or excessive thirst
- Avoidance of tension on the tubing and VAD
- Monitoring of the site

- Leaking at the site or pain and tenderness at the site
- Expected outcome

Patient/Family/Caregiver Discharge Teaching for Home TPN

- Assess ability and willingness to learn, availability of the caregiver, home environment, ability to assume self-care, and compliance with treatment regimen.
- Describe purpose and procedures for the parenteral nutrition regimen.
- Explain and demonstrate aseptic technique; stress that sterile technique is essential, and be consistent in all demonstrations and instructions to the patient and family; allow patients and families to handle equipment as much as possible.
- Break each procedure into small tasks and guide the patient through each task; have the patient and the caregiver talk each other through each procedure to enhance learning.
- Validate aseptic technique and skills of both the patient and the caregiver for initiation and discontinuation of therapy.
- Instruct the patient and caregiver in signs, symptoms, and self-management interventions specific to each complication, such as lethargy, fluid retention, increased urine output, and catheter complications.
- Instruct the patient and caregiver in the management of infusion devices.
- Provide information and a list of resources for obtaining home care services.

Guidelines for Home Care
TPN

Multiple factors need to be considered for the patient and family/caregiver when the patient receives TPN in the home setting. The initial assessment process includes knowing the patient's medical stability, presence of a knowledgeable and capable caregiver, and a home care agency that provides comprehensive services. A home care visit before discharge should be made to ensure that all elements of TPN infusion and monitoring are in place and to assess the home care setting for potential safety issues (e.g., steps between frequently used rooms may interfere with patient/pump mobility). Because of the requirements for TPN infusion and management, the following requirements are essential for safe TPN administration.

- Assess and determine the availability and type of refrigeration for the TPN product.
- Verify that all types of equipment (infusion pumps, VAD, glucose monitoring device) and the usual self-care monitoring equipment (e.g., weight scale, thermometer, and TPN infusion record for documentation) are in place and working efficiently.
- Confirm and document the patient's/caregiver's knowledge and/or skill level in the following:

  Able to obtain and record accurate measures for weight, temperature, and blood glucose levels

  Knows when and how to report signs and symptoms of infection, such as fever, chills, and shortness of breath; altered glucose level, such as excessive thirst, irritability, or shaky feeling inside; catheter/port malfunction, such as leaking at the exit site or inability to infuse TPN; and fluid retention, such as cough, difficulty breathing, or swelling of the lower extremities

  Can demonstrate aseptic technique for venous access management, can connect/disconnect the TPN infusion, and can troubleshoot problems with the infusion pump

  Knows how to order and store TPN supplies: type, amount, schedule for frequency of replacements

  Know names, contact resources, schedule appointments for home care agency staff, and how/when to contact for an emergency

Geriatric Considerations

Parenteral nutrition may be prescribed as an adjunct therapy for an elderly person for multiple medical reasons, for example, postoperatively for a surgical procedure that interferes with GI nutrient absorption, complications resulting from chemotherapy and radiation therapy for patients with cancer, and/or a chronic illness that requires short-term nutritional intervention. Similar factors, listed in Chapters 5 through 8, are likewise pertinent in parenteral nutrition administration. The elderly patient may have a compromised status related to homeostasis, reduced capacity of the various body systems (cardiac, respiratory, and renal systems; endocrine and liver functions; and neuromuscular deficits), and altered sensory functions. Refer to the previously listed chapters for those specific interventions.

In addition, consider other more intense and/or frequent assessments with interventions for the elderly patient regarding the following (topics listed in this chapter):

- Nutritional status indications
- Fluids and electrolyte additives
- Administration, continuous monitoring, and/or discontinuing parenteral nutrition
- Hyperglycemia and hypoglycemia assessment and intervention
- Potential complications of parenteral nutrition that may be more subtle in the elderly patient

Resources

Calculations Commonly Used in Nutritional Assessment

Harris-Benedict Equation
Step 1:

Male: BEE: $66 = (6.3 \times \text{wt}) + (12.7 \times \text{Ht}) - (6.8 \times \text{age})$

Female: BEE: $655 + (4.3 \times \text{wt}) + (4.7 \times \text{Ht}) - (4.7 \times \text{age})$

where *BEE* stands for basal energy expenditure, *Wt* stands for patient weight in pounds,* and *Ht* is patient height in inches.

Step 2:

Multiply BEE by activity/stress factor:
Bedrest: 1.2
Ambulatory: 1.3
Anabolic: 1.5

---

*Adjust formula for obesity (0.125% of IBW):

$[(\text{ABW} - \text{IBW}) \times 0.25 + \text{IBW}] = \text{Weight for BEE}$

where *ABW* is actual body weight and *IBW* is ideal body weight.

Total Lymphocyte Count

Total lymphocyte count = Percent lymphocytes × (WBC ÷ 100)

Creatinine/Height Index

Creatinine/height index = Actual urinary creatinine/Ideal urinary creatinine × 100

Nitrogen Balance

Nitrogen balance = Nitrogen intake − Nitrogen excretion = Protein intake in grams/6.25 = (UUN + 4)

where *UUN* is the urine urea nitrogen.

Clinical Competency—TPN Administration

	Yes	No	NA
1. Verify physician's TPN orders with the labeled TPN container contents.			
2. Verify TPN bag with patient's identification band at the patient's bedside.			
3. Verify rate and volume to be infused. Is rate to be gradually increased or tapered?			
4. Verify time period of infusion: 24 hours versus cycled.			
5. Wash hands.			
6. Use infusion pump, tubing, and 1.2-*μ* filter per agency guidelines.			
7. Use aseptic technique to spike the TPN bag with the IV administration set.			
8. Prime tubing and filter use per agency guideline.			
9. Clamp TPN IV tubing.			
10. Prepare VAD per agency guideline.			
11. Use aseptic technique for all connections and disconnections.			

Clinical Competency—TPN Administration—cont'd

	Yes	No	NA
12. Connect directly to the lumen of the catheter using a Luer-Lok connection. Do not use a needleless system connector.			
13. Ensure that the TPN tubing and VAD connection are secure.			
14. Unclamp the TPN tubing/and VAD line.			
15. Set rate and volume to be infused on the infusion pump. Start the TPN infusion.			
16. Label tubing with date/time.			
17. Document date, time, and vital signs at the initiation of the each bag of TPN solution.			
18. Follow agency guidelines for dressing changes of the VAD.			
19. Discard TPN solution and tubing after 24 hours.			

Study Questions

1. Clinical indications that usually require total parenteral nutrition include:
   a. Cancer, renal failure, hepatic dysfunction, postoperatively for 3 to 5 days
   b. Cancer, Crohn's disease, pancreatitis, postoperatively for 5 to 7 days
   c. Cancer, sepsis, trauma, postoperatively for 7 to 10 days
   d. Cancer, short bowel syndrome, dialysis, postoperatively for 10 to 21 days

2. Nutritional status indicators for the patient's nutritional assessment include:
   a. Diet history, BIA, SGA, prothrombin level
   b. Diet history, BEE, SGA, potassium level
   c. Diet history, BEE, BIA, sodium balance
   d. Diet history, BIA, BEE, SGA

3. The CNS requires about _____ g of glucose per day.
   a. 100
   b. 150
   c. 200
   d. 300

4. Fat emulsion products provide essential fatty acids as a major source of energy; these products are available in varied concentrations that include:
   a. 10%, 20%, and 30% concentrations
   b. 15%, 25%, and 30% concentrations
   c. 10%, 25%, and 50% concentrations
   d. 10%, 30%, and 50% concentrations

5. Adjustments for the amount of protein in TPN usually are made for patients with:
   a. Heart, hepatic, and/or liver disease/dysfunction
   b. Hepatic, renal, and/or liver disease/dysfunction
   c. Liver, renal, and/or reproductive disease/dysfunction
   d. Liver, hepatic, and/or CNS disease/dysfunction

6. The fat-soluble vitamins include:
   a. Vitamins A, B, D, E
   b. Vitamins A, C, D, K
   c. Vitamins A, D, E, K
   d. Vitamins A, B, C, D

7. Suggested laboratory monitoring parameters for parenteral nutrition include:
   a. CBC, creatinine, capillary glucose, serum iron
   b. CBC, creatinine, immunoglobulins, electrolytes
   c. CBC, DIC screen, creatinine, electrolytes
   d. CBC, PT/PTT, creatinine, electrolytes

8. Patient and family education topics for TPN administration include:
   a. Infection symptoms, sterile technique procedures, monitoring therapy, complications
   b. Infection symptoms, clean technique procedures, monitoring therapy, complications
   c. Infection symptoms, sterile technique procedures, discontinuing therapy, complications
   d. Infection symptoms, clean technique procedures, tapering therapy, complications

9. Critical elements for documentation of TPN in the acute care setting include:
   a. Infusion solution, VAD and site, intake and output, daily weight
   b. Infusion solution, glucose level, urinary output, home care nurse visit
   c. Infusion solution, VAD and site, intake and output, weekly weight
   d. Infusion solution, VAD and site, intake, family/caregiver visit

10. Benefits for nutritional status indicators: albumin and prealbumin levels reflect:
    a. Albumin levels reflect 10-day half-life; prealbumin reflects short 2-day half-life
    b. Albumin levels reflect 15 -day half-life; prealbumin reflects short 3-day half-life
    c. Albumin levels reflect 20-day half life; prealbumin reflects short 2-day half-life
    d. Albumin levels reflect 30-day half-life; prealbumin reflects short 5-day half-life

Answers   1. c   2. d   3. b   4. a   5. b   6. c
7. d   8. a   9. a   10. c

Vascular Access in Adult Critical Care

10

Objectives

1. Describe the difference between zero referencing, leveling, and verifying the dynamic response of the pressure transducer system.

2. List and discuss the clinical significance of each hemodynamic parameter monitored with the pulmonary artery catheter.

3. Discuss nursing responsibilities related to the insertion and care of hemodynamic pressure lines.

4. Discuss nursing interventions for potential complications associated with hemodynamic monitoring, including pressure transducer systems, arterial line catheters, and pulmonary artery catheters.

5. State the nursing responsibilities related to fluid resuscitation and drug administration in the critical care setting.

Critically ill patients require intravenous (IV) therapy for resuscitation, fluid and electrolyte maintenance, medication administration, and nutritional support. These patients often have injuries or illnesses that require vascular access for advanced hemodynamic monitoring. The tools available to the health care team for continuously monitoring the hemodynamic status of the patient in the critical care setting include arterial lines, central venous catheters, and pulmonary artery catheters (PACs). Arterial blood pressure, pulmonary artery pressures (PAPs), right atrial/central venous pressures, pulmonary artery wedge pressure, and cardiac output information provided by these tools help guide cardiac resuscitation, titration of medications, and oxygen delivery at a cellular level. Clinical assessment, laboratory values, and trends in hemodynamic variables provide information for the health care team to adjust therapy to improve patient outcome.

Pressure Transducer Systems and Nursing Care Considerations

Definitions

The *pressure transducer system* is a device that changes a physiologic pressure into an electric signal and displays the waveform and the digital pressure value on the bedside monitor. This direct monitoring reflects the patient's hemodynamic status.

Leveling is achieved by using a leveling tool to level the zero reference stopcock of arterial lines, central venous catheters, and PACs to the reference point of the phlebostatic axis. The phlebostatic axis is the intersection of imaginary lines drawn from the fourth intercostal space (vertical) and the midaxillary line (horizontal) (Fig. 10-1). Leveling to the phlebostatic axis prevents the influence of the patient's hydrostatic pressure on the monitoring system. The zero reference stopcock should be maintained at the phlebostatic axis reference point at all times.

Zero referencing eliminates the effect of atmospheric and hydrostatic pressure. The nurse should turn the zero reference stopcock off to the patient and open to air and should depress the zero key on the monitor. Zero referencing should be done before insertion, with significant changes in hemodynamic pressures, with changes in the patient's position, any time the transducer has been disconnected from the pressure cable, and whenever the accuracy of the hemodynamic values are questioned. Minimally, zero referencing would be done once per shift.

Dynamic compliance is achieved by performing the square-wave or fast-flush test to assess the ability of the transducer to accurately produce a waveform on the monitor. This should be done every 8 to 12 hours, when the system has been opened to air, or when the accuracy of the hemodynamic variables is questioned.

Disposable pressure transducer systems are packaged to meet specific hospital preferences and practices. Two transducers may be used with one bag of flush solution. One pressure transducer is used

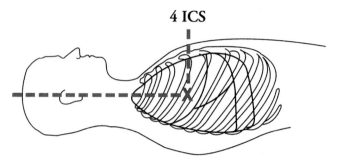

4 ICS

**Mid-Point
A-P Chest Wall**

Fig. 10-1
Phlebostatis axis.
(From Peter Lichtenthal MD: *Baxter quick guide to cardiopulmonary care,* Baxter Healthcare Corporation, 1998.)

to monitor the arterial pressure. The second transducer monitors the central venous pressure and/or pulmonary artery pressures.

Pressure Transducer System Procedure

Supplies are usually contained in the system packing or are stored in the patient care area.

1. Prepare and set up the pressure transducer system for hemodynamic monitoring of an arterial line, central venous line, and/or PAC by reviewing the patient's history and physical examination results, nursing assessment, and laboratory results (Fig. 10-2).
2. Obtain supplies.
   a. A pressure bag (These pressures bags may recycled—a cost-effective strategy.)
   b. 500-ml. bag of flush solution (Use heparinized normal saline [NS] to maintain the patency of the system; label the infusion bag with heparin units/concentration [Fig. 10-3].)

CLINICAL ALERT: Heparin may be contraindicated for patients with bleeding disorders or thrombocytopenia or for those who are receiving anticoagulants or thrombolytic agents. Verify patient

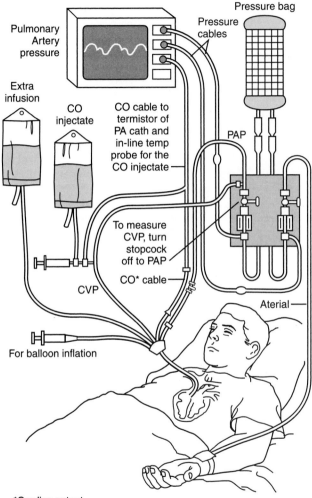

Pressure bag

Pressure cables

Pulmonary Artery pressure

Extra infusion

CO injectate

CO cable to termistor of PA cath and in-line temp probe for the CO injectate

PAP

To measure CVP, turn stopcock off to PAP

CVP

CO* cable

Aterial

For balloon inflation

*Cardiac output

Fig. 10-2
Invasive blood pressure monitoring system used for monitoring systemic arterial pressure, right arterial pressure (CVP), and pulmonary pressure.

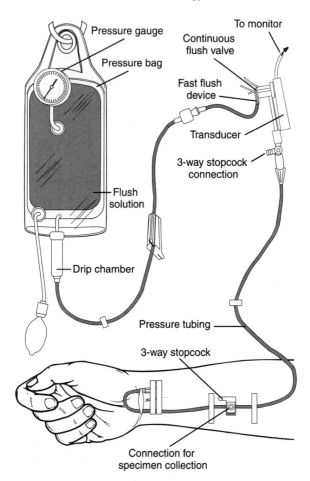

Fig. 10-3

Components of a pressure monitoring system.

(In Lewis SM, Heitkemper MM, Dirksen SR: *Medical surgical nursing: assessment and management of clinical problems,* ed 5, St Louis, 2000, Mosby. Redrawn from Gardner PE: *Hemodynamic pressure monitoring,* Redmond, Wash, 1994, Spacelabs Medical.)

history for bleeding disorders and/or anticoagulant use. Verify laboratory values for hemoglobin, hematocrit, and platelet count.

Always change the flush solution and pressure transducer system simultaneously. Label the flush solution bag and pressure transducer system with the date and time. Document the units/ml of heparin on the IV label. The Centers for Disease Control and Prevention (CDC) recommends changing the flush solution and the pressure transducer system at least every 96 hours. Follow hospital policy regarding changing the flush solution and pressure transducer system.

    c. IV tubing used to spike the bag of flush solution

CLINICAL ALERT: To prevent the possibility of air emboli, remove all air from the flush solution bag, drip chamber, and tubing in the pressure transducer system. Spike the flush solution bag. Remove the air from the flush solution bag and the drip chamber by holding the bag upside down and squeezing the bag to remove the air.

3. Zero reference the stopcock to return the pressure transducer system to the phlebostatic axis.
4. Flush the device. The pressurized system will continuously deliver 2 to 5 ml/hr. The system can be fast-flushed, which allows intermittent rapid flushing of the system. Flushing is also used to verify the dynamic response of the system.
5. Noncompliant pressure tubing is used from the transducer to the vascular access to prevent absorption of the transmitted pressure wave by the tubing.
6. Stopcocks permit access of the arterial line or PAC lumens. To prevent contamination of the system and the potential for hemorrhage, dead-end caps should *cover all open ends* of the stopcocks. If a stopcock is inadvertently opened without a dead-end cap present, the patient can hemorrhage and *exsanguinate*. Replace the dead-end cap each time the system is opened.

    NOTE: Stopcocks are some of the most confusing devices in the pressure transducer system for the novice critical care nurse. Think of the pressure transducer system as a road and the stopcocks are potential roadblocks. Ask yourself, can the monitor see the patient? Is the road blocked?

7. Secure all connections to prevent entry of air into the system, leakage of fluid from the system, and possible contamination of the system.

8. Prime the system, including all stopcocks. All air bubbles must be removed because their presence in the system can produce inaccurate information.

9. Maintain pressure in the system at 300 mm Hg via the pressure infuser bag to produce accurate and consistent waveforms and adequate flushing of the system.

10. Connect the pressure transducer systems to the arterial line, central venous catheter, or PAC.

11. The zero reference stopcock should be level with the phlebostatic axis (fourth intercostal space, midaxillary line) for arterial, central venous, and PACs.

12. If the patient has changed position since the previous variables were obtained, level the zero reference stopcock to the phlebostatic axis.

13. Verify the dynamic compliance of the pressure system. Activate the fast-flush. Perform the square-wave test. The square-wave test ensures that the transducer and the monitoring system will produce accurate physiologic values (Fig. 10-4).

14. Assess all hemodynamic waveforms for appropriate reference points. Troubleshoot the system if waveforms are not optimal.

15. Set alarm limits. Alarms should be *on. NEVER TURN OFF THE ALARM SYSTEM*. Adjust alarm limits based on the condition of the patient or per physician's orders.

16. Obtain baseline hemodynamic monitoring variables.

17. Monitor trends in hemodynamic variables.

CLINICAL ALERT: Maintain aseptic technique during assembly of the pressure transducer system. Manipulation of the equipment or access to the arterial line, central venous access device, or PAC requires aseptic technique to reduce the potential for infection. To minimize the potential for contamination of the arterial system, use an in-line blood reservoir system such as the Abbott Safeset (Fig. 10-5). An in-line blood reservoir system is a blood conservation strategy for the patient with a complex condition.

Troubleshooting Pressure Transducer Systems

Many factors can influence the pressure transducer system and catheters. Troubleshooting tips are noted in Table 10-1. Adding extra stopcocks and noncompliant tubing in the pressure transducer system is not recommended because the accuracy of the system may be compromised.

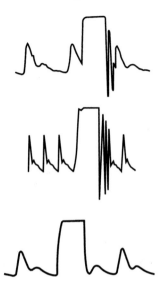

Optimally Damped:
1 - 2 oscillations before returning to tracing. Values obtained are accurate.

Underdamped:
> 2 oscillations. Overestimated systolic pressure, diastolic pressures may be underestimated.

Overdamped:
< 1 ½ oscillations. Underestimation of systolic pressures, diastolic may not be affected.

Fig. 10-4
Square-wave testing.
(From Peter Lichtenthal MD: *Baxter quick guide to cardiopulmonary care*, Baxter Healthcare Corporation, 1998.)

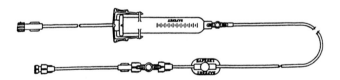

Fig. 10-5
Safeset, in-line blood reservoir system.
(Courtesy Abbott, Salt Lake Operations, Graphics, 1999.)

Arterial Line Catheter

An arterial line is a means of continuous direct monitoring of the arterial blood pressure. Direct monitoring of blood pressure is considered to be the most accurate. An arterial line also provides access for obtaining frequent blood samples to monitor arterial blood gases (ABGs) and perform other laboratory tests as ordered. Systems are available that can do point-of-care testing at the

Table 10-1 Troubleshooting tips for pressure monitoring systems

Problem	Causes	Interventions
Absence of waveform	Monitor turned off	Verify monitor on.
	Disconnection	Tighten all connections.
	Improper positioning of stopcocks	Verify position of all stopcocks.
	Inappropriate scale	Select appropriate scale.
	Faulty transducer	Assess dynamic response.
		Replace transducer.
Dampened waveform	Presence of air bubbles, blood, clot, or kink	Assess system and correct.
	Catheter tip against vessel wall	Activate fast-flush, briefly.
	Inadequate fluid or pressure in pressure infuser	Ensure adequate fluid and pressure at 300 mm Hg.
	Hypovolemia	Assess patient and report.
Significant change in parameter unrelated to status change	Improper transducer level: too high causes low reading; too low causes high reading	Perform level-zero dynamic response process.
Backup of blood in pressure line	Inadequate pressure or fluid in bag infuser	Ensure adequate fluid pressure >300 mm Hg.
		Tighten all connections.

bedside. Some systems can be placed in-line to monitor ABGs and other laboratory values such as potassium. Most laboratory specimens, including those for ABGs, can be drawn from the arterial catheter.

Selection of Patients for Arterial Pressure Monitoring

- Hemodynamically unstable patients who require titration of medications for hypotension or hypertension
- Critically ill patients with vasoconstriction or vasodilation caused by injury such as multisystem trauma or illness such as systemic inflammatory response syndrome
- Patients requiring frequent ABG sampling: patients requiring mechanical ventilation, patients with severe acid-base disturbances, or patients in septic shock

Sites for Arterial Cannulation

1. *Radial artery* (Fig. 10-6): The most commonly used sites for an arterial line are radial or femoral arteries. Collateral circulation makes these the preferred sites for cannulation. A modified Allen's test should be done before inserting the catheter to assess patency of the ulnar artery and collateral circulation. To perform the Allen's test, the patient's hand is held overhead with fist clenched while direct pressure is applied to both the radial and ulnar arteries. The hand is lowered and opened, and pressure is released from the ulnar artery. A positive Allen's test is an erythematous blush in 6 seconds, indicating a patent ulnar artery. Pallor in 6 seconds is interpreted as a negative test. The radial artery should not be used if the test is negative.
2. *Femoral artery:* Access is easily obtained in urgent and emergency situations when the patient is severely injured, vasoconstricted, or hypotensive or is in cardiac failure. The line should be changed to the radial artery when the patient is hemodynamically stable to allow increased mobility in bed.
3. Other arterial sites such as axillary, dorsalis pedis, or brachial arteries are rarely used because of an increased risk of complications.

Arterial Line Insertion Procedure

1. Explain the procedure to the patient and family.
2. Ensure that informed consent has been obtained from patient and/or family.

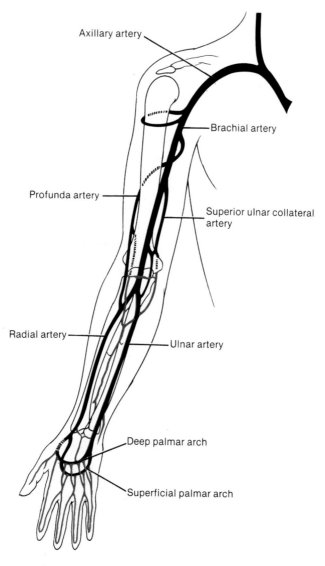

Fig. 10-6
Anatomic locations of the arteries of the arm.
(From Daily EK, Schroeder JS: *Techniques in bedside hemodynamic monitoring,* ed 5, St Louis, 1994, Mosby.)

3. Provide sedation and pain medication.
4. Obtain supplies for insertion of an arterial line: site preparation solution, 1% lidocaine (Xylocaine), 10-ml syringe, 14- to 18-gauge arterial line catheter, dressing supplies, and arm-board. Refer to the physician's procedure preference for other supplies.
5. Prepare the pressure transducer system and flush solution as previously described.
6. Label the arterial line, pressure transducer, and tubing to help prevent accidental disconnection or infusions into the site.
7. Assist with insertion of the arterial line. Obtain baseline vital signs and monitor during the procedure.
8. Apply a sterile dressing to the insertion site. The dressing should indicate the date and time of insertion.
9. Level and zero reference to the phlebostatic axis. The American Association of Critical-Care Nurses Protocol for Arterial Pressure Monitoring recommends the phlebostatic axis as the reference point. The tip of the arterial catheter as the zero reference point is under debate in the literature.
10. Document mean arterial pressure (MAP) as well as systolic/diastolic blood pressure. MAP is the perfusion pressure. It is calculated as follows:

$$MAP = 1 \text{ (systolic pressure)} + 2 \text{ (diastolic pressure)} \div 3$$

MAP should be more than 60 mm Hg to adequately perfuse vital organs and the brain. MAP should be used as a titration indicator for vasoactive medications.

Maintenance of the Arterial Line

1. Keep alarms *on* at all times.
2. Verify that line connections are secure to prevent disconnection. Perform verification during physical assessment of the patient and when recording arterial blood pressure values.
3. Assess pulse, capillary refill of the extremity, sensation, movement, color, and temperature distal to the insertion site at least every 2 hours. Follow agency guidelines.

CLINICAL ALERT: A decreased or absent pulse, cool or mottled skin, or changes in sensation or movement may indicate occlusion of the artery. Report changes promptly to the physician.

4. Assess the insertion site for tenderness, redness, or drainage.
5. Monitor trends in temperature.

6. Change the arterial insertion site per hospital policy. CDC guidelines recommend changing the arterial line site every 4 days if the patient's condition warrants continuous monitoring of the arterial blood pressure. Always change the tubing and flush solution simultaneously per hospital policy. The CDC recommends changing the flush solution and the pressure transducer system at least every 96 hours.

7. Assess the arterial pressure waveform.

8. Immobilize the cannulated extremity only when necessary. Flexion of the extremity may alter the waveform and blood pressure readings. Long-term hyperextension of the hand on an armboard can result in complications.

9. Relevel the zero reference stopcock to the phlebostatic axis if there has been a change in the patient's position.

10. Verify the dynamic response of the pressure transducer system according to hospital policy.

11. Change the dressing per hospital infection control policy.

12. Maintain aseptic technique when zero referencing the system or obtaining blood samples.

13. Notify the physician of changes in the patient's condition and response to therapy.

Potential Complications

Potential complications include hemorrhage, infection, vascular complications, and equipment-related complications. (See "Potential Complications of Invasive Hemodynamic Monitoring Lines" on page 350 and Table 10-2.)

Multilumen Central Venous Catheters

For insertion and care of the central venous catheter, see Chapters 3 and 4.

Central venous access is useful for rapid administration of fluids, blood, and blood products; titration of medications; and administration of total parenteral nutrition (TPN). To minimize the potential for infusion incompatibilities, the nurse should reserve one of the catheter lumens for TPN. In the critical care setting, use of the multilumen subclavian catheter is usually on a short-term basis. The multilumen subclavian catheter may be used to monitor right atrial pressure (RAP) and/or central venous pressure (CVP).

Table 10-2 Potential cardiac complications and interventions

Complication	Causes and Indications	Interventions
Arrhythmias Transient PVCs and short runs of VT	Irritation of myocardium	Observe ECG. Notify the physician. Physician may reposition.
Persistent ectopy	Kinking or looping in the RV	May require antiarrhythmics.
Spontaneous wedge	PAC tip migrates forward into "wedge" position	Ensure balloon is deflated. Flex/extend arm. Reposition (side to side). Encourage cough. Suction, if appropriate. Notify the physician. Pull the catheter back until PAP tracing observed.*
Risk of pulmonary infarction or rupture	PAP replaced by permanent PAWP tracing	Monitor ECG for lethal arrhythmias. Inflate balloon and monitor for return of PAP. Notify the physician. Pull the catheter back until the RA tracing is observed.*
Migration of the catheter tip backward into RV May cause lethal arrhythmias	PAP replaced by RV tracing (RV should only be seen during insertion)	

*Clinical Alert: Always deflate the balloon before withdrawing the catheter. Pulling the catheter back with the balloon inflated can cause severe valvular and myocardial damage. Hospital policy should be followed regarding manipulation of the pulmonary artery catheter. Some hospitals allow only physicians to manipulate these catheters.

ECG, Electrocardiogram; *PA,* pulmonary artery; *PAC,* pulmonary artery catheter; *PAP,* pulmonary artery pressure; *PAWP,* pulmonary artery wedge pressure; *PVC,* premature ventricular contractions; *RA,* right atrium; *RV,* right ventricle; *VT,* ventricular tachycardia. *Continued*

Table 10-2   Potential cardiac complications and interventions—cont'd

Complication	Causes and Indications	Interventions
Migration of RA port forward into RV	Often seen with cardiomyopathies Not serious RA replaced by RV tracing	Notify the physician to reposition catheter.
Overwedge	Overinflation of balloon Catheter advanced too far (inflated requires <1 ml to obtain PAWP tracing)	Inflate slowly and stop when PAWP tracing observed. Verify location with chest x-ray film. Notify the physician to reposition catheter.
Balloon rupture	Duration/frequency of use Manual deflation of balloon Indicated by loss of resistance to inflation, inability to obtain PAWP tracing, or lack of passive deflation	Limit frequency of inflations. Tape end of syringe to prevent further attempts. Label as "broken balloon." Report to physician.
Pulmonary infarct	Distal movement of catheter into "wedge" position Embolization of thrombus	Monitor waveform for spontaneous wedge. Maintain continuous flush of pressure lines.
Pulmonary artery rupture Death may occur owing to pulmonary hemorrhage	Arterial wall punctured by catheter tip Balloon overinflation in small branch of PA Sudden hemoptysis with bright red blood	Verify placement with chest x-ray film. Limit frequency of inflation. Stop inflation when PAWP tracing observed. If suspected, put in decubitus position (bleeding lung down). Notify the physician. Discontinue anticoagulant therapy as ordered.

- RAP/CVP is representative of the preload of the right side of the heart.
- RAP/CVP is an indicator of fluid status (preload): if inadequate, the value is low and if excessive, the value is high.

Pulmonary Artery Catheter

The basic multilumen, flow-directed, balloon-tipped PAC (Fig. 10-7) is preferably inserted through the right internal jugular vein for access to venous circulation. The PAC is guided through the right atrium (RA) and right ventricle of the heart and into the pulmonary artery (PA). Variables measured by the PAC are right- and left-sided heart pressures and thermodilution cardiac output (CO).

The PAC comes in various lengths, sizes, and types. Special PACs have pacing capability, continuously monitor venous oxygen saturation (Svo_2), right ventricular ejection fraction, or CO, or they may have an antimicrobial coating. Routine direct monitoring of right- and left-sided heart pressures include RAP, CVP, pulmonary artery systolic (PAS) pressure, pulmonary artery diastolic (PAD) pressure, and pulmonary artery wedge pressure (PAWP). Thermodilution CO and blood sampling to measure mixed venous oxygen saturation (Mvo_2) can be done via the standard PAC. Noninvasive hemodynamic monitoring is possible by impedance cardiography. Clinical research to demonstrate reliability and validity of this new technology continues.

The value of routine use of the PAC in the critical care setting was questioned in a published report in the *Journal of the American Medical Association*. The report suggested an increase in resource utilization and mortality related to PAC use. As a result of the report, the value of the PAC in improving outcomes was questioned. A consensus conference on PACs to address the issue has suggested the following general clinical indications for PAC use (Box 10-1).

Site Selection for PAC Insertion

The patient's diagnosis, mechanism of injury, surgical procedure, and/or physician preference may indicate the choice of insertion sites. The most commonly used sites are the right internal jugular, subclavian, or femoral arteries.

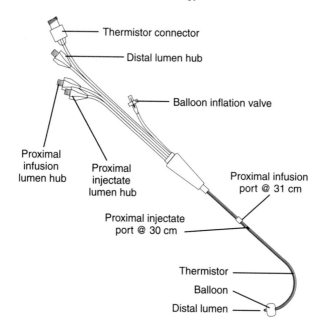

Fig. 10-7

Pulmonary artery catheter. The proximal injectate lumen hub is attached to a pressure line to measure right atrial CVP. This also is the hub where the solution will be injected to measure CO. The injectate solution will exit at the proximal injectate port, located in the right atrium.

(From Peter R, Lichtenthal MD: *Baxter quick guide to cardiopulmonary care,* Baxter Healthcare Corporation, 1998; in Swan-Ganz Catheter Reference Section. CCOmbo, Paceport, Swan-Ganz are registered trademarks of Baxter International, Inc. AMC THROMBOSHIELD and VIP are trademarks of Baxter International Inc.)

Pulmonary Artery Lumens and Ports

Ports of the PAC have specific uses depending on the port exit locations (see Fig. 10-7).

1. The PA (distal) port is used to measure systolic and diastolic pulmonary artery pressure.

   NOTE: The PA port is the blood sampling port for mixed venous gases to monitor Mvo_2.

Box 10-1   General Indications: Standard Pulmonary
Artery Catheter

General indications for using the pulmonary artery catheter
have been defined for patients in cardiac surgery. They
include

Patients Undergoing Coronary Artery Bypass Grafts, Who Have

- Poor LV function; LVEDP >18 mm Hg; LV ejection fraction <40%
- LV wall motion abnormalities
- Recent myocardial infarction (MI) (<6 months) or complications of MI
- Severe preoperative angina
- >75% left main coronary artery disease

Patients with

- Valvular disease
- Pulmonary hypertension
- Complex cardiac lesions
- Combined cardiac and valve procedures
- Older than 65 years
- Concomitant systemic diseases

Data from Hensley FA, Martin DE: *A practical approach to cardiac anesthesia,*
ed 2, Boston, 1995, Little, Brown; Controversies in pulmonary artery catheteriza-
tion. Pulmonary artery catheter consensus statement, *New Horizons* 175-194;
Lichtenthal PR: *Baxter quick guide to cardiopulmonary care,* Baxter Healthcare
Corporation, 1998; in Swan-Ganz Catheter Reference Section, pages 63-64.
Swan-Ganz is a registered trademark of Baxter International, Inc.

Continued

CLINICAL ALERT: Use of the distal PA lumen/port for
administration of IV fluids or medications may cause vasospasm
and PA rupture.

2. RA proximal (injectate) port assesses RAP/CVP and is used
   for administration of IV fluids or intermittent medications.
   The proximal injectate port should not be used to infuse
   vasoactive drugs or other continuous infusion drugs such as
   insulin. The proximal port is used for CO measurement. If the
   port has been used for continuous medication infusion,
   interrupting the infusion to obtain the CO would result in the
   patient receiving a bolus of medication.

Box 10-1   General Indications: Standard Pulmonary
Artery Catheter—cont'd

Cardiovascular Disease

- MI with hypotension or cardiogenic shock, mechanical complications, or right ventricular infarction
- Congestive heart failure
- Pulmonary hypertension
- Shock or hemodynamic instability

Perioperative Period

- Cardiac surgery, high risk
- Peripheral vascular surgery (reduced complications, reduced mortality)
- Aortic surgery, low or high risk
- Neurosurgery
- Trauma

Sepsis/Septic Shock

Supranormal Oxygen Delivery

- SIRS, high-risk surgery

Respiratory Failure

Pediatric Patients (Certain Patients and Conditions)

Data from Hensley FA, Martin DE: *A practical approach to cardiac anesthesia,* ed 2, Boston, 1995, Little, Brown; Controversies in pulmonary artery catheterization. Pulmonary artery catheter consensus statement, *New Horizons* 175-194, 1997; Lichtenthal PR: *Baxter quick guide to cardiopulmonary care,* Baxter Healthcare Corporation, 1998; in Swan-Ganz Catheter Reference Section, pages 63-64. Swan-Ganz is a registered trademark of Baxter International, Inc.

3. The balloon gate valve monitors PAWP by "floating" the catheter, via the balloon located at the distal tip of the PAC, into a small branch of the PA. Use the volume-limited, 1.5-ml syringe provided with the PAC. Use of another syringe is not recommended. A larger syringe would increase the amount of air used to inflate the balloon, which could cause balloon and/or pulmonary artery rupture.

4. The thermistor port is located approximately 3 cm from the catheter tip. The catheter measures CO by sensing the change in the temperature as the injectate flows over the thermistor.

The thermistor can continuously monitor core body temperature. A time saving tip is to keep the pressure cable connected to the thermistor connector. Core body temperature is considered the most accurate.

Insertion of the PAC

Follow hospital procedure for insertion of the PAC and use of fluoroscopy during the insertion of the catheter.

1. Explain the procedure to the patient and family.
2. Ensure that informed consent has been obtained.
3. Provide sedation and pain medication as appropriate.
4. Assemble supplies for PAC insertion. Refer to the physician's procedure preference for other supplies.
5. Assemble the pressure transducer system and flush solution for the PA distal and proximal injectate lumens. Prepare setup and flush solution per hospital policy. See pages 326 to 330 for specific steps to set up the pressure transducer system.
6. Prime the pressure transducer system. Eliminate all air bubbles in tubing and stopcocks.
7. Before insertion, the physician will prime the RA and PA ports of the PAC. The PA distal and RA proximal injectate ports are then connected to the transducer tubings.
8. The cordis is inserted into the subclavian, jugular, or femoral vein, and the PAC is advanced into the RA. The cordis (also known as the *introducer* or *bloodless port*) is a large-bore introducer through which the catheter is passed at the time of insertion. It is not part of the PAC. The exit of the cordis lumen terminates in the superior vena cava just above the RA. The lumen of the cordis may be used as an additional site to rapidly give fluid boluses or blood. Medications that are not compatible or need frequent titration such as nitroprusside or insulin infusion can be given via the cordis.
9. The balloon of the PAC is inflated in the RA. The catheter floats through the tricuspid valve into the right ventricle. Rapidly advancing the catheter through the pulmonic valve into the PA reduces the possibility of right ventricular irritation. The balloon is deflated, and PAP measurements are recorded.
10. The right atrial, right ventricular, PA, and PAWP waveforms will be displayed on the bedside monitor as the catheter is

advanced through the right side of the heart and to the PA (Fig. 10-8). The physician and the nurse should observe the waveforms to monitor progression and position of the catheter. Document waveforms per hospital policy.

CLINICAL ALERT: Ventricular arrhythmia may occur during insertion as the catheter passes through the right ventricle. Monitor the electrocardiogram (ECG) continuously during insertion. Keep emergency drugs at the bedside during the procedure.

11. Verify PAP waveforms.
12. Interpret all pressures at the end of expiration. The pressures can be altered by changes in intrapleural pressures during inspiration and expiration.
13. Obtain the PAWP.
    a. Detach the volume-limited syringe from the balloon port and draw up 1.5 ml of air. Reconnect the syringe to the balloon port.
    b. Slowly inflate the balloon until a PAWP tracing is observed.
    c. Obtain PAWP at end expiration. Place a bedside monitor to scale, freeze the waveform, and record a paper tracing. Determine PAWP after analysis of the waveform.
    d. The PAWP is obtained when the PA balloon is inflated, and the catheter floats to "wedge" in a small branch of the PA. While the balloon is inflated, transmission of pressure from the right side of the heart is blocked, permitting documentation of pressures on the left side of the heart. The PAWP is a left atrial tracing that is used as an indicator of left ventricular end-diastolic pressure (LVEDP).

CLINICAL ALERT: The waveform must be observed closely on the monitor throughout the procedure to prevent overinflation. Inflation is stopped as soon as the PAWP tracing is observed and should not exceed 15 seconds. Inflation should require 1.25 to 1.5 ml of air. Use only the amount of air needed to inflate the balloon and obtain a waveform. Document the volume of air needed to produce the waveform. If more or less air is required, assess the location of the catheter. If the PAWP is within 1 to 4 mm Hg of the PAD, monitor the trend of the PAD. Frequent inflation of the balloon could cause balloon and/or PA rupture.

    e. Detach the syringe from the balloon port and allow the balloon to passively deflate. Never aspirate the air

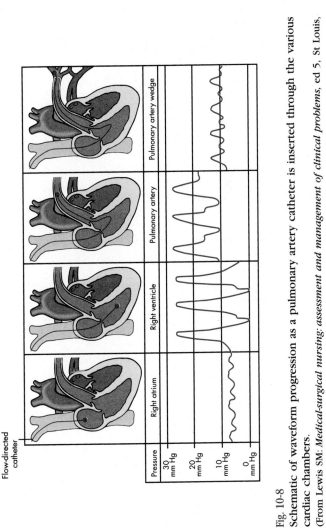

Fig. 10-8
Schematic of waveform progression as a pulmonary artery catheter is inserted through the various cardiac chambers.
(From Lewis SM: *Medical-surgical nursing: assessment and management of clinical problems*, ed 5, St Louis, 2000, Mosby.

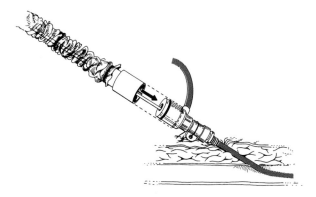

Fig. 10-9
After the sterile sheath has been secured to the catheter, the "sterile" portion can be distinguished from the "contaminated" portion of the catheter.
(From Butterworth JF: Pulmonary artery catheterization. In *Atlas of procedures in anesthesia and critical care*, Philadelphia, 1992, WB Saunders.)

    through the syringe as this may cause the balloon to rupture.

f. Verify return of the PAP waveform. The frequency of monitoring will depend on the hemodynamic stability of the patient.

g. The PAC is advanced through a sterile sheath (Fig. 10-9) and connected to the introducer. The catheter remains sterile inside the introducer. If at any time, fluid is noted inside the sheath or the integrity of the sheath is interrupted, contact the physician for replacement of the entire system.

h. Follow hospital policy regarding manipulation of the catheter after insertion.

i. A chest x-ray film is required after insertion to verify correct placement of the catheter.

j. Document the cm marking of the PAC as it exits the introducer. If the PAP and waveforms change in configuration, verify to see whether the cm marking is the same as previously noted. The catheter may have inadvertently been pulled back during patient repositioning.

Obtaining PAC Pressure Values

Protocols for Practice from the American Association of Critical Care suggest recording waveforms and determining pressure values from the paper strip recordings. Analysis of the waveform components provides the most accurate data versus recording the digital value on the monitor.

Maintenance

- Follow hospital policy regarding site care and dressing changes.
- Follow-up with chest x-ray films to verify placement is done according to hospital policy.
- Monitor PAP waveforms continuously.
- Monitor trends in hemodynamic variables. Note changes in titration of medications, therapy, and interventions to allow for assessment of their effect.
- Maintain aseptic technique when manipulating system. Keep dead-end caps on all ports at all times.
- Change pulmonary artery catheter per hospital policy. The CDC guidelines for prevention of intravascular device-related infections recommends tubing changes every 72 to 96 hours.

Potential Complications

The PAC is an invasive technology. Complications specific to PACs include arrhythmias, spontaneous wedge, catheter migration, overwedge, knotting or kinking of the catheter, balloon rupture, pulmonary infarction, and pulmonary rupture (see Table 10-2). Complications can be life-threatening and may require surgical intervention.

CLINICAL ALERT: Follow hospital policy regarding removal of the PAC. After competency validation, a registered nurse may be permitted to remove the catheter. Always allow the balloon to passively deflate before withdrawing the catheter. Pulling an inflated balloon through a valve can cause severe valvular and myocardial damage.

Thermodilution Cardiac Output

Obtaining a thermodilution CO measurement is the method most commonly used in critical care. A bolus of room temperature or iced fluid is injected into the proximal injectate port of the PAC. The thermistor located at the distal end of the PAC registers the change in blood temperature over time, and the CO waveform is displayed on the monitor. Continuous monitoring of CO can be done with a special thermodilution catheter and computer equipment. Research continues to establish the reliability and validity of continuous CO monitoring.

Equipment

1. CO pressure cable with the injectate temperature probe
2. Sterile, prepackaged, closed CO injectate system
3. IV solution for injectate, per hospital policy
    a. Verify with the physician the amount of the CO injectate to use for the patient receiving fluid restriction. Dextrose 5% in water (D_5W) is recommended because the specific gravity of D_5W is a constant in the formula used to determine the CO by the thermodilution method. Consider use of NS if the patient is hyponatremic or has an elevated blood glucose.
    b. Verify injectate solution with the physician. Use of a consistent amount of injectate and type of injectate solution promotes good technique.
4. Label for IV fluid and tubing
5. Ice slush (if using iced injectate)

Procedure

1. Record a complete set of vital signs and hemodynamic parameters before beginning the CO sequence.
2. Ensure that height and weight have been entered correctly on the bedside monitor.
3. Level the zero reference stopcock at the phlebostatic axis. Document patient position.
4. Explain the procedure to the patient/family.
5. Assemble the injectate system according to the package insert.
6. Label the IV bag with solution type, amount, date, and time.
7. Spike the IV bag with the injectate system tubing.
8. Remove all the air from the bag and the drip chamber by squeezing the bag while holding it upside down.
9. Prime the tubing.
10. Hang the bag on the IV pole.
11. If using iced injectate, place the coiled portion of the tubing in the ice slush solution.

12. Attach the injectate syringe to the proximal injectate port of the PAC.
13. Connect the CO pressure cable to the bedside monitor, injectate syringe, and thermistor port.
14. Follow the manufacturer's procedure for measuring CO on the bedside monitor.

CLINICAL ALERT: Ensure that the computation constant is correct for the catheter in use, the amount of the injectate, and room temperature or iced injectate. A computation constant must be entered into the monitor before obtaining the CO. The computation constant is a correction factor for variances noted earlier. Computation constants may be noted on the package insert of the PAC or are available from the manufacturer.

15. Record three CO waveforms. Assess the waveforms. CO values within 10% are considered acceptable. Delete waveforms and values outside the acceptable range. It may be necessary to perform additional measurements. The acceptable CO waveforms are averaged.
16. Perform calculation step per monitor guidelines. Verify physician preference for indexed values. Turn index *on* or *off* as appropriate. Indexed values account for the patient's body size.
17. Print a copy of waveforms and calculations. Document per hospital policy.
18. Document patient position, amount of injectate and medications, and other therapies at the time of the CO.

Potential Complications

Potential complications specific to the thermodilution CO procedure include fluid overload, arrhythmias caused by irritation from the cold injectate, and inadvertent bolus of medications if this injectate port is used for continuous medication infusion.

CLINICAL ALERT: Poor technique results in inaccurate data. Use the same injectate volume. Verify the dynamic compliance of the pressure transducer system. Level to the phlebostatic axis before obtaining PAP. Verify the computation constant, height, and weight.

PAPs, PAWP, and CO are affected by high levels of positive end-expiratory pressure (PEEP) (>10 cm H_2O) during mechanical ventilation. Inform the physician of the use of a high level of PEEP when communicating hemodynamic variables.

Potential Complications of Invasive Hemodynamic Monitoring Lines

- *Hemorrhage:* The most common complication associated with arterial lines is hemorrhage. A hematoma may be the result of insufficient pressure applied for an adequate time after removal of the arterial line. Pressure must be applied a minimum of 5 to 10 minutes after removal of the radial arterial catheter. Closely observe the insertion site in patients with bleeding disorders and those receiving anticoagulants or thrombolytics. Exsanguination can occur if the tubing becomes disconnected or the catheter is dislodged. Rapid exsanguination can be fatal.
- *Infection:* Strategies to prevent infection include the use of aseptic technique with manipulation of the system, maintenance of a closed system with dead-end caps on all stopcocks, and use of in-line blood reservoir systems. Surgery, trauma, disease processes, medications, and treatments often suppress the immune system of critically ill patients. Multiple invasive lines also place them at a high risk for infection. Signs and symptoms of infection at the insertion site include tenderness, erythema, swelling, and purulent drainage. Infection may become systemic. Monitor trends in temperature elevation and laboratory values for an elevated white blood cell count. If the catheter (arterial catheter, multilumen central venous catheter, or PAC) is suspected to be the cause, catheter use must be discontinued and the catheter tip sent to the laboratory for culture and sensitivity. Also, obtain culture and sensitivity of the insertion site if there is drainage present.
- *Vascular complications:* Vessel occlusion caused by thrombosis or embolism can result in ischemia or necrosis of the cannulated extremity. Evidence of ischemia is a diminished or absent distal pulse, pain, paresthesias, and/or pallor. If the ischemia continues, the skin color will become progressively mottled.

Clinical Significance of Hemodynamic Parameters (Table 10-3)

The pressures measured by the PAC can assess right- and left-sided heart function and fluid volume status. CO and cardiac index (CI) provide information about overall cardiac function. CI is considered a better indicator of cardiac function because it is based on the

Table 10-3   Hemodynamic parameters

Hemodynamic Parameter	Normal Range*	Method of Obtaining or Calculation
Mean arterial pressure (MAP)	70-105 mm Hg	$\dfrac{(2 \times \text{Diastole}) + \text{Systole}}{3}$
Right atrial pressure (RAP)	2-6 mm Hg	Measured by RA port of PAC as a mean pressure
Pulmonary artery systolic pressure (PAS)	15-25 mm Hg	Measured by distal lumen of PAC
Pulmonary artery diastolic pressure (PAD)	8-15 mm Hg	Measured by distal lumen of PAC
Pulmonary artery mean pressure (PAM)	10-20 mm Hg	$\dfrac{(2 \times \text{PAD}) + \text{PAS}}{3}$
Pulmonary artery wedge pressure (PAWP)	6-12 mm Hg	Measured by distal lumen of PAC with balloon inflated
Cardiac output (CO)	4-8 L/min	Heart rate (HR) $\times$ SV Measured with thermodilution method
Cardiac index (CI)	2.5-4.0 L/min/m^2	$\dfrac{\text{CO}}{\text{Body surface area (BSA)}}$

*The normal range for hemodynamic parameters varies slightly between references. The values provided are meant only as a guide. Consult hospital policy for standard values.

Continued

Table 10-3   Hemodynamic parameters—cont'd

Hemodynamic Parameter	Normal Range*	Method of Obtaining or Calculation
Stroke volume (SV)	60-100 ml/beat	$\dfrac{CO}{HR} \times 1000$
Stroke volume index (SVI)	33-47 ml/beat/m^2	$\dfrac{SV}{BSA}$
Systemic vascular resistance (SVR)	800-1400 dynes/s/cm^{-5}	$\dfrac{MAP - RAP}{CO} \times 80$
Systemic vascular resistance index (SVRI)	1970-2390 dynes/s/cm^{-5}	$\dfrac{MAP - RAP}{CI} \times 80$
Pulmonary vascular resistance (PVR)	<250 dynes/s/cm^{-5}	$\dfrac{PAM - PWP}{CO} \times 80$
Pulmonary vascular resistance index (PVRI)	255-285 dynes/s/cm^{-5}/m^2	$\dfrac{PAM - PWP}{CI} \times 80$
Right ventricular stroke work index (RVSWI)	5-10 g-m/m^2/beat	$SVI \times (PAM - RAP) \times 0.0136$
Left ventricular stroke work index (LVSWI)	50-62 g-m/m^2/beat	$SVI \times (MAP - PWP) \times 0.0136$

patient's body size. It is vital that the height and weight, computation constant, and recorded PAPs are accurate before beginning a thermodilution CO.

Monitoring patterns and trends of vital signs and hemodynamic variables in relationship to medications and interventions provides the clinician a picture of the patient's condition, which is either improving or deteriorating.

Preload, Afterload, and Contractility

Phrases you may hear in a critical care unit are "filling pressures" or "we need to unload the patient." What do they mean?

Preload is the amount of blood in the ventricles at the end of diastole. This is the filling pressure. It is the amount of blood available for the stroke volume (SV) of the CO. *Right ventricular (RV) preload* is obtained by monitoring the RAP/CVP. It is a variable that indicates fluid volume status and right-sided heart function. *Left ventricular (LV) preload* is obtained by monitoring the PAWP and PAD. When a PAD gradient is greater than 4 mm Hg, factors other than preload should be considered as the etiology. The cause may have a respiratory component such as hypoxia, chronic obstructive pulmonary disease, or adult respiratory distress syndrome. Under these conditions, PAD would not be of value in determining LV preload. The PAWP is not affected by these conditions.

Afterload is the amount of resistance to ejection of blood from the ventricles. Afterload is increased with vasoconstriction. In conditions of vasodilation, the afterload resistance is less. *RV afterload* is measured by a pulmonary vascular resistance (PVR) calculation on CO. *LV afterload* is measured by a systemic vascular resistance (SVR) calculation on CO.

Contractility is the force the heart muscle is able to generate to produce myocardial contraction. *Right ventricular stroke work index* (RVSWI) is a calculated value for right-sided contractility. *Left ventricular stroke work index* (LVSWI) is a calculated value for left-sided contractility. The nurse should verify the physician's preference regarding whether the index is off or on when calculating cardiac output variables. Indexed values account for the patient's body size.

Cardiac output is calculated as follows:

$$CO = HR \text{ (heart rate)} \times SV$$

CO is the amount of blood ejected from the heart over time. It is measured in liters per minute. Preload, afterload, and contractility affect SV.

Fluid and Drug Therapy in Critical Care

Fluid resuscitation and initiation and titration of IV medications are part of the management of a patient in a critical care unit. Complications may include cardiac or respiratory arrest, cardiogenic shock, systemic inflammatory response syndrome (SIRS), sepsis, or multiple organ dysfunction syndrome (MODS). Patients may require fluid resuscitation and/or drug therapy. To maximize oxygen delivery and oxygen consumption at the cellular level, consideration is usually given to administration of fluids first. Second, based on the patient's hemoglobin value, administration of blood may be necessary. Finally, initiation and titration of drug therapy will be based on the hemodynamic variables and laboratory results. The goal of therapy is to prevent the development of MODS.

The ongoing nursing assessment would include determination of the patient's volume status. Is there inadequate or excess preload? Can the patient tolerate fluid resuscitation?

The nurse should assess hemodynamic parameters, RAP/CVP, PAP, PAWP, and CO, which reflect both volume and cardiovascular status. The pattern and trend of these parameters should be monitored and the patient's physical assessment and laboratory results reviewed. The nurse should monitor ABGs, electrolytes, complete blood count, and coagulation status as appropriate. The information should be shared with the physician to help guide fluid resuscitation, administration of blood and/or blood components, and drug administration in the critically ill patient.

Actions of IV medications administered in critical care include vasoconstriction, vasodilation, affects on the force of myocardial contractility, changes in heart rate, or treatment of arrhythmias, which affect cardiac output. The following IV medication categories are some of the most common used in critical care (Table 10-4).

■ Antiarrhythmic drugs slow conduction through the atrioventricular (AV) node, can interrupt reentry pathways through the AV node, and decrease the rise of the depolarization phase of the action potential. Drugs in this category include adenosine, amrinone, atropine, bretylium, digoxin, isoproterenol HCl, lidocaine, procainamide, and quinidine.

Text continued on p. 370

Table 10-4 Selected cardiovascular drugs

Drug	Dosage	Infusion	Dilution/ Concentration	Therapeutic Monitoring	Comments
Adenosine (antiarrhythmia)	IV bolus 6 mg; may give 12 mg IV bolus × 2	IV bolus over 1 min; flush IV access with 10 ml NS	Follow manufacturer's guidelines.	Half-life 30 sec	*Contraindications:* second- or third-degree heart block, AV block, atrial flutter/fibrillation, ventricular tachycardia. Monitor BP continuously for fluctuations or ECG changes.

ALT, Alanine aminotransferase; *AST,* aspartate aminotransferase; *BP,* blood pressure; *CNS,* central nervous system; *CVC,* central venous catheter; D_5R, dextrose 5% in Ringer's solution; $D_5NS,$ dextrose 5% in normal saline; $D_5W,$ dextrose 5% in water; *EENT,* eyes, ears, nose, and throat; *GI,* gastrointestinal system; *LR,* lactated Ringer's solution; *NS,* normal saline; *P,* pulse; *PVC,* polyvinyl chloride; *R,* respirations.
Continued

Table 10-4   Selected cardiovascular drugs—cont'd

Drug	Dosage	Infusion	Dilution/ Concentration	Therapeutic Monitoring	Comments
Amrinone (Inocor) (cardiac inotropic)	IV bolus 0.75 mg/kg given over 2-3 min; then infusion 5-10 µg/kg/ min	IV bolus then IV infusion via IV pump	Follow manu-facturer's guidelines; do not mix with glucose directly.	Onset 2-5 min, peak 10 min; half-life 4-6 hr	Incompatible with furosemide and dextrose solution for direct dilution; monitor BP, P, Q5min during the drug infusion. Monitor hypotension cardiac glyco-sides, ALT, AST, bilirubin daily.
Atropine (antiarrhythmia and bradycar-dia)	IV bolus 0.5-1 mg every 3-5 min; dose not to exceed 2 mg	IV bolus	May administer undiluted in urgent need; may dilute in 10 ml NS at rate of 0.5 mg/ min.	IV peak 2-4 min; half-life 2-3 hr	Incompatible with multiple medica-tions. Evaluate ther-apeutic effects; monitor vital signs, cardiac status, and rhythm continu-ously during IV dosing.

| Bretylium tosylate (antiarrhythmia agent for ventricular fibrillation, ventricular tachycardia) | Initial dose 5-10 mg/kg up to 30 mg/kg; continuous IV infusion 1-4 mg/min (1 g/250 ml) | IV bolus over 10 minutes; repeat as needed 15-30 min up to 30 mg/kg. If continuous infusion use IV pump. | Dilute 500 mg in 50 ml NS or D₅W. Infuse over 10-30 min. Continuous infusion: dilute 1 g/250 ml; infuse 1-4 mg/min. | Onset 5 min | Monitor cardiac status/rhythm and vital signs continuously during drug dosing. Drug may cause severe nausea and vomiting, respiratory depression, or rebound hypertension after 1-2 hr. |
| Digoxin (antiarrhythmia) | IV bolus 0.5 mg over 5 min | IV bolus | Use in IV undiluted or 1 mg of drug in 4 ml NS or D₅W. | Onset 5-30 min; 0.8-2.0 ng/ml immediately before next dose every 7 days | Assess apical pulse for 1 min before drug administration. Monitor CNS (headache), GI (nausea and vomiting, anorexia, diarrhea), EENT (blurred vision, diplopia, and muscle weakness); intake and output, daily weights, and therapeutic drug level. |

Continued

Table 10-4   Selected cardiovascular drugs—cont'd

Drug	Dosage	Infusion	Dilution/ Concentration	Therapeutic Monitoring	Comments
Diltiazem (Cardizem) (calcium channel blocker)	Usual IV bolus dose 0.25 mg/kg body weight; second bolus 0.35 mg/kg in 15 min; infusion 5-15 mg/hr based on patient response	Continuous infusion via infusion pump, after bolus therapy	Dilute 250 mg (50 ml)/250 ml in D_5W or NS. Verify agency policy.	Onset 3 min; peaks 2-7 min	Monitor ECG and BP (hypotensive side effect).
Dobutamine HCl (vasopressor)	Infusion 2.5-10 µg/kg/min up to 40 µg/kg/min	Continuous infusion via IV pump	Dilute 250 mg/10 ml of D5W or NS, then further dilute in 50 ml or more. Titrate dose.	Onset 1-5 min; peak 10 min	Incompatible with acyclovir, amphotericin B, cephalothin, gentamicin, and sodium bicarbonate. Monitor vital signs, cardiac status/

					rhythm continuously during drug infusion. Evaluate therapeutic response.
Dopamine HCl (vasopressor)	Begin infusion at 10 μg/kg/min for severe hypotension or 0.5-2 μg for renal perfusion	Continuous infusion via IV pump	Use NS, D_5W, LR, 2 g in 500 ml solution for 4 mg/ml.	Onset 5 min; duration <10 min	Incompatible with acyclovir, amphotericin B, cephalothin, gentamicin, and sodium bicarbonate. Monitor vital, cardiac status/rhythm Q5min during initial infusion; thereafter, on a scheduled frequency. Evaluate therapeutic response. Monitor CVP initial infusion.

Continued

Table 10-4   Selected cardiovascular drugs—cont'd

Drug	Dosage	Infusion	Dilution/ Concentration	Therapeutic Monitoring	Comments
Epinephrine HCl (Adrenalin chloride) (cardiac stimulant, bronchodilator, vasopressor)	IV bolus dose for cardiac arrest 1.0 mg of 1:10,000 IV solution, may repeat q3-5min, follow each dose with 20 ml IV infusion, flush to ensure drug delivery; intermediate dose 2-5 mg q3-5min; escalating dose 1, 3, 5 mg dosing 3 min apart; high dose 0.1 mg/kg body weight q3-5min	Usually used as vasopressor or maintenance, 1-10 µg/min titrated to desired patient response	1 mg in 500 ml $D_5W = 2$ µg/ml 2 mg in 500 ml $D_5W = 4$ µg/ml (1 mg in 250 ml = 4 µg/ml)	Onset immediate; duration short	Monitor BP q5min. Infusion during cardiac arrest must be administered via CVC. Use cardiac monitor.

Esmolol HCl (Brevibloc) (beta-adrenergic blocker)	IV loading dose 500 µg/kg/min for 1 min; maintenance 50 µg/kg for 4 min. Increase maintenance infusion by 50 µg/kg/min; titrate to patient response.	Continuous infusion via IV pump	Dilute 5 g/20 ml, then dilute in the remaining 480 ml NS, D₅W, D₅R; D₅NS, or 0.45% NaCl.	Onset—rapid; duration—short; half-life 9 min	Incompatible with furosemide and sodium bicarbonate. Do not mix with any drug before full dilution. Monitor vital signs, continuously on initial dosing then on a scheduled frequency. Monitor respiratory status, hypotension, and intake and output. Evaluate therapeutic outcome.

Continued

Table 10-4   Selected cardiovascular drugs—cont'd

Drug	Dosage	Infusion	Dilution/ Concentration	Therapeutic Monitoring	Comments
Isoproterenol HCl (Isuprel) (antiarrhythmia)	IV 0.02-0.06 or 5 μg/min	5-10 μg continuous infusion via IV pump	Infuse 1 mg/250 ml D_5W.	Onset rapid; duration ~10 min	Incompatible with aminophylline, barbiturates, carbenicillin, epinephrine, lidocaine, and sodium bicarbonate. Monitor BP, P, R continuously; monitor for cardiac arrest or bronchospasms.
Labetalol (Nomodyne, Trandate) (antihypertensive)	Usual IV bolus dose 20 mg over 2 min; may repeat 40-80 mg q10min, *not* to exceed 300 mg	Continuous infusion via infusion pump 200 mg/160 ml D_5W. Infuse at 2 ml/min; stop infusion at desired response; repeat q6-8h as needed.	200 mg of drug in 160 ml solution = 1 mg/ml; 300 mg/240 ml = 1 mg/ml; 200 mg/259 ml = 2 mg/3 ml.	Onset 2-5 min; peaks 8 min	Monitor ECG and BP.

Lidocaine (antiarrhythmia)	Initial dose 1-1.5 mg/kg; then 0.5 mg/kg to maximum 3 mg/kg	Continuous infusion 2-4 mg/min via IV pump	2 g/500 ml D_5W = 4 mg/ml 1 g 500 ml D_5W = 2 mg/ml 2 g/250 ml D_5W = 8 mg/ml concentration	Onset 2 min; duration 20 min 6-12 hr after starting continuous IV infusion; 1.5-5 µg/ml	Monitor ECG and BP continuously for fluctuations. Incompatible with ampicillin, cefazolin, phenytoin, and blood. Evaluate therapeutic response; monitor intake and output, respiratory depression, and cardiovascular response.

Continued

Table 10-4   Selected cardiovascular drugs—cont'd

Drug	Dosage	Infusion	Dilution/ Concentration	Therapeutic Monitoring	Comments
Mannitol (osmotic diuretic)	IV 300-400 mg/kg of 20%-25% solution up to 100 g of a 15%-20% solution for oliguria; IV 1.5-2 g/kg of 15%-25% solution over 30-60 min for intracranial pressure; 50-200 g/24 hr for renal failure to maintain output 30-50 ml/hr	IV 15%-25% solution with filter over 30-90 min; *test dose in severe oliguria;* 0.2 g/kg over 3-5 min; may repeat ×2; if no urine response, reassess patient	Follow manufacturer's guidelines.	Onset 30-60 min for diuresis; 30-90 min for intraocular pressure	Incompatible with whole blood, potassium, and sodium chloride. Monitor CNS status, vital signs, and intake and output. Evaluate therapeutic response.

Drug	Dosage	Administration	Dilution	Onset/Peak	Considerations
Milrinone (Primacor) (cardiac inotropic, similar to Inocar)	IV bolus 0.375-0.75 µg/kg/min. Loading dose may be given undiluted.	Continuous infusion via infusion pump	Verify drug resource for diluent/desired infusion concentration information.	Onset 5-15 min; peaks 1-2 hr	Monitor ECG. Use with caution in impaired renal function. Monitor platelets and potassium and response to therapy: CO/CI, PAWP, CVP, and BP.
Nitroglycerin (vasodilator)	IV 5 µg/min; then increase by 5 µg/min q3-5min; if no response after 20 µg/min, increase by 10/20 µg/min until desired response	Continuous infusion via IV pump; use glass bottle and non-PVC tubing; no filters	50 mg/250 ml D_5W = 0.2 mg/ml concentration; 50 mg/500 ml D_5W = 0.1 mg/ml concentration; 100 mg/250 ml = 0.4 mg/ml	Onset—immediate	Incompatible with any drug in solution or syringe; monitor vital signs continuously during initial dosing, then as scheduled. Assess cardiovascular and CNS status.

Continued

Table 10-4 Selected cardiovascular drugs—cont'd

Drug	Dosage	Infusion	Dilution/Concentration	Therapeutic Monitoring	Comments
Nitroprusside (antihypertensive)	5-8 µg/kg min IV continuously	Continuous IV via IV pump	Dissolve 50 mg in 2-3 ml of D_5W; then dilute in 250-1000 ml D_5W.	Onset 1-2 min; duration 1-10 min; half-life 4 days	Incompatible with any drug in solution or syringe. Monitor vital signs, BP, P q5-15min. Assess intake and output, daily weight, and electrolytes. Evaluate therapeutic response.
Norepinephrine (Levophed) (vasopressor)	Initial dose 0.5-1 µg/min; usual range 2-12 µg/min; larger doses up to 30 µg/min if patient remains hypotensive, and blood volume corrected	Continuous infusion via infusion pump	Dilute 4 mg/l L = 4 µg/ml in D_5W; do not use NS	Monitor response q1-2min until stable. Use lowest rate possible; gradually discontinue.	

Phenylephrine (Neo-Synephrine) (vasopressor)	100-180 µg/min initially to stabilize BP; maintenance 20-80 µg/min	Continuous infusion via infusion pump	Dilute 10 mg/500 ml in NS or D_5W.	Immediate; peak unknown	Monitor response q2min until stable; titrate to effect.
Procainamide (Pronestyl) (antiarrhythmia)	IV bolus 100 mg q5min given 20-50 mg/min; not to exceed 500 mg; then IV infusion	Continuous IV infusion via IV pump 2-6 mg/min	Dilute 100 mg/ml D_5W; give 20 mg or less for 1 minute; then dilute 1 g in 250-500 ml D_5W; run at 2-6 mg/min Half-life 3 hr 16-24 hr after starting continuous IV infusion, at 4-8 µg/ml.		Monitor vital signs, BP, and P continuously for fluctuations; monitor ECG to determine increased PR or QRS segments. If these develop, discontinue drug immediately. Monitor intake and output and electrolytes; potential exists for heart block, cardiac arrest.

Continued

Table 10-4 Selected cardiovascular drugs—cont'd

Drug	Dosage	Infusion	Dilution/ Concentration	Therapeutic Monitoring	Comments
Propranolol HCl (Inderal) (antihypertensive)	IV bolus 0.5-3 mg over 1 mg/min; may repeat in 2 min for arrhythmia	Bolus and/or short term (10-15 min) only	Dilute drug in 50 ml NS and infuse 1 mg over 10-15 min	Onset 2 min; peak 15 min; duration 3-6 hr; half-life 3-5 hr	Incompatible with any drug in solution or syringe. Monitor vital signs, BP, and P continuously during IV dosing. Assess intake and output, ECG, and daily weight; watch for hypotension and bronchospasm. Evaluate therapeutic response.
Quinidine (antiarrhythmia)	IV infusion 800 mg in 40 ml D_5W run at 16 mg/min	Continuous infusion via IV pump	Dilute 800 mg into 40 ml or more D5W; give 16 mg or less over 1 min as infusion.	Immediately before next dose, 2-5 μg/ml	Considered incompatible with any drug in solution or syringe. Monitor vital signs, BP, and P continuously for fluctuations; watch ECG to determine

Drug	Dose	Route	Administration	Onset/Peak/Duration	Comments
					increased PR or QRS complex. If these develop, discontinue or reduce drug dose. Evaluate therapeutic response.
Verapamil HCl (calcium channel blocker)	IV bolus 5-10 mg over 2 min; repeat if necessary in 30 min	IV bolus only	Follow manufacturer's guidelines.	Onset 3-5 min; peak 3-5 min; duration 10-20 min	Incompatible with albumin, amphotericin B, ampicillin, dobutamine, hydralazine, mezlocillin, nafcillin, oxacillin, and sodium bicarbonate. Monitor cardiac status BP, P, and ECG; evaluate therapeutic response.

- Antihypertensive drugs directly relax arteriolar and venous smooth muscle, resulting in a reduction in cardiac preload and afterload. Drugs in this category include labetalol, nitroprusside, and propranolol HCl.
- β-Blockers block stimulation of β-adrenergic receptors in the myocardium (which decreases the rate of sinoatrial node discharge, slows conduction of the AV node, and decreases O_2 consumption in the myocardium) and reduce cerebral flow and cerebral perfusion. Esmolol HCl is a β-blocker.
- Calcium channel blockers inhibit calcium ion influx across the cell membrane during cardiac depolarization, produce relaxation of coronary vascular smooth muscle, and dilate coronary arteries. Drugs in this category include diltiazem and verapamil HCl.
- Osmotic diuretics act by increasing osmolarity of the glomerular filtrate, which raises the osmotic pressure of fluid in the renal tubules; by decreasing reabsorption of water and electrolytes; and by increasing urinary output and sodium and chloride excretion. Drugs in this category include mannitol and urea (Ureaphil, Carbamex).
- Vasodilators decrease preload and afterload, which is responsible for decreasing LVEDP and SVR. Drugs in this category include amrinone, milrinone, and nitroglycerin.
- Vasopressors cause increased contractility and increased coronary blood flow and heart rate by acting on β-receptors in the heart. Drugs in this category include dobutamine HCl, dopamine HCl, epinephrine HCl, norepinephrine (Levophed), and phenylephrine (Neo-Synephrine).

CLINICAL ALERT: Consult with the physician, pharmacist, or agency guidelines for drug administration protocols (infusion, solution, dilution/concentration, dosing amounts and frequency, and patient monitoring requirements). The patients' medical diagnosis may require staff competency in advanced drug administration requirements (including staff advanced cardiac life support certification), intensive care patient status, and continual ECG monitoring of the patient during drug dosing/infusion.

Nursing responsibilities for critical care drug administration include the following:

- For safe administration of continuous infusion IV medications in the critical care setting, the nurse should understand actions, indications, dosage, drug compatibility, and method of administration. Review the patient's history for drug allergies. Continue to assess for possible medication side effects.

- Know and practice drug and infusion dose and rate calculation (see Chapter 13).
- Use an infusion pump to administer all vasoactive drugs. Infusion pumps designated for critical care have the capability of dose calculation and allow for careful titration of the drug therapy.
- Document the name of the drug, concentration, rate, and dosage at the time of initiation.
- Document drug titration changes. *Always* document new interventions and the patient's response.
- At all times, the nurse should be able to communicate the dosage of the IV medication the patient is receiving.
- Evaluate the effectiveness of drug therapy based on vital signs, hemodynamic variables, laboratory values, and physical assessment. Communicate these variables to members of the health care team.
- Remember the five rights of medications. They are always the best practice.

CLINICAL ALERT: Always verify the concentration of the new bag of IV medications. If the infusion pump maintains the drug concentration, verify the pump settings. The medication concentration may have been doubled or quadrupled in concentration because of the patient's total fluid intake or fluid restriction.

Documentation of Hemodynamic Monitoring

- The practice of recording the digital values from a bedside monitor may not provide accurate information. *Analyze hemodynamic waveforms.*
- Leveling, patient position, the amount of injectate, medication rates, and ventilator changes can have an impact on the next set of hemodynamic measurements. Do not just fill in the boxes on the flow sheet. *Assess the patient, pressure transducer system, catheters, and waveforms.*
- Record hemodynamic values according to hospital policy. When the patient's condition changes, obtain a complete set of vital signs and hemodynamic measurements, determine intake and

output and rate of all medications, and then call the physician.
- Follow protocol or standing orders for initiation or titration of medications.
- Document the cm marking of the PAC on every shift.
- Document insertion site assessment and pulses as appropriate.

Nursing Diagnoses

- Infection, risk for, related to break in skin integrity, multiple invasive lines, and altered immune function
- Cardiac output, decreased, related to decreased volume, altered vascular tone, impaired contractility
- Pain, related to catheter insertion, immobilization
- Tissue perfusion, altered, related to decreased cardiac output and presence of catheter in vascular bed
- Hemorrhage, risk for related to use of heparinized flush solution, coagulopathies, tubing disconnection
- Fluid volume excess, related to fluid resuscitation, excess fluid maintenance, impaired renal function
- Fluid volume deficit, risk for related to decreased fluid intake, gastrointestinal loss of fluid, pharmacological agents
- Injury, risk for, related to complications of hemodynamic monitoring

This chapter provides a brief introduction to hemodynamic monitoring in critical care. The reader is encouraged to refer to more comprehensive texts on hemodynamic monitoring, and treatment of specific illnesses, injury, and/or complications. The author of this chapter would like to acknowledge and thank Shirley Otto for being a mentor and friend.

Resources

Clinical Competency—Vascular Access in Adult Critical Care

	Yes	No	NA
1. Explain procedure to patient and family.			
2. Verify that informed consent has been obtained.			
3. Review the patient's laboratory values and anticoagulation status for variations from normal limits.			
4. Assemble supplies for the specific invasive line insertion. Refer to the physician's specific procedure supply list.			
5. Prime invasive lines with heparinized saline in preparation for insertion.			
6. Assist the physician with the procedure.			
7. Zero, level, and verify dynamic compliance of the pressure transducer system.			
8. Monitor and verify waveforms for arterial blood pressure and hemodynamic monitoring.			
9. Document invasive line insertion, flush solution, concentration volume, and time of infusion and/or other intermittent medications infused.			
10. Apply pressure to the arterial site at least 5 minutes after the arterial line has been discontinued.			
11. Verify concentration of the drug and calculate drug dose.			

Continued

Clinical Competency—Vascular Access in Adult Critical Care—cont'd

	Yes	No	NA
12. Set up the infusion pump and verify pump settings, drug, concentration, time, and volume for infusion.			
13. Monitor vital signs every 5 to 15 minutes and/or per unit guidelines until the patient is hemo-dynamically stable.			
14. Monitor hemodynamic parameters every hour unless the condition of the patient changes.			
15. Report changes regarding the patient's condition promptly to the physician.			

Study Questions

1. Before collecting a set of hemodynamic variables, it is necessary to:
   a. Level to the patient's position
   b. Rezero the transducer system
   c. Verify the dynamic compliance of the system
   d. Flush the line with heparinized solution

2. Nursing measures that reduce the risk of nosocomial infection in patients receiving hemodynamic monitoring include:
   a. Opening stopcocks to air, ensuring line patency
   b. Cleansing all ports with alcohol three times a day
   c. Using dead-end caps and in-line blood reservoir systems
   d. Changing the flush solution every shift

3. The function of the PA port of the PAC is to:
   a. Monitor PAS and PAD and site for drawing mixed venous blood sample
   b. Serve as an infusion port for intermittent medications
   c. Serve as a port for cardiac output injectate
   d. Monitor core body temperature

4. Nursing practice for safe administration of IV medications via an infusion pump in the critical care setting includes:
   a. Ensuring the five rights of medication administration, verifying drug concentration and dose calculation
   b. Administering medication after bag/concentration is verified by pharmacy personnel to ensure immediate infusion of solution
   c. Ensuring the five rights of medications, verifying drug concentration and drug calculation, validating infusion pump for correct infusion settings
   d. Administering bag/drug concentration verified by pharmacy personnel after validating infusion pump settings

5. The hemodynamic variable that accounts for body size is:
   a. Cardiac index
   b. Cardiac output
   c. Systemic vascular resistance
   d. Pulmonary artery wedge pressure

6. To obtain correct hemodynamic values, the zero reference stopcock should be level with the:
   a. Phlebostatic axis
   b. Catheter insertion site
   c. Head of the bed
   d. Femoral artery

7. Verifying the dynamic compliance of the pressure transducer system ensures that:
   a. Atmospheric and hydrostatic pressure will not affect the system
   b. Patient position and hydrostatic pressure will not affect the system
   c. Patient position changes have not affected the square-wave test
   d. The transducer system will produce an accurate waveform

8. The preferred site for arterial cannulation is the:
   a. Brachial artery
   b. Radial artery
   c. Carotid artery
   d. Femoral artery

9. Clinical features that may indicate occlusion of an artery include:
   a. Absent pulse, erythema
   b. Cool or mottled skin and pulse
   c. Changes in sensation and pulse
   d. Absent pulse, cool or mottled skin

10. Steps to obtain PAWP include:
    a. Using a 5-ml syringe, injecting air, recording digital value on the monitor
    b. Using a volume-limited 1.5-ml syringe, injecting air until PAWP appears on the monitor, recording the value at end expiration, allowing the balloon to passively deflate
    c. Using a volume-limited 1.5-ml syringe, injecting air until PAWP appears on the monitor, recording the value at end expiration
    d. Using a 5-ml syringe, injecting air, recording the value at end expiration

Answers   1. a   2. c   3. a   4. c   5. a   6. a
7. d   8. b   9. d   10. b

Pediatric Intravenous Therapy

11

Objectives

1. Discuss the developmental stages of childhood that influence the practice of pediatric intravenous (IV) therapy.

2. Differentiate between the principles of pediatric and adult fluid and electrolyte balance.

3. Identify the clinical findings that correlate with varying grades of dehydration in pediatric patients.

4. List the criteria used for selecting an intravenous site in pediatric patients.

5. Describe the nursing interventions recommended for pediatric chemotherapy administration.

Providing care for pediatric patients can be a rewarding and challenging experience. IV therapy for these patients presents its own unique challenges. Children require IV therapy for many of the same reasons as adults:

- Medication administration
- Fluid and electrolyte maintenance
- Parenteral nutrition
- Chemotherapy
- Blood transfusions
- Pain management

However, unlike most adults, pediatric patients have not yet developed the cognitive or coping skills necessary to prepare them for many aspects of IV therapy. A basic knowledge of the child's growth and developmental process is a crucial step for nurses to prepare themselves, the patient, and the patient's family for all IV therapy procedures. Table 11-1 lists guidelines for child and family preparation, correlated with the child's age, developmental level, and psychologic characteristics.

The nurse should keep in mind that chronologic age and the stage of psychosocial development in children might not always coincide. Children often temporarily regress to an earlier developmental stage during an illness or hospitalization. It is important to remember that every child is unique, with different life experiences and different reactions to various life events. In the provision of care, safety must prevail as the main concern through every age and stage of the developmental process.

Similarly, the nurse should establish a good rapport with the family and the child, using good communication techniques. Well-informed parents are more likely to remain calm, and the child will cue into this behavior and be less apprehensive about the therapy. Following are recommendations to use when initiating or maintaining pediatric intravenous therapy:

- Explain the procedure and its purpose.
- Encourage questions.
- Allow the parents to decide whether they wish to be present for the procedure.
- Allow the child to remain in a parent's arms as long as possible, for those parents who chose to be present for the procedure.
- Encourage parents to remain close to the child throughout the procedure and to comfort the child by touching, caressing, talking, or singing to the child.
- Avoid doing procedures in the child's room, and opt for a procedure room or neutral room.

CLINICAL ALERT: Never ask the parent to assist with restraining the child for the procedure. Enlist the assistance of a coworker to restrain the child.

The previous chapters in this text have discussed the theoretic and clinical components required for each topic. Fundamental guidelines presented in those chapters for all the various therapies should be followed in providing IV therapy for the child. Additional practice guidelines related to the child's growth and developmental process with physiologic rationale are presented in this chapter. Patient and family teaching for self-care management are incor-

Table 11-1 Guidelines for preparation of child and family for intravenous therapy

Age	Developmental Level	Characteristics	Child/Family Preparation
Infants (birth–1 yr)	Trust versus mistrust: consistent response to needs allows infant to predict responses and develop trust	Fear of separation Fear of strangers Behavior is under reflexive control Uses cry to communicate	Attempt to provide consistent caregivers. Prepare equipment out of view. Avoid feeding child immediately before procedure. Decrease parental anxiety by keeping parents well informed. Minimize parental separation. Never use parents or family members to assist with restraining the child. If feasible, use a procedure room. If parents choose to remain during procedure, encourage tactile and verbal soothing during and after procedure (i.e., cuddling the child).

Continued

Table 11-1 Guidelines for preparation of child and family for intravenous therapy—cont'd

Age	Developmental Level	Characteristics	Child/Family Preparation
Toddlers (1-3 yr)	Autonomy versus shame and doubt; desire to do things independently	Fear of injury Fear of loss of control Fear of the dark Separation anxiety Egocentricity Ritualistic behavior helps to master skills and decrease anxiety Magical thinking Lack of concept of time	Keep security objects close (i.e., teddy bear, blanket). Minimize parenteral separation. Explain only shortly before procedure. Use a calm, quiet tone with simple and honest explanations. If feasible, allow child to handle equipment. Use immediate and concrete rewards (i.e., stickers).
Preschool (4-6 yr)	Initiative versus guilt	Short attention span Tend to mimic behavior Involved in parallel play Developing body image Fears concerning body integrity, loss of control, the dark, being alone	Use pictures, models, dolls, and actual equipment to demonstrate procedure. Emphasize that the procedure will help make the child healthy. Reinforce that the procedure is not punishment for bad behavior. Encourage choices (i.e., which arm) and assistance (i.e., opening alcohol wipes) when possible. Use simple terms and prepare only shortly before procedure. Praise cooperation and provide rewards (i.e., stickers).

Age	Developmental Stage	Characteristics	Interventions
School age (6-12 yr)	Industry versus inferiority: using hands to make things, being helpful and mastering tasks	Fears loss of control, death, bodily injury, and failure to meet expectations of significant others Plays with peers Developing a sense of belonging, cooperation, and compromise Engages in fantasy play Enjoys learning Peer group becoming increasingly important	Prepare in advance so child has a greater sense of control. Use pictures, models, and videos. Allow time to handle equipment, if possible. Have child explain what he or she already knows of procedure. Include the child in decision-making (i.e., which arm) to increase sense of control. Give immediate tactile and verbal praise for cooperation.
Adolescents (13-19 yr)	Identity versus identity diffusion: defining self related to others, vacillating between dependence and independence	Fears loss of control, altered body image, and separation from peer group Developing maturation and independence Strong need for privacy Peer acceptance is important May use noncompliance as a means of exerting independence and control	Advance preparation is vital for adolescent's coping, cooperation, and compliance. Explain the procedure using adult terms. Include adolescent in decision making. Models, diagrams, and videos are useful. Encourage participation in self-care (i.e., monitoring IV site). Coping/relaxation techniques may be useful.

Table 11-2   Body water in proportion to age and weight

Age/Weight	Total Body Water	Extracellular Fluid	Intracellular Fluid
		Percentage of Body Water	
Premature infant (1.2 kg)	81	59	22
Term infant (3.6 kg)	69	42	27
1-year-old child (10 kg)	60	32	28
Adult male (70 kg)	54	23	31
Adult female (60 kg)	49	23	26

From Terry J and others: *Intravenous therapy: clinical principles and practice,* Philadelphia, 1995, WB Saunders.

porated into all the topics, and a section at the end of this chapter addresses the issues related to home care and the discharge process.

Fluid and Electrolyte Balance

Fluid and electrolyte balance in the child has a different physiologic rationale than it does for the adult patient. The significant differences are as follows:

- Children have proportionally more body water than adults. Water constitutes approximately 75% to 80% of the term infant's weight, compared with 60% to 70% of the adult's weight. The proportion of the body water to body weight decreases with increasing age, development of body fat, and growth of the solid body structures. Table 11-2 shows body water in proportion to age and weight.
- The distribution of body water in the child also differs from that in the adult. Infants have more total body water in the extracellular compartment (42% to 45%) compared with adults (20%) (Fig. 11-1). Because of the increased percentage of water in the extracellular fluid (ECF), the child's water turnover rate is two to three times greater than that of the adult. Fifty percent of the infant's ECF is exchanged every day, compared with only 20% of the adult's. In addition, the smaller the child, the less fluid volume there is in each compartment, specifically in the intracellular fluid. Lower fluid volume results in less fluid reserve.

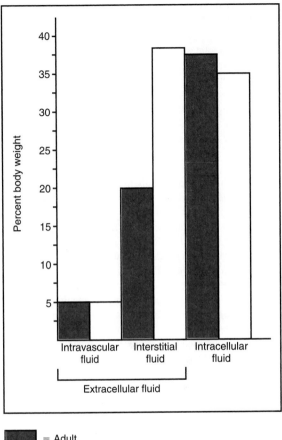

Fig. 11-1
Distribution of fluid in body compartments.
(From Pillitteri A: *Child health nursing: care of the child and family,*
Philadelphia, 1999, Lippincott.)

- A child's metabolism is two to three times greater than an adult's. A higher pulse and higher respiratory and peristaltic rates result in a greater proportion of insensible water loss and more metabolic waste. Therefore a child requires more water per kilogram of body weight than an adult does.
- Children have more body surface area (BSA) in proportion to body mass. This increased BSA ratio results in greater fluid loss through the skin by evaporation.
- An infant's kidneys do not concentrate urine at an adult level until after age 2; as a result, infants are less able to conserve water in the event of excessive fluid loss or diminished fluid intake.
- Children have a greater daily fluid requirement (per kilogram of body weight) than adults. Following are the three common methods used to determine the child's fluid requirements:
    1. *Meter-squared method:* A nomogram is used to calculate the child's BSA; then 1500 to 1800 ml of fluid/m^2 is calculated for the fluid replacement (Table 11-3).
    2. *Calorie method:* The usual fluid expenditure is approximately 150 ml for every 100 calories metabolized. Table 11-4 lists the daily caloric requirements by age.
    3. *Weight method:* The child's weight in kilograms is used to estimate the fluid requirements. Table 11-3 provides maintenance fluid requirements in children.

The weight method is used most often, but it tends to be less accurate than other methods when the child weighs more than 10 kg. The most accurate method is based on the child's BSA using the meter-squared formula.

Monitoring Fluid Replacement

Although the fluid requirement per kilogram of body weight is greater for a child than for an adult, the actual fluid volume amount required by the child is minimal. The following are recommendations to avoid fluid volume overload in the child:

- Regulate all pediatric infusions with volumetric chambers (e.g., Buretrol sets).
- Use volume-controlled infusion pumps to ensure accurate fluid delivery.
- Use microdrop tubing (60 drops/ml) to administer small-volume infusions and help prevent bolus infusions.

Table 11-3   Calculation of daily maintenance fluid
and electrolyte requirements for children

Weight	Formula
Body Weight Daily Maintenance Formula	
Neonate (<72 hr)	60-100 ml/kg
0-10 kg	100 ml/kg (may increase up to 150 ml/kg to provide caloric requirements if renal and cardiac function is adequate)
11-20 kg	1000 ml for the first 10 kg + 50 ml/kg for each kg over 10 kg
21-30 kg	1500 ml for the first 20 kg + 25 ml/kg for each kg over 20 kg
Body Weight Hourly Maintenance Formula	
0-10 kg	4 ml/kg/hr
11-20 kg	40 ml/hr for first 10 kg + 2 ml/kg/hr for kg 11-20
21-30 kg	60 ml/hr for first 20 kg + 1 ml/kg/hr for kg 21-30
Body Surface Area (BSA) Formula	1500 ml/m^2 BSA/day
Insensible Water Losses	300 ml/m^2 BSA/day
Electrolytes	
Sodium (Na$^+$)	3-4 mEq/kg/24 hr
Potassium (K$^+$)	2-3 mEq/kg/24 hr
Calcium (Ca$^+$)	50-100 mg/kg/24 hr
Magnesium (Mg^{++})	0.4-0.9 mEq/kg/day

Modified from Hazinski MF: *Manual of pediatric critical care,* St Louis, 1999, Mosby;
and Whaley LF, Wong DL: *Nursing care of infants and children,* ed 6, St Louis, 1999,
Mosby.

Table 11-4   Nutritional requirements for infants and children

Age	Daily Caloric Requirement
Up to 6 mo	120 cal/kg
6-12 mo	100 cal/kg
12-36 mo	90-95 cal/kg
4-10 yr	80 cal/kg
>10 yr, male	45 cal/kg
>10 yr, female	38 cal/kg

Nutrient	% Total Calories
Carbohydrates	40-45
Fat	40 combined 85-88
Protein	20

From Hazinski MF: *Manual of pediatric critical care,* St Louis, 1999, Mosby.

- Measure and evaluate intake and output with fluid balance every 4 to 8 hours.
- Monitor IV site, infusion, and equipment at least hourly.

Dehydration

The younger the child, the more rapid fluid and electrolyte imbalances develop. Children become dehydrated more quickly than adults and require more urgent replacement for these losses. The most common type of dehydration is isotonic dehydration. This occurs when water and sodium are lost in proportion to each other (e.g., from diarrhea and/or vomiting). Common dehydration symptoms for children and adults include dry mucous membranes, weight loss, poor skin turgor, and decreased urine volume with increased urine concentration. Specific dehydration characteristics found in the dehydrated infant include a sunken anterior fontanel, lethargy, irritability, high-pitched weak cries, creases on the soles of the feet, and an increased basal body temperature.

Oral intake is often compromised during a child's illness and can expedite the dehydration process, requiring IV fluids to maintain the fluid and electrolyte balance. It is a common practice to grade the severity of dehydration and prescribe fluid replacement accordingly. Table 11-5 lists the clinical signs and grades of pediatric dehydration. Table 11-3 and Box 11-1 address fluid therapy for dehydration and routine maintenance fluid therapy for pediatric patients.

Table 11-5   Clinical signs associated with isotonic dehydration in pediatric patients

Symptoms	Mild	Moderate	Severe
Weight loss (<10 yr) (%)	3-5	5-10	10-15
Weight loss (>10 yr) (%)	3-5	5-7	7-9
Fluid volume loss (ml/kg)	<50	50-90	>100
Blood pressure	Normal	Normal-low	Low
Pulse	Rapid	Rapid	Rapid/weak
Capillary filling time (sec)	<2	2-3	>3
Eyeball	Normal	Sunken	Sunken
Fontanel	Flat	Sunken	Sunken
Tears	Normal	Absent	Absent
Mucous membranes	Dry	Dry	Dry
Skin turgor	Normal	Decreased	Tenting
Skin color	Normal	Normal-pale	Pale-mottled
Urine output	Normal	Decreased	Decreased-absent
Mental status	Normal	Normal-lethargic	Lethargic-coma

Data from Rogers JS, Soud TE: *Manual of pediatric emergency nursing*, St Louis, 1998, Mosby; and Whaley LF, Wong DL: *Nursing care of infants and children*, ed 6, St Louis, 1999, Mosby.

Box 11-1   Guidelines for Fluid
Therapy—Dehydration

1. Administer bolus therapy of 20 ml/kg normal saline or lactated Ringer's solution as necessary to maintain perfusion.
2. Calculate maintenance requirements (see Table 11-3).
3. Calculate fluid deficits
    3%-5% body weight loss = 30-50 ml/kg
    7%-10% body weight loss = 70-100 ml/kg
    11%-15% body weight loss = 110-150 ml/kg
4. Calculate electrolyte requirements based on deficit and maintenance requirements (Table 11-3).
5. Estimate abnormal ongoing losses (e.g., fever, vomiting, diarrhea).
    ▪ Fever = 10%-12% increase in maintenance water requirements for each degree (Celsius) of temperature elevation (8% increase for each degree of Fahrenheit)
    ▪ Emesis and diarrhea = ml for ml replacement
6. Replace half of the fluid deficit and one third of the daily maintenance requirements over the first 8 hours of therapy with dextrose 5% in ½ normal saline.
7. Add supplemental potassium to parenteral fluids once renal function has been established.
8. Replace the remaining fluids (one half of the deficit and two thirds of the maintenance) over the next 16 hours.

From Rogers JS, Soud TE: *Manual of pediatric emergency nursing,* St Louis, 1998, Mosby.

Depending on the type of fluid and electrolyte imbalance, a hypertonic, hypotonic, or isotonic IV solution will be indicated for the management of the dehydration. Dextrose water is an isotonic solution and may be administered to children, but it should be used with *extreme caution.* If dextrose water is administered in large amounts, it can alter the child's extracellular osmolarity, resulting in cerebral edema.

Table 11-6   Pediatric intravenous site access

Age	Site	Example
Neonates and premature infants	Upper arms Inner thighs Scalp	Upper arms: axilla Scalp: superficial temporal, frontal, occipital, postauricular, supraorbital, posterior facial areas Inner thighs: popliteal vein
Infants and toddlers	Scalp Antecubital area Foot Hand	Antecubital area: cephalic, basilic veins, median areas Foot: saphenous vein, median, marginal areas; dorsal arch Hand: metacarpal, dorsal venous arch, tributaries of cephalic and basilic veins
Preschool through adolescents	Hand Forearm	Forearm: cephalic, basilic veins, median, antebrachial areas

Intravenous Site Selection and Maintenance

The following principles are guidelines for IV site selection:

1. Always select a site at the most distal point on the extremity.
2. Avoid previously used sites.
3. Avoid joints and areas that may restrict extremity movement (potential increased risk for infiltration).
4. Consider age, hand dominance, and mobility when selecting an IV site (Table 11-6 and Figs. 11-2 and 11-3).

Venipuncture Procedure Recommendations

- Apply topical anesthetic cream 1 to 4 hours before the IV access procedure.
- Wrap the extremity in a warm compress for 10 minutes before IV access to assist in vein dilation.
- Use a cannula gauge (20 to 24 gauge), depending on the infusion solution.
- Apply a Penrose drain or rubber band for a tourniquet in a small child or use a blood pressure cuff inflated to just below the

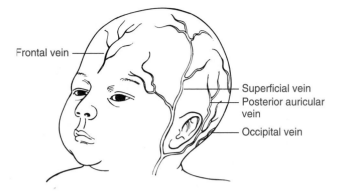

Fig. 11-2
Scalp veins of an infant.
(From Wheeler C, Frey AM: Intravenous therapy in children. In Terry J and others, editors: *Intravenous therapy: clinical principles and practice,* Philadelphia, 1995, WB Saunders.)

patient's diastolic blood pressure. This allows greater control over the pressure and makes veins more visible.

- Consider placing a flashlight or transilluminator device beneath the extremity to outline the vein and improve vein visualization.
- Insert the needle or catheter following the direction of blood flow. In scalp veins, the venous blood generally flows from the head toward the neck but should be assessed before IV insertion.
- Insert the cannula with the bevel pointed downward to prevent puncturing the far wall of the vessel and minimize occurrence of fluid extravasation in small veins.
- Never attempt to start an IV access on an infant or young child alone or without a passive restraining device.
- Consider using appropriate-size armboards and footboards to secure the IV site.
- Never tape all the way around the extremity because of the potential for blood flow obstruction (Fig. 11-4).
- Ensure that the ID band is not placed on the same extremity as the IV access.
- Consider using commercially available IV site protectors or plastic medication cups to cover and protect the IV site in young, active children (Fig. 11-5).

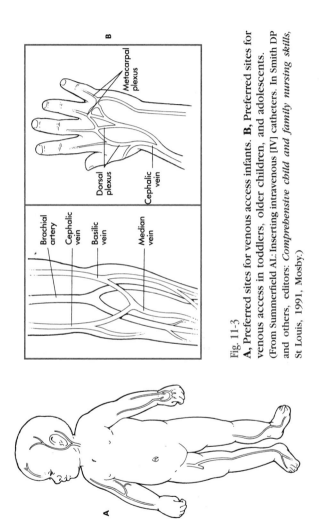

Fig. 11-3
A, Preferred sites for venous access infants. **B,** Preferred sites for venous access in toddlers, older children, and adolescents. (From Summerfield AL: Inserting intravenous [IV] catheters. In Smith DP and others, editors: *Comprehensive child and family nursing skills,* St Louis, 1991, Mosby.)

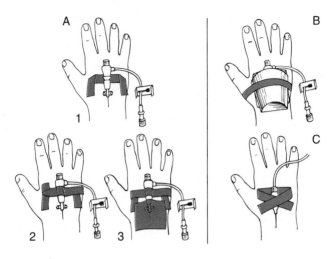

Fig. 11-4

Taping techniques for keeping IV devices in place. **A1,** Foundation tape. **A2,** Bridge tape. **A3,** Cover with occulsive dressing. **B,** Complete with protective shield or, **C,** Secure dressing with tape.

(From Wheeler C, Frey AM: Intravenous therapy in children. In Terry J and others, editors: *Intravenous therapy: clinical principles and practice,* Philadelphia, 1995, WB Saunders.)

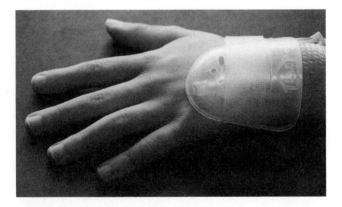

Fig. 11-5

Example of a commercial IV shield.

(From Whaley LF, Wong DL: *Nursing care of infants and children,* ed 6, St Louis, 1999, Mosby.)

- Protect the IV site from accidental dislodgment with stretch netting in older children.

CLINICAL ALERT: Monitor the IV site for pain, redness, edema, phlebitis, and infiltration every 30 to 60 minutes.

Central Venous Catheters

Intravenous access is often achieved through the peripheral veins in the pediatric patient's hand, forearm, foot, leg, or scalp. When inadequate peripheral access is present or long-term or aggressive IV therapy is required, central venous access becomes a viable option. Central venous access provides options for drug and fluid delivery and blood sampling for diagnostic testing. Needlesticks are a source of fear and pain in the child, and the central venous access offers a less traumatic approach to IV therapy. Using central venous catheters (CVCs) also eliminates the invasive procedure of peripheral IV site rotation every 48 to 72 hours. Regardless of which device is used, it is vital that the patient (if appropriate) and caregivers are taught the proper care and management of their child's device.

Central venous access devices commonly used in pediatric patients include umbilical, percutaneous, tunneled, and peripherally inserted central catheters and implantable ports. The appropriate device depends on vein access, prescribed type and duration of therapy, disease process, and patient/family preference. In addition, the device selection criteria should include the child's age and size, cognitive ability, body image considerations, and self-care management requirements. The Centers for Disease Control and Prevention also recommends that catheter selection be based on knowledge of potential complications and the general experience of the institution. The anatomic placement and potential advantages and disadvantages of each device follow.

Umbilical Catheter

Use of the umbilical catheter is common practice in neonatal and intensive care units for the acutely ill infant. The umbilical vein is the anatomic placement.

- *Advantages:* Easy route for IV fluid or drug administration; can be used for central venous pressure measurements, venous blood sampling, and exchange blood transfusions. Catheter can be removed as soon as an alternate IV access is established.

- *Disadvantages:* Site is not accessible after the fourth day of life. Potential complications include thrombosis, embolism, vasospasm, vascular perforation, infection, and hemorrhage.

Percutaneous Central Venous Catheter

Catheter placement for the neonate and infant is the jugular vein. The site of choice for older children is the subclavian vein. The femoral vein with catheter tip placement in the vena cava can be used; however, this site should be used with caution if the child is in diapers because of the potential increased infection risk.

- *Advantages:* Venous access is obtained without needlestick to the child. It can be used for short-term intermittent or continuous infusion therapy.
- *Disadvantages:* Prudent daily aseptic site care, dressing change, and heparinization are required; alteration in body image.

Tunneled Catheters

Device options include single- or double-lumen Broviac and Groshong catheters. Catheter placement for infants and children younger than 5 years of age is access through the facial vein threaded into the superior vena cava (Figs. 11-6 and 11-7); for older children, the catheter is inserted percutaneously into the subclavian vein. When the chest is not a viable access site, the catheter can be inserted into the inferior vena cava through the femoral vein with the catheter exit site on the abdomen, thigh, or back. To avoid catheter dislodgment, the nurse should loop the external "tail" of the catheter under the dressing and secure it with tape to the chest. T-shirts, stretch netting, and binders are also recommended to secure the catheter. As a precaution, any connections should be secured with tape.

CLINICAL ALERT: Never use a tie or string around the child's neck to secure the catheter because of the potential risk of strangulation. Instead, opt for a T-shirt, stretch netting, or a binder cut to the appropriate size to prevent pulling on the catheter.

- *Advantages:* Catheter longevity (months/years); easy access by patient or caregiver, catheter repair options; clean dressing technique use after tissue healing; IV access possible without needlestick; swimming in chlorinated water allowed after tissue site healing, based on the child's immune status and physician's order

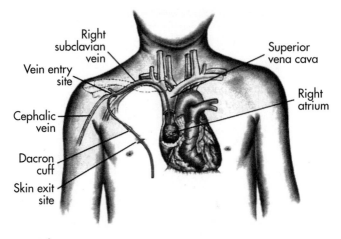

Fig. 11-6
Central venous catheter insertion and exit site.
(From Whaley LF, Wong DL: *Nursing care of infants and children,*
ed 6, St Louis, 1999, Mosby.)

- *Disadvantages:* Daily to weekly catheter heparinization and
  site care; alteration in body image; risk of accidental catheter
  dislodgment or puncture (e.g., infant may bite catheter during
  teething, or toddler may pull out catheter); central venous
  catheter thrombosis; avoidance of vigorous contact sports

Peripherally Inserted Central Catheter

Catheter placement is in the antecubital fossa through the basilic,
cephalic, or median cubital veins in older children. The saphenous,
superficial temporal, external jugular, popliteal, or axillary veins are
used most often in newborns, infants, and toddlers. A radiograph
must confirm verification of tip location before initiating therapy.

- *Advantages:* Insertion by specially trained nurses; allows
  repeated venous access without needlestick; a safe and
  less-expensive option than tunneled catheters; catheter size is
  French 2, 3, or 4, depending on the child's size and type or
  duration of therapy; currently no known limitations for the
  duration of use; as with any invasive device, prompt removal
  when the peripherally inserted central catheter (PICC) is no
  longer necessary.

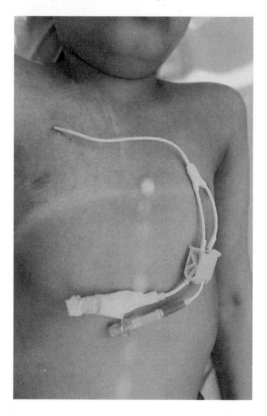

Fig. 11-7
External venous catheter.
(From Whaley LF, Wong DL: *Nursing care of infants and children,*
ed 6, St Louis, 1999, Mosby.)

- *Disadvantages:* Requires daily catheter heparinization and
  site care; PICC site should not be submerged in water; should
  avoid blood pressures and venipuncture in affected extremity;
  small-gauge PICCs not recommended for blood sampling;
  avoidance of repetitive movements in the affected extremity;
  alteration in body image

Implantable Port

Device placement is the anterior chest under the skin via the
subclavian vein, with the catheter tip in the superior vena cava.

Alternative site placement is the anterior fossa of the arm, with the catheter threaded via the basilic/cephalic vein into the superior vena cava.

- *Advantages:* Ideal for the child who requires intermittent therapy or long-term therapy for a child aged 3 and older (before age 3, the lack of sufficient subcutaneous tissue may allow the port to erode through the skin); requires minimal site care and maintenance; intact body image; device longevity (2 to 3 years); bathing or swimming allowed when port is not accessed; no external components to break or malfunction
- *Disadvantages:* Needlestick is required for IV access; potential pain associated with needle aspiration; restriction of vigorous contact sports because of the potential risk for port displacement; requires monthly heparinization with needle access

Clinical Guidelines for Pediatric Central Venous Devices

- Only qualified nurses experienced in the care of CVCs should be responsible for teaching and management of these devices.
- It is recommended that nurses knowledgeable in the scope and the practice of IV therapy have input into the selection of vascular access devices.
- All IV tubing and catheter connections should be secured with tape to help prevent disconnection.
- Heparin concentration, volume of flush per lumen, and frequency of catheter maintenance need to be correlated with the child's body requirements, fluid balance, and medical diagnosis.
- Three-way stopcocks may be used during blood sampling procedure, and the discarded blood sample is returned to the patient. Follow the institution or agency guidelines for this procedure.
- Blood sampling discard volume should be limited in volume (e.g., 5 ml or less).
- Normal saline flush volume is 5 ml or less; *calculate* the total volume of these flushes in the child's daily intake.
- Consult the manufacturer's recommendations for device flush protocols and site/dressing requirements.
- Assess the child, parent, or caregiver's ability and compliance for catheter/device management.
- Include in the teaching strategies for catheter/device man-

agement the child's growth, developmental, and psychosocial status.

Intraosseous Route

Use of the intraosseous route (into the bone) is an emergency measure in infant and child resuscitation when immediate vascular access is required. This route is used only when conventional IV access is unobtainable. A needle is inserted into the bone marrow of a long bone, and blood, fluid, or drugs are then infused.

The fluid injected into the bone marrow cavity is rapidly drained into the central venous channel and then into systemic circulation. The intraosseous route is as effective as the central venous route for delivering IV solutions. The optimal sites for intraosseous needle placement in infants and children include the distal tibia, proximal tibia, and distal femur (Fig. 11-8). Other sites include the iliac crest and the humerus. The sternum is never used in children. Complications are rare but can include osteomyelitis, sepsis, cellulitis, abscess, local necrosis, and fat embolism.

CLINICAL ALERT: The intraosseous route is intended for short-term use only, and once the child's condition is stabilized, an alternative IV access route must be obtained.

Intravenous Medication Administration

The pediatric patient is susceptible to drug and fluid overload with various IV therapy infusions. To diminish this occurrence, minimal fluid amounts should be used for drug dilution and flushing the IV access. Additional precautions follow:

- Use preservative-free solutions for the neonate.
- Use small-volume infusion tubing with pumps and controllers to infuse drugs and solutions.
- Use pumps and controllers that have alarms and tamper-proof or locking features.
- Preferably, use microinfusion pumps that can infuse fluids in increments of 0.1 ml/hr for medication delivery in the neonate and infant.
- Have knowledge of the child's body weight (kg/BSA/m^2) for accurate drug dose calculations.
- Adhere to the prescribed or recommended infusion rates.

Table 11-7 lists common IV medications by drug, with indications and dosing guidelines with nursing considerations.

Text continued on p. 406

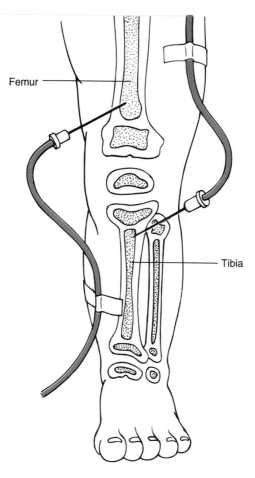

Fig. 11-8
Intraosseous access sites for IV infusion.
(From Wheeler C, Frey AM: Intravenous therapy in children. In Terry J and others, editors: *Intravenous therapy: clinical principles and practice,* Philadelphia, 1995, WB Saunders.)

Table 11-7   Common intravenous medications

Drug	Indications	Dosage	Nursing Considerations
Antibiotics			
Ampicillin Amcil Ampicin	Systemic infections Acute and chronic urinary tract infections caused by susceptible organisms Meningitis Uncomplicated gonorrhea	100-300 mg/kg IV daily, divided into 6-hr doses	Drug should be discontinued if immediate hypersensitivity reaction occurs. Use cautiously in patient with other drug allergies. Dosage should be altered in patients with impaired renal functions. Follow manufacturer's directions for stability data. IV dose should be mixed in D_5W or saline solution.
Sulfamethoxazole Bactrim Septra sulfamethoxazole-trimethoprim (SMX-TMP)	Urinary tract infections Shigellosis Otitis media *Pneumocystis carinii* pneumonia	8 mg/kg TMP per 40 mg/kg SMX to 20 mg/kg TMP per 100 mg/kg SMX for serious infections daily, divided into 12-hr doses	Not recommended for children <2 mo old. Infuse slowly over 60-90 min. Use solution within 2 hr after preparation. Check solution carefully for precipitate.

Drug	Indications	Dosage	Comments
Cefazolin Ancef Kefzol	Serious respiratory, genito-urinary, skin and soft tissue, bone, and joint infections Septicemic endocarditis	8-16 mg/kg IV every 8 hr or 6-12 mg/kg every 6 hr	Monitor renal functioning. IV infusion must be diluted in D_5W. Dose may be reduced for patients with impaired hepatic or renal function. Patients with altered renal functioning should be monitored closely. Monitor carefully for superinfections.
Ceftazidime Fortaz Tazicef	Bacteremia Septicemia Serious respiratory, urinary, gynecological, intraabdominal, CNS, and skin infections	30-50 mg/kg IV every 8 hr	
Cefuroxime Kefurox Zinacef	Serious lower respiratory, urinary tract, skin, and skin structure infections Septicemia Meningitis	50-100 mg/kg IV per day, divided into 6- or 8-hr doses	

BUN, Blood urea nitrogen; *CNS*, central nervous system; *CMV*, cytomegalovirus; *D_5W*, dextrose 5% in water; *SGOT*, serum glutamic-oxaloacetic transaminase; *SGPT*, serum glutamate pyruvate transaminase.

Continued

Table 11-7   Common intravenous medications—cont'd

Drug	Indications	Dosage	Nursing Considerations
Antibiotics—cont'd			
Clindamycin Cleocin	Infections caused by streptococci, pneumococci, *Bacteroides* species, *Fusobacterium* species, and *Clostridium perfringens*	15-40 mg/kg IV divided into 6-hour doses	Culture and sensitivity (C & S) testing should be done prior to starting IV. Administer no faster than 30 mg/min or 1.2 g/hr. Monitor renal, hepatic, and hematopoietic functions during prolonged therapy. Monitor closely for diarrhea.
Gentamicin Garamycin	Serious infections caused by susceptible organisms Meningitis Endocarditis prophylaxis External ocular infections caused by susceptible organisms Primary and secondary bacterial infections Superficial burns Skin ulcers and infected lacerations Abrasions, insect bites, or minor surgical wounds	2.0-2.5 mg/kg IV every 8 hr	Use cautiously in patients with impaired renal function. Monitor renal function (output, specific gravity urinalysis, BUN, and creatine levels). Keep patient well hydrated. Monitor drug levels as ordered.

Oxacillin Bactocill Prostaphlin	Systemic infections caused by susceptible organisms	100-200 mg/kg IV per day, divided into every 4- to 6-hour doses	Monitor renal and hepatic function. Watch for elevated SGOT and SGPT. IV infusion should be mixed with D_5W. Monitor for superinfection. Infuse over 20-60 min.
Tobramycin Nebcin	Serious infections caused by susceptible organisms	3 mg/kg-5 mg/kg, divided into 8-hr doses	Impaired renal function will require adjusted doses. Serum levels should be monitored. Obtain C & S tests before starting therapy. Infuse over at least 60 min.
Vancomycin Vancocin	Severe staphylococcus infections Enterocolitis Endocarditis prophylaxis	20-40 mg/kg IV daily, divided into 6-hr doses	Monitor BUN, creatine, and serum drug levels. If patient develops maculopapular rash on face, neck, trunk, and upper extremities, slow infusion rate. Monitor patient for ringing in the ears. Monitor renal function.

Continued

Table 11-7   Common intravenous medications—cont'd

Drug	Indications	Dosage	Nursing Considerations
Antivirals			
Acyclovir Zovirax	Initial and recurrent mucocutaneous herpes simplex virus Severe initial genital herpes in immunocompromised patients	For children >12 yr, 5 mg/kg over 1 hr every 8 hr For children <12 yr, 250 mg/m^2 over 1 hr IV every 8 hr	Infuse slowly over at least 1 hr to prevent renal tubular damage. Patients must be adequately hydrated.
Ganciclovir Cytovene	Treatment of CMV infections in immunocompromised patients	7.5-10 mg/kg IV divided in 2 to 3 doses for induction, then 2.5-5 mg/kg/day	Monitor blood counts.
Antifungals			
Amphotericin B Fungizone	Systemic fungal infections caused by susceptible organisms Meningitis Coccidioidal arthritis	0.25 mg/kg daily by slow infusion over 6 hr to start; increase as tolerated to 1 mg/kg daily to a maximum of 1.5 mg/kg	If drug has been discontinued for >1 wk, then initial dose must be given and increased gradually. C & S testing must be completed. Mix with D_5W. Use an in-line filter membrane with a mean pore diameter larger than 1 μ.

Do not mix or piggyback with other antibiotics.

Monitor hepatic and renal function studies.

Patients often premedicated with aspirin, antihistamines, antiemetics, or corticosteroids.

Monitor vital signs every 30 min for at least 4 hr after starting IV infusion.

Fever may appear within 1-2 hr of starting infusion but should subside in 4 hr of discharging drug.

Monitor input and output closely and report changes.

Monitor K^+, Ca^+, and Mg^{++} levels closely.

Antiemetic

Ondansetron
Zofran

Nausea and vomiting induced by chemotherapy

For children >4 yr, 0.15 mg/kg over 15 min, 30 min before emetogenic chemotherapy.
Repeated at 4 and 8 hr after the first dose.

Blood and Blood Component Administration

Blood product administration for children requires precautions and monitoring guidelines similar to those used with adult patients. However, there are differences related to circulating blood volume, infused blood volume, red cell life span, hemoglobin level, and maturation of the hematopoietic system. Children have a much greater circulating blood volume per unit of body weight than adults do, yet their absolute blood volume is very small (Table 11-8).

Indications for transfusion therapy in children include acute hemorrhage, anemia, abnormal blood component function or deficiency, and removal of harmful elements such as bilirubin during an exchange transfusion. Blood replacement should be considered when the blood loss is greater than 5% to 7% of the total circulating volume. Reduction in the child's blood volume by 30% to 40% produces evidence of clinical shock (Table 11-9).

Consider the following factors in transfusion therapy for children:

- Explain the transfusion procedure to the parents, obtain their consent, and review the transfusion history of the child. Include the child in all the instructional preparations.
- Consider the child's and family's perspective of the transfusion process, their prior experiences, and their cultural and religious views related to transfusion therapy.
- Blood from the newborn is usually crossmatched against the mother's serum, which contains equal or greater quantities of antibodies present in the infant at birth.
- Neonates with severe hyperbilirubinemia or ABO incompatibility receive exchange transfusions by withdrawing small amounts of the infant's blood and infusing the same amount

Table 11-8   Calculation of circulating blood volume in children

Age	Circulating Blood Volume (ml/kg)
Neonates	85-90
Infants	75-80
Children	70-75
Adolescents	65-70

From Rogers JS, Soud TE: *Manual of pediatric emergency nursing,* St Louis, 1998, Mosby.

Table 11-9 Blood component therapy for pediatric patients

Blood Product	Indication	Dosage/Rate
Red blood cells (packed)	Treatment of anemia without volume expansion	10 ml/kg, not to exceed 15 ml/kg at 2.5 ml/kg/hr
Platelets	To control bleeding associated with deficiency in platelet number or function	1 unit (50-70 ml)/7-10 kg body weight run over 30 min to a maximum of 4 hr; IV push or drip
Fresh frozen plasma	To increase levels of clotting factors in children with demonstrated deficiency Occasionally volume expansion in acute blood loss	Acute hemorrhage: 15-30 ml/kg as indicated Clotting deficiency: 10-15 ml/kg at 1-2 ml/min

From National Blood Education Program, Public Health Service, National Institutes of Health, US Department of Health and Human Services: *Transfusion therapy guidelines for nurses*, Washington, DC, 1990, US Government Printing Office.

of plasma and red cells from one or more donors via an umbilical catheter. The neonate's blood is typed and cross-matched before the transfusion process, and the blood transfusion is cleared of the offending antigen.

- Intrauterine blood exchange transfusion is believed to prevent kernicterus, severe anemia, brain damage, and death when an amniocentesis test indicates increasing bilirubin levels in the amniotic fluid of a fetus with Rh incompatibility or if the mother's indirect Coombs' test is strongly positive.
- *Only* qualified personnel (physicians and nurses) with advanced skills should perform exchange transfusions in newborns or intrauterine transfusions. These transfusions should take place only in an appropriate clinical environment.
- Blood transfusion volume in children varies according to age and weight. The volume is calculated in milligrams per kilogram of body weight.
- Pediatric blood units are prepared in special units (e.g., Pedipacks) and usually equal half the volume of a conventional adult unit.
- Red cell transfusions require strict infusion times (e.g., calculate 5% of the total blood product to be transfused, and infuse this amount over the initial 15 minutes). This method facilitates early detection of a potential hemolytic reaction.
- Microaggregate filters are not routinely required in neonatal transfusions because the blood neonates receive is usually younger than 7 days old and rarely contains the microaggregate component; when microaggregate filters are used, they must be changed every 2 to 4 hours according to the manufacturer's recommendations.
- Blood warmers prevent hypothermia, which could result in potential cardiac arrhythmia. The blood temperature should be maintained between 32° and 37° C.
- Infusion pumps capable of infusing blood are recommended for all transfusion therapies in children. The blood may be prefiltered and infused via a syringe pump for the neonate and infant.
- Blood and blood products may be administered via 27-, 26-, or 24-gauge peripheral IV access in the neonate and via 24- or 22-gauge peripheral IV access in older children.
- Straight-line IV tubing should be used to minimize the volume of saline infused. Small amounts of normal saline

(1 ml) should be used for flushing the IV line to prevent fluid overload.

Chemotherapy Administration

Childhood cancers are treated with a combination of surgery, radiation therapy, chemotherapy, and biologic response modifiers. Treatment of diseases seen in pediatric oncology, such as leukemia, lymphoma, neuroblastoma, Hodgkin's disease, Wilms' tumors, and brain tumors, usually requires intermittent chemotherapy. The aggressive chemotherapy protocols used for many of these diseases often require long-term venous access to deliver the prescribed drugs. The venous access devices used to deliver the various chemotherapy drugs are tunneled catheters, PICCs, and implantable ports.

The chemotherapy drug side effects, duration of therapy, and maintenance of long-term venous access devices result in many physical and psychosocial changes for the child. Maintaining a child's developmental status to enable achievement of normal milestones throughout the course of chemotherapy can be challenging. A change in body image (e.g., hair loss, weight changes) can have a significant impact on the child's self-concept, especially in the adolescent years. Focusing on the child's strengths and providing the child with as much autonomy as possible promotes a positive self-concept. Allowing children who are cognitively able to participate in decisions regarding their course of therapy also contributes to a positive outlook. The nurse should consider age-related diversionary activities selected by the child or parent to minimize distress associated with invasive procedures in the treatment regimens.

Clinical practice interventions recommended for pediatric chemotherapy administration include the following points:

- Consider the child's cognitive level, developmental level, and chronologic age in preparation of instructional and recreational materials and resources. Chronically ill children often have developmental delays, and the child's response to the treatment may not be age appropriate; interventions need to be based on the child's developmental level, not chronologic age.
- Include caregiver education in all components of the chemotherapy (e.g., drug side effects and toxicities, administration route, schedule). Encourage caregivers to actively participate in the child's care.

- Instruct the caregiver regarding safe handling precautions (e.g., wearing latex gloves when changing diapers; handling chemotherapy-contaminated linen; disposing of vomit, urine, or stool; disposing of chemotherapy drug and infusion supplies; managing a chemotherapy drug spill).
- Anticipate potential drug side effects such as nausea and vomiting; include age-appropriate assessments and interventions. Small children have an increased risk for aspiration; position children appropriately and monitor them according to a scheduled frequency.
- *Calculate* the prescribed drug dose with each course of chemotherapy. The child's height and weight will change throughout the treatment process.
- Keep an accurate, up-to-date, cumulative drug dose record for all children receiving drugs that have maximum dose limits.
- Intrathecal drug dosages may be based on age as an estimate of cerebrospinal fluid volume rather than on the BSA or weight.
- *Never* apply heat to suspected or actual drug infiltration sites because tissue necrosis and sloughing may occur.

Parenteral Nutrition

Parenteral nutrition in the pediatric population is highly specialized. This therapy needs to sustain the child's life and weight and allow for the child's normal growth and developmental needs. Total parenteral nutrition (TPN) and partial parenteral nutrition (PPN) are most often used as supportive therapy for infants and children with complex illness and structural gastrointestinal anomalies.

Pediatric Indications for TPN and PPN

Gastrointestinal obstruction	Inflammatory bowel disease
Cystic fibrosis	Hirschsprung's disease
Crohn's disease	Congenital heart disease
Short bowel syndrome	Necrotizing enterocolitis
Pancreatitis	Cancer
Renal failure	Acquired immunodeficiency syndrome (AIDS)
Gastroschisis (a congenital fissure in the wall of the abdomen that remains open)	

Criteria used to determine whether a child is a potential candidate for TPN or PPN include the following:

- Greater than 5% weight loss
- Height-to-weight ratio below the fifth percentile when plotted on a growth chart
- Serum albumin level less than 3 g/dl
- Total lymphocyte count less than 1000/mm^3 (excluding granulocytopenia)

In the past several years, it has been common practice to discharge the child to home care with TPN or PPN. Home parenteral nutrition allows the child a greater degree of normalcy in the growth and development process. Portable infusion pumps allow relative freedom, do not require an IV pole, and can be contained in an unobtrusive carrying case. Many children receive the TPN or PPN over 8 to 12 hours during the night, which allows the child a normal lifestyle of school and activities. TPN or PPN in the home setting requires individually tailored education and instruction for the child and parent or other caregiver. All educational components should be tailored according to the child's growth and developmental process and the prescribed TPN or PPN therapy.

Clinical Guidelines for TPN or PPN in Children

The initial rate of infusion and glucose concentration must be low and increased gradually to allow the child's insulin production to accommodate the continuous glucose load. Similarly, the glucose concentration and rate of infusion must be decreased gradually to wean the child from TPN or PPN. *Hypoglycemia* and *hyperglycemia* occur more rapidly in children than in adults.

Dextrose provides the main calorie source and should be concentrated to provide enough energy requirements. However, the fluid volume required to dilute very concentrated dextrose is prohibitive to the *fluid balance* for infants and small children. The higher concentrations of dextrose (≥25%) can be administered via a central venous access device using less diluent.

Fats are essential for the neurologic development in the infant. The fatty acids in the TPN solution may displace the bilirubin from the albumin, causing a rise in the bilirubin level and an increased risk of kernicterus. Bilirubin levels should be obtained 4 hours after the fat emulsion has been infused.

- Children have higher metabolic rates than adults and require more calories per kilogram of body weight (see Table 11-4).

The active child needs to maintain caloric intake to provide the necessary energy requirements for basal metabolism, growth and development, and tissue healing. Children receiving long-term therapy (months or years) must be monitored continuously to ensure that these nutritional requirements are met to allow a normal growth pattern.

- Infants receiving TPN are usually acutely ill and are deprived of maternal contact. It is important to hold and cuddle the child to help meet the emotional needs. If no oral intake is provided to the infant, ensure that the infant's sucking need is met.

- Children may develop adverse reactions to lipid infusions (e.g., dyspnea, flushing, nausea, headache, dizziness, chest pain, back pain). Therefore lipids should be administered only three to four times a week, over a portion of the day, such as 8 hours. The *maximum* lipid infusion is 4 g/kg/24 hr and *should not exceed* 3 ml/kg/hr.

- Adjust the TPN or PPN rate by 10% increments, and never adjust the lipid infusion rate.

- Weigh children daily and infants every shift while they are receiving TPN or PPN.

- Maintain strict intake and output records. Obtain glucose level every 4 to 8 hours when initiating TPN or PPN, then every 4 hours for infants and every 8 hours for children. Obtain vital signs at least every 4 hours.

- Monitor liver function studies and serum liver enzymes on a scheduled frequency; abnormalities and elevations in these tests occur often in children.

Home Care

As the cost of health care continues to rise, the expectation to care for patients in the home setting increases. Pediatric home infusion therapy is a positive alternative to the traditional hospitalization process for the payer, physician, parent, and patient. Home infusion therapy allows the child to participate in normal activities related to school, family, and friends that the hospital setting often hinders.

Common pediatric infusion therapies administered at home include antibiotics, chemotherapy, parenteral nutrition, blood sampling for laboratory tests, and therapeutic drug monitoring. Review Boxes 11-2 and 11-3 for the levels that are often monitored

Box 11-2   Therapeutic Drug Levels

Carbamazepine (Tegretol)	4-12 µg/ml
Clonazepam (Klonopin)	15-70 µg/ml
Digoxin (Lanoxin)	0.8-2.0 µg/ml
Gentamicin/tobramycin	Peak 4-10 µg/ml; trough 2 µg/ml
Phenobarbital	15-30 µg/ml
Phenytoin (Dilantin)	10-20 µg/ml
Theophylline (Marax)	10-20 µg/ml
Valproic acid (Depakene)	50-150 µg/ml
Vancomycin (Vancocin)	Peak 25-40 µg/ml; trough 10 µg/ml

in children. Refer to "Pediatric Infusion Therapy" under "Guidelines for Home Care" on page 415.

Discharge Teaching Process

Once the discharge criteria are met, the nurse must educate the family and child on the specific home infusion therapy prescribed. The following are important aspects to consider in the discharge teaching plan:

- Psychosocial aspects, growth, and development of the child
- Therapy effects on the child's body image
- The child's participation in certain sports or desired activities
- The child's peers' reactions to home infusion therapy
- The type, complexity, and duration of home infusion therapy
- The ability of the child and parent or other caregiver to meet the care requirements
- Home environment factors (e.g., patient care in a multiple-level home, need for refrigeration for parenteral nutrition, phone availability)
- Self-care processes such as catheter site care and medication administration, with return demonstration of learned techniques to ensure prudent technique and accuracy in dosing
- Instructional materials tailored to age and comprehension
- Verbal and written instructions regarding who, when, where, and how to call for assistance in an emergency or with significant concerns about the home infusion therapy

Box 11-3   Normal Term Newborn Blood Values and Urinalysis Values

Blood Values

Hemoglobin	15-20 g/dl
Hematocrit	43%-61%
WBCs	10,000-30,000/mm^3
Neutrophils	40%-80%
Immature WBCs	3%-10%
Platelets	100,000-280,000/mm^3
Reticulocytes	3%-6%
Blood volume	82.3 ml/kg (third day after early cord clamping)
	92.6 ml/kg (third day after delayed cord clamping)
Sodium	124-156 mmol/l
Potassium	5.3-7.3 mmol/l
Chloride	90-111 mmol/l
Calcium	7.3-9.2 mg/dl
Glucose	40-97 mg/dl
IEM-PKU	<4 mg
Bilirubin	Bilirubin level peaks 3-5 days and should not exceed 13 mg/dl
Capillary heel stick*	4-6 mg/dl
Cord blood	1.0-1.8 mg/dl

Urinalysis Values

Protein	<5-10 mg/dl
WBCs	<2-3
RBCs	Negative
Casts	Negative
Bacteria	Negative
Specific gravity	1.001-1.025
Color	Pale yellow

IEM, Inborn errors of metabolism; *PKU*, phenylketonuria; *RBCs*, red blood cells; *WBCs*, white blood cells.

*Breast-milk jaundice: bilirubin rises the fourth day after mature breast milk comes in; a bilirubin peak level of 20 to 25 mg/dl is reached at 2 to 3 weeks of age.

Documentation Recommendations

- Document exact placement of all peripheral IV devices and gauges, IV site management, and IV access securing.
- Document type, placement, site care, and maintenance for all central venous access devices.
- Document all drugs, solution types, volume and tubing, dose, time, date, weight/drug/solution calculations, and type of IV filter used.
- Document all infusion devices, type, infusion rate; alarm function, tubing, and volume.
- Document all therapeutic drug and laboratory diagnostic monitoring levels and blood sampling volumes.
- Document all chemotherapy, blood and blood products, and parenteral solutions (type, dose, volume, and weight/dose calculations such as kg/wt or m^2), and the type and number of product filters used.
- Document all educational strategies related to the child and parent or other caregiver; note their understanding of the instructions, techniques in drug dosing, catheter maintenance, chemotherapy precautions, emergency procedures.
- Document all assessment parameters related to fluid volume deficit or overload; pain, vital signs, and weight/BSA calculations.

Nursing Diagnosis

Table 11-10 lists potential nursing diagnoses and results of proper treatment.

Guidelines for Home Care
Pediatric Infusion Therapy

- Monitor prudently to maintain therapeutic drug levels.
- Administer prescribed drug at the schedule times.
- Peak drug levels should be obtained 30 to 60 minutes after the drug has been infused.
- Trough drug levels should be obtained just before the next scheduled drug dose.
- Communicate to the physician promptly variations from normal regarding vital signs, intake and output, drug peak and trough levels, and laboratory test results (e.g., serum electrolytes, creatinine level, hematology values, bilirubin levels).

Table 11-10 Nursing diagnoses and desired patient outcomes in children receiving intravenous therapy

Nursing Diagnosis	Patient Outcome
Fluid volume deficit, risk for, because of vomiting, diarrhea, burns, hemorrhage, wound drainage, or diabetic ketoacidosis	The child's hydration status will demonstrate improvement by improved skin turgor, moist mucous membranes, stable weight, 1 ml/kg/hr of urine output, serum electrolyte values within normal limits. Oral fluids will be tolerated. Urine specific gravity will be between 1000 and 1010.
Fluid volume excess, because of fluid overload, cardiac or renal disease, inappropriate secretion, or fluid shift	The child's weight will return to preillness status, edema will decrease, vital signs will return to normal, and no audible rales will be present.
Sensory/perceptual alteration (visual, auditory, gustatory, tactile), because of electrolyte imbalance, cerebral edema, or fever	The child will respond appropriately for age (e.g., smile at parents, suck from bottle).
Skin integrity impaired, risk for, because of diarrhea, edema, or dry skin	The child's skin will be free of signs of breakdown, excoriation in diaper area will decrease, and skin turgor will return to normal.
Diversional activity deficit, because of environmental lack of activity; frequent, lengthy treatments; or long-term hospitalization	The child will participate in chosen activities and will express interest in surroundings and activity.
Fear, because of separation from parent, unfamiliar environment, treatment, IV equipment, or normal developmental phobias	The child will demonstrate reduced fear behaviors (e.g., crying, wide-eyed gaze, tension, or hiding).

From Terry J and others: *Intravenous therapy: clinical principles and practice,* Philadelphia, 1995, WB Saunders.

Table 11-10   Nursing diagnoses and desired patient outcomes in children receiving intravenous therapy—cont'd

Nursing Diagnosis	Patient Outcome
Knowledge deficit (self-care, central venous catheter site care), because of lack of exposure, information misinterpretation, cognitive limitation	The child and family will verbalize understanding of what was taught and will demonstrate ability to perform new skills.
Mobility, impaired physical, because of restraints and IV support boards and decreased endurance and strength	The child will achieve maximum mobility within age and medical restrictions and have no skin breakdown, no contractures, and maximum joint range of motion.
Nutrition, altered; less than body requirements, because of nausea, vomiting, diarrhea, and inability to absorb nutrients	The child will tolerate feedings via oral route, feeding tube, or IV line without side effects; will gain a predetermined amount of weight per day; will experience an increased energy level; and will participate in diet decisions, if age appropriate.
Self-esteem disturbance/body image disturbance, because of venous access device, illness, and effects of treatment (e.g., alopecia)	The child will participate in decision-making process about self-care, will take initiative to do tasks, will make eye contact, and will interact freely with peers.
Urinary elimination altered, because of fluid shift, diarrhea, inadequate intake, and chronic illness	The child will have adequate output that is in balance with intake and will have urine specific gravity between 1000 and 1010.

From Terry J and others: *Intravenous therapy: clinical principles and practice,* Philadelphia, 1995, WB Saunders.

- Physician's order may vary the prescribed times for obtaining the peak and trough level blood sample. It is crucial to document the medication infusion dose and time with the time that the peak and trough levels were obtained.
- Review Boxes 11-2 and 11-3 for the levels that are often monitored in children.

Resources

Clinical Competency—Pediatric Intravenous Therapy

	Yes	No	NA
Initiating Infusion Therapy (Fluid or Medication)			
1. Use basic knowledge of pediatric growth and development.			
2. Explain the procedure using a calm and age-appropriate manner.			
3. Allow the parent/caregiver the option to remain present for the procedure.			
4. Encourage the parent/caregiver to provide comfort measures throughout the procedure.			
5. Use a neutral/procedure room to perform the procedure.			
6. Enlist the help of passive restraints or coworkers for restraining the patient.			
7. Consider age, hand dominance, and mobility when selecting an IV site.			
8. Use aseptic technique for needle or catheter insertion.			
9. Use appropriate protective and securing devices.			
10. Use minimal fluids for drug dilution and flushing.			
11. Use preservative-free solutions for neonates.			

Clinical Competency—Pediatric Intravenous Therapy—cont'd

	Yes	No	NA
12. Select appropriate volume infusion tubing and pumps for medication delivery.			
13. Ensure infusion pumps are tamper proof with locking devices.			
14. Verify drug dosages/fluid volumes by using the appropriate calculations/formulas.			

Blood Product Administration

1. Verify the volume of blood product to be transfused by calculating ml/kg of body weight.
2. Adhere to strict infusion times.
3. Use blood warmers as needed.
4. Use appropriate infusion pumps.
5. Minimize the volume of saline solution used to flush IV lines.

Chemotherapy Administration

1. Verify correct dosage of chemotherapy drug using appropriate calculations/formulas.
2. Instruct parent/caregiver in safe handling/precautionary procedures with regards to their child's specific chemotherapy.
3. Anticipate chemotherapy side effects and take age-appropriate action.

TPN Administration

1. Ensure that initiation or cessation is done in a gradual manner to avoid hyper/hypoglycemia.
2. Ensure that bilirubin levels are monitored 4 hours after a lipid infusion.

Continued

Clinical Competency—Pediatric Intravenous Therapy—cont'd

	Yes	No	NA
3. Maintain lipid infusions at a maximum rate of 3 ml/kg/hr.			
4. Ensure that infants' need for sucking is met.			
5. Maintain strict routine intake and output records.			
6. Monitor weight accordingly (infants every shift and children every day or as ordered).			
7. Adjust the rate of TPN by no more than 10% increments as ordered.			
8. Monitor vitals signs and glucose levels at least every 4 hours or as ordered.			
9. Monitor liver function studies and serum liver enzymes routinely.			

Study Questions

1. When initiating pediatric intravenous therapy the nurse should:
   a. Ask the parent to assist with restraining the child for the procedure
   b. Ask the parent to leave the room for the duration of the procedure
   c. Opt for doing the procedure in a neutral/procedure room
   d. Discourage questions or discussion until the procedure is complete

2. Fluid and electrolyte balance in children differs from that in adults because:
   a. Children have proportionally more body water than do adults
   b. Children have a greater BSA in proportion to body mass
   c. A child's metabolism is greater than an adult's
   d. All of the above

3. Nursing interventions for monitoring fluid replacement in pediatric patients include:
   a. Using volumetric chambers to regulate infusions only in infants younger than 12 months

b. Measuring intake and output every 12 to 24 hours
c. Using microdrop tubing to prevent bolus infusions
d. Monitoring IV sites, infusions, and equipment daily

4. Common symptoms of dehydration in infants and children may include the following:
   a. Dry mucous membranes, sunken fontanels, and weight loss
   b. Poor skin turgor, increased urine concentration, and low blood pressure
   c. Decreased urine volume, rapid pulse, and decreased tearing
   d. All of the above

5. Recommended IV sites for school-aged children include the:
   a. Hand or forearm
   b. Scalp
   c. Inner thigh
   d. Foot

6. One advantage of central venous catheters is:
   a. Daily aseptic site care
   b. Insertion that can be performed by any nursing personnel
   c. Most can be submerged in water for bathing or swimming
   d. They allow for long-term or aggressive IV therapy

7. Indications for transfusion therapy in children include:
   a. Increase in the child's blood volume by 35
   b. Acute hemorrhage
   c. Amniocentesis
   d. Wilms' tumors

8. Clinical interventions recommended for pediatric chemotherapy administration include all of the following *except*:
   a. Applying heat to suspected drug infiltration sites to increase tissue absorption
   b. Educating caregivers
   c. Calculating drug dosage with each course of chemotherapy
   d. Anticipating potential side effects

9. Indications for pediatric parenteral nutrition include the following *except:*
   a. Cystic fibrosis, AIDS, pancreatitis
   b. Hirschsprung's disease, gastritis, Crohn's disease
   c. Short bowel syndrome, cancer, renal failure
   d. Gastrointestinal obstruction, gastroschisis

10. Principles of pediatric IV medication administration include:
    a. Knowledge of the child's body surface area
    b. Use of preservative-free solutions for the neonate
    c. Adhering to prescribed infusion rates
    d. All of the above

Answers   1. c   2. d   3. c   4. d   5. a   6. d
7. b   8. a   9. b   10. d

Home Care Infusion Therapy

Objectives

1. Identify components of safety assessment that must be completed before accepting a patient for home care infusion.

2. Discuss the focus of staff education for management of infusion in the home setting.

3. Discuss the focus of patient/caregiver teaching for management of infusion in the home.

4. Identify crucial areas of assessment and documentation in home care infusion therapy.

5. Discuss the major areas of responsibility for home infusion therapy that will involve the home care agency.

Providing infusion therapy in the home setting has become increasingly common as high-tech care is moving out of the inpatient setting and into the arena of community health. Therapies provided in the home include infusions for hydration, parenteral nutrition, chemotherapy, and antibiotic, antiviral, and antifungal treatment. Cardiac care management drugs, biologic response modifiers, and continuous heparin therapy have also been added to the growing list of infusion treatments now being given in patients' homes. In addition, pain control and comfort measures for a variety of acute and chronic disease processes are now managed by in-home infusion therapy and patient controlled analgesia devices.

The growth of home care infusion has also brought with it an increasing number of legal, ethical, and quality care concerns that need to be addressed in the policies and procedures of each home care agency. The main issues for risk management involve patient safety and adequate information related to the electronic, mechanical, and vascular access devices and the medications or solutions used for intravenous (IV) therapy. Therefore discharge planning to the home and the initial and ongoing assessment of in-home infusion must include complete and accurate information about the home environment, the patient and caregiver abilities, and the competency of the professional health care provider.

Discharge Planning
Home Environment

It is critical that the planning for a home care infusion include an adequate assessment of the patient's living arrangements and home setting. It may be difficult to obtain a complete assessment without an actual visit to the patient's home. However, before the patient leaves the hospital or clinic the following areas should be covered:

- Does the patient currently live alone or with others?
- Does the home have adequate facilities and utilities to support home infusion (e.g., electricity, running water, refrigeration, space to safely store infusion equipment)?
- Can the patient and/or caregiver learn the infusion procedures and precautions and be able to manage home infusion therapy?
- Are the primary caregiver and additional caregivers available to perform the required monitoring and procedural tasks?

The home care agency uses this information to determine the eligibility of the patient to receive IV therapy in the home. Once a referral is accepted by the home care agency, the home care nurse is responsible for making a complete assessment on the initial home visit. This assessment includes the same areas as listed previously. The home environment is determined to be adequate to support the infusion or deficient. If any deficiencies are noted, the home care nurse guides the patient and caregivers in the correction process.

Potential issues that may impede safe management of a home infusion include the following:

- Sanitation problems that could increase the risks of infection secondary to an infusion procedure
- Patients/caregivers who are not physically, mentally, or emotionally prepared to manage treatment or assist with the management of treatment

- Limited availability of safe and appropriate storage areas in the home especially in the presence of children or pets, including consideration for medications or solutions requiring refrigeration or other storage precautions and adequate means for safe disposal of sharps and hazardous materials

If any deficiencies identified are not correctable, the physician responsible for the home infusion orders is notified and arrangements are made for the IV therapy to be provided in another setting. If the home environment is deemed safe to support the infusion, the home care nurse proceeds with other areas of teaching and assessment. It is the nurse's responsibility to continue evaluation of home safety throughout the duration of infusion therapy.

Patient/Caregiver

Discharge planning also includes assessing whether it is appropriate for the patient to receive home infusion therapy. This includes consideration of the type of therapy and potential complications. The areas of assessment include the following:

- The patient's homebound status (regulations limit home care services to those who meet the criteria for being homebound)
- The laboratory tests required and arrangements for obtaining them after the patient's discharge to the home
- The type of vascular access device (VAD) the patient currently has in place and the adequacy and safety of the device related to home infusion
- The patient's ability and willingness to accept and manage therapy in the home

Home care regulations require skilled intermittent care, which places limitations on duration and frequency of visits. In general, home care visits should be completed within 2 hours, and the number of visits required must take place in a specified time period. Therefore, for infusions requiring longer than 2 hours or treatments without a definite ending date, the patient and caregivers must be prepared to demonstrate sufficient independence with the infusion to manage it safely without the direct supervision of the nurse once they have been taught the necessary procedures. Specific infusions such as chemotherapy, parenteral nutrition, pain management, or selected antibiotics may require use of an electronic pump to ensure safe administration in the home. An infusion is not appropriate for the home setting if it cannot be managed either independently by the patient/caregiver or managed with home care support within the intermittent care parameters.

In addition, the patient and caregiver need to be prepared to manage the care of the particular VAD in use, which encompasses heparinization and normal saline flushing procedures, dressing changes, and knowledge of signs and symptoms of complications to report. The patient and/or caregiver must be able to perform any required tasks related to the connection and disconnection of IV therapy equipment. This includes the ability to operate and monitor electronic or mechanical infusion pumps.

CLINICAL ALERT: Patients sent home with a peripheral IV access site may be at an increased risks for complications related to therapy, particularly when the infusion therapy is expected to be of long-term rather than short-term duration. If the infusion is continuous rather than intermittent, the possibility of infiltration, phlebitis, and dislodgment of the catheter is present at times when the home care nurse may not be immediately available. It is preferable to place a central VAD or midline catheter before discharge to the home for continuous or longer duration therapies.

Coordination of Home Care Services

Once it is determined that a patient meets all criteria to receive home infusion services, steps need to be taken to ensure a smooth transition to the home setting.

1. Patients and caregivers should be given initial teaching about infusion therapy in the clinic or hospital before discharge.
2. Arrangements need to be made with a provider of home infusion therapy pharmaceuticals and equipment. At times, the infusion therapy provider will also provide home nursing care. However, nursing support is often provided by a separate home care agency.
3. It is important to determine the time frame for delivery of equipment and the initial nursing visit.

CLINICAL ALERT: Many home care agencies have policies prohibiting or restricting the administration of first-dose medication in the home. If the IV therapy to be given is a first dose, arrangements may need to be made to give the initial treatment at the inpatient facility or clinic. If a first dose will be done in the home, the physician should provide specific orders related to management of potential complications, including anaphylaxis.

Home Care Infusion Therapy Staff Education

The focus of staff education for home care infusions should be on accepted standards of practice. The amount and variety of home infusion protocols and products make it necessary to ensure that staff are adequately prepared for all home infusion services. Therefore orientation and staff education must be comprehensive. Some agencies prefer to have high-tech or infusion therapy teams, but in most cases, the primary home care nurse is responsible for managing all aspects of patient care. Agencies should have advanced practice and certified nursing staff available for education and consultation. The necessary components of education include the following:

- Knowledge of the home care agency's pertinent policies and procedures
- Demonstration of technical skills used in home infusion procedures (see "Clinical Competency—Home Care Infusion Therapy" on page 430)
- Knowledge of regulatory, legal, and ethical issues related to home IV therapy
- Knowledge of infusion products and equipment and manufacturer's recommendations for use
- Knowledge of infusion therapy drugs and solutions and their potential side effects, complications, and interactions

Documentation Recommendations

- All findings related to safety of the home environment to support safe administration of IV therapy
- Physician's orders for the prescribed infusion therapy, including dose, amount, and frequency
- Times and dates of all care provided to manage VAD and infusion
- Patient/caregiver responsibilities and goals related to home infusion
- Patient/caregiver abilities and readiness to learn
- Laboratory reports and results
- Information related to blood sampling in the home, including site, amount of blood obtained, and disposition of specimens
- VAD assessment, including description of site and patency
- Care of the VAD, including dressing changes and heparinization and/or normal saline flush

- Administration procedures, including connection and disconnection of infusion
- Operation of electronic and manual pumps with specific information on the programming required for the IV therapy ordered
- Disposal procedures for sharps and hazardous materials
- Availability of 24-hour assistance for patient/caregivers related to infusion and devices, including recording of necessary phone numbers
- Delineation of responsibilities of professional care providers, including information regarding which agency or provider to contact for specific issues related to the infusion equipment, products, services, and clinical care and whether an agency has sole or shared responsibility

$^{n}d_{x}$ Nursing Diagnosis

- Knowledge deficit related to purposes and side effects of intravenous therapy
- Knowledge deficit related to administration procedures for intravenous therapy
- Knowledge deficit related to care of the VAD
- Potential alteration in safety related to home infusion therapy
- Potential for effective or ineffective coping related to home infusion management

Patient/Family Teaching for Self-Management

- Instruct the patient and family regarding the purposes, potential side effects, and complications associated with the prescribed infusion therapy.
- Instruct the patient and family regarding the types of IV supplies and equipment and their management, which includes storage, preparation of the infusion, inventory and ordering information, and the correct procedures for disposal.
- Provide written instructions for every aspect of the infusion procedure for which the patient and family are responsible.
- Provide manuals and troubleshooting guidelines for all electronic pumps or mechanical infusion devices.
- Instruct verbally and provide written instructions for the care of the VAD, such as dressing change, heparinization and/or normal saline flush, and cap/injection port change.

- Instruct on and reinforce the importance of monitoring the VAD for signs and symptoms of infection, infiltration, occlusion, or phlebitis, depending on the device in use.
- Instruct on and reinforce the importance of reporting any adverse effects, complications, problems, or concerns related to the infusion, VAD, or equipment, including operation and/or malfunction of mechanical or electronic pumps.
- Provide telephone numbers for 24-hour service and emergencies.
- Instruct the patient and family regarding safety in the home and precautions to support effective home infusion treatment and prevent complications.
- Require return demonstrations for all procedures and continue supervision and teaching until the patient and family achieve independence.
- Continue assessment and evaluation of infusion therapy management by patient and family until therapy is completed or the patient meets the criteria for discharge from home care services.
- Coordinate arrangements for ongoing assessment and evaluation by the physician and/or outpatient clinic upon discharge from home care services.

Geriatric Considerations

The type of IV therapy along with the physical condition and mental health status of an elderly patient will determine the appropriateness of infusion in the home setting. Increased safety risks potentially exist for many geriatric patients related to their ability to manage the tasks associated with an infusion if their medical condition includes functional limitations or memory deficits. The designated caregiver in a household often is the spouse, and if the patient and spouse are both elderly with observable deficits, it is imperative that caregiving support be provided by others. Because many geriatric patients may be more vulnerable to the adverse effects of certain IV therapies, it may also be necessary to provide more frequent nursing visits to the home.

Resources

Clinical Competency—Home Care Infusion Therapy

Nurses providing infusion care in the home should be able to demonstrate skills related to the initiation, administration, and discontinuation of IV therapy. They must be prepared to provide all necessary assessment, intervention, and evaluation, including management of emergency situations. Certain advanced skills may be reserved for nursing staff with advanced clinical education or specialized certifications. The following lists provide guidelines for the nursing skills required.

	Yes	No	NA
General Skills			
1. Peripheral IV site management, including site selection, insertion of catheter, postinsertion site care, and assessing for infiltration			
2. Peripheral blood sampling techniques			
3. Central venous catheter device care, including dressing changes, heparinization and/or normal saline flush procedures, and blood sampling procedures			
4. IV administration techniques, including priming, connection, and disconnection of tubing; use of manual devices to control rate and flow; bag and cassette changes; use of filters; and use of injection ports/caps and needleless access devices			
5. Calculation of infusion and/or medication drip rates			
6. Preventive and emergency management care related to first-dose administration, adverse reactions and anaphylaxis, and management of infiltration			

Clinical Competency—Home Care Infusion Therapy—cont'd

	Yes	No	NA
7. Infusion pump management, both general principles and specific operating procedures for the types of pumps in use			
8. Fluid and electrolyte balance assessments			
9. Nutritional assessments			
10. Pain/comfort assessments			
11. Handling and disposal of sharps and hazardous waste materials			
Intermediate Skills			
12. Implanted central venous access port care and management, including site care, accessing of port, securing of noncoring needle or specialized catheter after port access, irrigation/flush procedures, and blood drawing techniques			
13. Admixture of solutions including total parenteral nutrition (TPN), chemotherapy, and other solutions that require preparation in the home			
14. IV bolus and/or continuous administration of medication and/or infusion solution with precautions specific to therapy provided			
15. Implanted infusion pump access and administration procedure			
16. Removal of midline catheters and peripherally inserted central catheter (PICC) lines			
17. Preventive and emergency management care related to vesicant administration including measures for extravasation			
18. Measures for chemotherapy spills			

Continued

Clinical Competency—Home Care Infusion Therapy—cont'd

	Yes	No	NA
19. Measures for repair of a central venous catheter			
20. Management of non-IV infusions, including epidural ports and catheters and intraarterial lines			
Advanced Skills			
21. Measures for declotting of occluded central venous catheters and ports			
22. Insertion of PICC			
23. Management of intrathecal infusions			

Home Care Considerations for Specific Types of Infusion Therapy

The following are additional considerations for home care infusion therapy. Please refer to the designated chapters in this book for more extensive information on the specific types of infusions and/or related procedures. See Chapter 14, "Professional Resources," for product, device, and infusion pump manufacturer and professional and government agency listings.

General Practices for Home Care Infusion Therapy

For each topic, specific home care guidelines are included in the appropriate chapter.

Infusion Therapy	Home Care Considerations
Fluid and Electrolyte Replacement (Chapter 5)	Have results of most recent serum electrolyte values available.
	Review orders for continued monitoring of electrolytes.
	Document cardiovascular and fluid volume status assessments.
	Provide measures to prevent fluid overload.

Infusion Therapy	Home Care Considerations
Antibiotic and Antiinfective Therapy (Chapter 6)	Obtain patient history of adverse drug and allergic reactions.
	Provide information on dose-related adverse reactions.
	Provide additional support for patient and family if therapy requires more than one infusion of a certain drug or infusion of multiple drugs in a 24-hr period with starting and stopping of infusion and repeated disconnections and reconnections.
	Consider electronic infusion pump for intermittent dosing to ensure safety and decrease risks of infusion-related complications.
	Document all assessment related to infection or condition being treated and responses to therapy including pertinent laboratory values, body systems affected by therapy, particularly gastrointestinal and urinary function changes, rashes, and sensitivities.
	Assess for changes in mental status.
	Be prepared for possibility of anaphylactic reaction.
Blood and Blood Components (Chapter 7)	Many home care agencies do not administer blood or blood products in the home due to issues of intermittent skilled care limitations and the risks to patient safety. If you are employed by an agency that provides this therapy in the home setting be sure you are aware of all of your agency policies and procedures regarding delivery of care and emergency management of blood and blood component administration.

Infusion Therapy	Home Care Considerations
Chemotherapy (Chapter 8)	Assess and prepare home environment to support proper storage, preparation, and handling of chemotherapy agents, including properly ventilated room away from areas of food preparation and storage.
	Take measures to protect the patient and family from accidental contact with the agent, including provision of acceptable means of disposable and plastic-backed absorbent pads large enough to place on the patient and to protect countertops or other surfaces during preparation and administration.
	Follow all guidelines and recommendations related to protective gear and disposal of chemotherapy waste.
	Provide patient/caregiver with instructions related to chemotherapy spills and place spill kit in the home.
	Inform patient/caregiver that chemotherapy agent may be present in body fluids for up to 2 days (48 hr).
	Instruct patient/caregiver that universal precautions should be used for at least 2 days after administration when handling clothing or linen soiled with a patient's body fluids and these articles should be washed twice in hot water and detergent separate from other laundry.
	Instruct patient/caregiver to make sure toilet is flushed completely after use by patient.
	Instruct patient/caregiver to treat disposable items contaminated with patient bodily fluids in the first few days as hazardous waste material.
	Advise extreme caution if administering a vesicant in the home setting; home agencies may have policies limiting the types of chemotherapy agents they will provide in the home.

Infusion Therapy	Home Care Considerations
Chemotherapy (Chapter 8)—cont'd	Document all pertinent assessment including complete blood count and electrolytes, functional level and fatigue, responses to therapy, and potential side effects of all body systems especially signs and symptoms of infection.
	Be prepared for events and provide interventions for anaphylaxis, allergies, hypersensitivities, infiltrations, and extravasations.
Parenteral Nutrition (Chapter 9)	More storage capacity than needed with other types of infusions, including adequate refrigeration space.
	Many TPN treatments are scheduled for 12- to 16-hr administration to allow the patient free time without a pump; *focus initial teaching* on the disconnection procedures as this is the easiest area for the patient/caregiver to master independently.
	Teach patient/caregiver how to accurately measure and record weight and temperature.
	Obtain and document all necessary laboratory test results, as ordered by physician.
	Assess and document the nutrition/hydration status, cardiovascular and fluid volume status, and presence or absence of signs and symptoms of infection.

Infusion Therapy	Home Care Considerations
Pediatric Intravenous Therapy (Chapter 11)	Refer to Chapter 11 for all topics regarding pediatric infusion therapy, for example, infusion guidelines, fluid and electrolyte balance with recommendations for replacement regarding losses, venipucnture, central venous and peripherally inserted catheters, implantable ports, blood products, medication, and parenteral nutrition administration, and home care considerations with definitive discharge instructions. Refer to Chapter 13, "Calculations for Infusion Therapy."

Study Questions

1. Which components are necessary to make a complete assessment of the safety of the patient's home environment to support home infusion therapy?
   a. The patient's medical history and type of infusion required
   b. Patient and family reports of living conditions and available home support
   c. A home visit by the nurse to assess the caregiver and home environment
   d. All of the above

2. The home care staff education for management of home care infusion therapy should include the following issues:
   a. Legal, ethical, and moral issues of care
   b. 24-hour recall of all telephone numbers for infusion procedures
   c. Technical competencies related to infusion management
   d. Patient's physician home phone number

3. Which of following indicates that a patient and family are ready to manage a home infusion safely?
   a. Patient and family are able to verbalize knowledge of adverse reactions, complications to report to the physician, and an understanding to report changes as soon as possible.
   b. Patient and family are aware of 24-hour numbers for

emergencies, but did not report a significant symptom or problem.

c. Patient and family are able to perform all infusion procedures and verbalize potential complications with assistance or direction from the nurse.

d. Patient and family are able to contact product and device companies to obtain troubleshooting guidelines for infusion procedures.

4. Which is the best way to ensure that patients and families will be able to understand and adhere to teaching when the nurse is *not present*?

a. Multiple return demonstrations completed on the same home visit

b. Provision of written instructions for all infusion-related procedures

c. Verbalization of all the product, device, and infusion companies' phone numbers

d. Performance of required blood sampling procedure with disposition of specimen

5. Which of the following infusion therapy procedures is considered an advanced skill?

a. VAD heparinization, dressing, and/or blood sampling

b. PICC heparinization, dressing, and/or infusion pump alarm

c. PICC insertion

d. Pain management and drug titration according to protocol

6. Risk management issues for patients receiving home infusion therapy include:

a. Patient safety, home care status eligible days, VAD and infusion solution

b. Patient safety, VAD and infusion pump interventions and infusion solution

c. Patient safety, medications and infusions, home care eligible days

d. Patient safety, VAD information, immunization history

7. Home care infusion services usually *restrict* the following services *except:*

a. First-dose medication infusion, blood products, pain management, TPN

b. First-dose medication infusion, blood sampling, pain management, TPN

c. Vesicant chemotherapy infusions, blood sampling, hydration infusions, TPN

d. Chemotherapy, antimicrobial therapies, hydration infusions, TPN

8. Issues that potentially impede safe management of home infusion therapy include:

a. Sanitation, patient caregiver status, safe disposal of sharps and hazardous materials

b. Sanitation, insurance reimbursement, safe disposal of sharps and hazardous materials

c. Patient caregiver status, refrigeration for medications/TPN, physician office location

d. Patient caregiver status, refrigeration for medications/TPN, infusion agency location

9. Geriatric patients receiving home infusion therapy have unique issues regarding _____ and require _____ home visits.

a. Potential increased safety risks and spouse/caregiver status; fewer

b. Potential decreased safety risks and spouse/caregiver status; more

c. Potential increased safety risks and spouse/caregiver status; more

d. Potential decreased safety risks and spouse/caregiver status; fewer

10. Home care considerations for infusion therapy with fluid and electrolyte replacement, monitoring, and intervention require tests availability and results for:

a. Results of serum electrolyte values over the past 30 days

b. Results of serum electrolyte values over the past 21 days

c. Results of serum electrolyte values over the past 14 days

d. Results of serum electrolyte values of most recent specimen

Answers   1. d   2. c   3. a   4. b   5. c   6. b
7. d   8. a   9. c   10. d

Calculations for IV Infusions

13

Objectives

1. Calculate IV flow rates using 10-, 12-, 15-, and 60-drop infusion sets.

2. Calculate drug dosage requirements for microgram and kilogram for the child and adult patient.

3. Calculate body surface area drug doses for the child and adult patient.

4. Calculate the pediatric IVs infusion rate using the rule of six.

Flow Rate Calculations

Flow rate calculations are integral to the safe delivery of IV fluids and medications. Information necessary to calculate the flow rates includes the following:

1. Volume of fluid to be infused
2. Total infusion time
3. Calibration of the administration set used (number of drops per milliliter it delivers; this information is found on the IV tubing package)

Manufacturers of IV tubings use 10, 12, 15, or 60 drops (gtt) to deliver a milliliter of fluid. To calculate an hourly IV rate, use the following formula:

$$\frac{\text{gtt/ml of set}}{60 \text{ min}} \times \text{Total hourly volume} = \text{gtt/min} \qquad \text{Equation 1}$$

1000 ml over 8 hr = 125 ml/hr; 10 gtt/ml infusion set

$$\frac{10 \text{ gtt/ml}}{60 \text{ min}} \times 125 \text{ ml/hr} = \frac{1 \text{ gtt}}{6 \text{ min}} \times 125 \text{ ml/hr}$$

$$\frac{1}{6} \times \frac{125 \text{ ml/hr}}{1} = \frac{1}{6} \times \frac{125}{1} = 20 \text{ gtt/min}$$

Because $^{10}/_{60}$ reduces to $^1/_6$, any hourly volume may be divided by 6 to determine the drops per minute of an IV set that delivers 10 drops/ml.

1000 ml over 10 hr = 100 ml/hr; 15 gtt/ml infusion set   Equation 2

$$\frac{15 \text{ gtt/ml}}{60 \text{ min}} \times 100 \text{ ml/hr} = \frac{1 \text{ gtt}}{4 \text{ min}} \times 100 \text{ ml/hr}$$

$$\frac{1}{4} \times \frac{100 \text{ ml/hr}}{1} = \frac{1}{4} \times \frac{100}{1} = 25 \text{ gtt/min}$$

CLINICAL ALERT: Calculations for other IV tubing sets include the following: gtt/ml/set

$$\frac{12 \text{ gtt}}{60 \text{ min}} = \frac{1}{5} \text{ or divide by 5}$$ Equation 3

$$\frac{15 \text{ gtt}}{60 \text{ min}} = \frac{1}{4} \text{ or divide by 4}$$

$$\frac{20 \text{ gtt}}{60 \text{ min}} = \frac{1}{3} \text{ or divide by 3}$$

$$\frac{60 \text{ gtt}}{60 \text{ min}} = 1 \text{ or divide by 1}$$

Often a 24-hour volume is prescribed by a physician. Divide the desired volume by 24 before using the preceding formula.

3000 hr   Equation 4

$3000 \div 24$

$$\frac{3000}{1} \times \frac{1}{24} = 125 \text{ ml/hr}$$

To calculate drops per minute for fluid volume that is prescribed in milliliters per hour, proceed to the step of

$$\frac{\text{gtt/ml of set}}{60 \text{ min}} = \text{Total hourly volume} = \text{gtt/min}$$ Equation 5

When small-volume IV piggyback medications are administered through the same IV line as a continuous infusion, the IV infusion will not stay on time unless the time needed to infuse the piggyback medications is included in the total calculations. Subtract the time required for the piggyback infusion from the 24-hour period before calculating the drops per minute for the continuous IV.

IV fluid 3000 ml 24 hr   Equation 6

Piggyback medication

50 ml over 20 min × 3 in 24 hr = 1 hr

24 hr − 1 hr = 23 hr

3000 ml ÷ 23

$$\frac{3000}{1} \times \frac{1}{23} = 130 \text{ ml/hr}$$

This consideration is important for very ill patients receiving triple antibiotic therapy, especially if each drug dose is diluted in 50 to 100 ml of IV fluid.

Monitoring IV flow rate is facilitated by recording the milliliters per hour by hourly increments on each IV container. This information may be recorded on the IV time-tape affixed to the outside of the container.

Flow Rate (ml)	Time
	8 AM start
125	9
250	10
375	11
500	12 PM
625	1
750	2
875	3
1000 ml	4 PM end

Subsequent rate adjustments can be made throughout the IV fluid delivery by observing the desired milliliters to be infused at the scheduled time and adjusting the flow rate.

Drug Dose Calculations—Adult

IV drug dosage may be prescribed in micrograms per kilogram per minute, milligrams per hour, or units of drug per hour, or by body surface area (BSA) requirements. Calculations of micrograms per kilogram per minute include conversion of pounds to kilograms and milligrams to micrograms. Drug units per hour and milligrams per hour are determined by the concentration of a drug in a volume of solution. BSA requirements are calculated via a nomogram. The following formulas and examples describe a step-by-step process for each method.

Micrograms per Kilogram per Minute

Convert weight in pounds to kilograms (divide the weight by 2.2):

132 lb ÷ 2.2 = 60 kg

Convert total milligrams of medication dose to micrograms (multiply the milligrams by 1000 or move decimal three places to the right):

100 mg × 1000 = 100,000 µg

In most instances, a microdrop IV tubing will be used, and 60 µgtt/min equal 1 ml.

Patient—176 lb   Equation 7

Medication—dopamine 200 mg in 250 ml dilute strength (DS)/0.45 normal saline

Dose—dopamine 5 µg/kg/min

1. Convert 176 lb to kg:

   176 ÷ 2.2 = 80 kg

   Dopamine 200 mg to µg

   200 mg × 1000 = 200,000 µg

2. Determine µg/min dose based on kg weight:

   5 µg/kg/min × 80 kg = 400 µg/min

3. Determine µg/ml dosage:

   200,000 µg : 250 ml = x µg : 1 ml

   $$\frac{200,000}{250} = \frac{x}{1}$$

$$x = \frac{200,000}{250}$$

$x = 800 \ \mu g/ml$

4. Determine μgtt/min:

Microdrop tubing 60 μgtt/ml

800 μg: 60 μgtt/ml = 400 μg/min

$$\frac{800}{60} = \frac{400}{x} : 800 \ x = 24,000$$

$$x = \frac{24,000}{800}$$

$x = 30 \ \mu gtt/min$

Milligrams per Hour

Drug concentration in milligrams per milliliter will vary according to the dilution factor. Note the drug concentration in milligrams per milliliter of each drug before calculation of flow rate.

Morphine—50 mg in 100 ml = 1 mg/20 ml   Equation 8

Dose—morphine 4 mg/hr

Infusion set—60 gtt/min

1 mg = 20 ml

4 mg = x ml/hr

4 × 20 = 80

80 ml/hr

$$\frac{60 \ \mu gtt}{60 \ min} \times 80 \ ml/hr = \mu gtt/min$$

$$\frac{60}{60} \times 80$$

1 × 80 = 80 μgtt/min

Units of Drug per Hour

Heparin—20,000 units in 500 ml of dextrose in water (D/W)

Dose—heparin 1000 units/hr   Equation 9

Infusion set—60 gtt/ml

20,000 units of heparin ÷ 500 ml infusion

20,000 ÷ 500 = x units/ml

$$x = \frac{20,000}{500}$$

$x = 40$ units/ml

$$\frac{1000 \text{ units/hr}}{40 \text{ units/ml/solution}}$$

$$\frac{1000}{40} : 1 \times \frac{1000}{40} = x \text{ ml/min}$$

$$\frac{1000}{40} = 25 \text{ ml/hr}$$

$$\frac{60 \text{ } \mu\text{gtt}}{60 \text{ min}} \times 25 \text{ ml/hr} = \mu\text{gtt/min}$$

$$\frac{60}{60} \times \frac{25}{1} = 25 \text{ } \mu\text{gtt/min}$$

Drug Dose Calculations for Critical Care Medications*

Calculating Micrograms per Kilogram per Minute

To convert pounds into kilograms: divide pounds by 2.2 = kilograms

To calculate micrograms per kilogram per minute

Step One: $\dfrac{\text{Total amount of medication}}{\text{Total Volume}} \times 1000 \div 60 \div \text{kg} =$

constant

A. Multiply by 1000 μg (to convert from mg to μg)
B. Divide this by 60 minutes (to convert from hours to minutes)
C. Divide this by patient weight in kg (these are weight-based medications)

This number is your *constant*.

Step Two: If μg/min is known, use step A. If ml/hr is known, use step B.

A. Total μg/min ÷ constant = ml/hour
B. Constant × ml/hr = total μg/min

---

*Courtesy Via Christi Regional Medical Center, Wichita, Kans.

Medication Calculations*
Units per Hour and Milligrams per Hour

Step One: $\dfrac{\text{Total amount (units or mg)}}{\text{Total volume (ml)}} = \dfrac{\text{units}}{\text{ml}}$ or $\dfrac{\text{mg}}{\text{ml}}$

Step Two: $\dfrac{\text{Medications (units or mg)}}{\text{units or mg}} \times \dfrac{\text{ml}}{1 \text{ hr}} = \text{ml/hr}$

Milligrams per Minute

Step One: $\dfrac{\text{Total amount (mg)}}{\text{Total volume (ml)}} = \text{mg/ml}$

Step Two: $\dfrac{\text{Desired amount (mg/min)}}{\text{On-hand amount in (mg/ml)}} \times 60 \text{ min} = \text{ml/hr}$

Micrograms per Minute

Step One: Calculating your constant

$\dfrac{\text{Amount of drug}}{\text{Total volume (ml)}} \times 1000 \div 60 = constant$

Step Two: If µg/min is known, use step A. If ml/hr is known, use step B.

    A. Total µg/min ÷ constant = ml/hr

    B. Constant × ml/hr = total µg/min

BSA Requirements

The dosages of some drugs are calculated proportionally to the BSA of the patient. BSA is calculated in square meters. A nomogram is used to correlate height (centimeters or inches) with weight (kilograms or pounds) to determine BSA in square meters. The drug dose is ordered in milligrams per square meter.

Height—68 in   Equation 10

Weight—150 lb

$m^2 = 1.80$ BSA

Dose 75 mg/m^2

$1.80 \times 75 = x$ dose

    $x = 135$ mg dose

Drug Dose Calculations—Pediatric

There are several methods for calculating pediatric dosage based on age, weight, or BSA. The usual means of calculating pediatric

---

*Courtesy Via Christi Regional Medical Center, Wichita, Kans.

dosage is the milligrams-per-kilogram or micrograms-per-kilogram methods. These methods require conversion of pounds to kilograms before determining the desired dose. Drug literature giving the recommended dose per kilogram or pound of body weight should be consulted before measuring the desired dose.

Milligrams per Kilogram Body Weight

Convert weight in pounds to kilograms (divide the weight by 2.2).

Child—22 lb

Equation 11

Medication—phenytoin 5 mg = (child's body weight)

Required dose—mg

1. Convert 22 lb to kg:

   $22 \div 2.2 = 10$ kg

2. Determine dose based on 1 kg = 5 mg of phenytoin (Dilantin):

   1 kg (child) = 5 mg (drug)

   10 kg (child) = x mg (drug)

   10 kg × 5 = 50 mg

   50 mg = drug dose

Micrograms per Kilogram Body Weight

Convert weight in pounds to kilograms (divide the weight by 2.2):

Child—33 lb

Equation 12

Medication—actinomycin 15 μg = 1 kg (child's body weight)

Required dose—μg

1. Convert 33 lb to kg:

   $33 \div 2.2 = 15$ kg

2. Determine dose based on 1 kg = 15 μg of actinomycin:

   1 kg (child) = 15 μg

   15 kg (child) = x μg (drug)

   15 kg × 15 μg = 225 μg

   225 μg = drug dose

Other Methods

If the dosage is not given in terms of milligrams per kilogram, the pediatric dose is calculated from the standard adult dose. These methods are referred to as rules, and the dosage is calculated by weight in pounds, age in months, age in years, or surface area in square meters compared with an adult dose.

Clark's rule (child of 2 years and older)

This method is based on weight in pounds. The adult dose is multiplied by the following fraction:

$$\frac{\text{Weight (in pounds)}}{150 \text{ lb}} \times \text{Adult dose} = \text{Approximate child dose}$$

$$\frac{50 \text{ lb}}{150 \text{ lb}} \times 150 \text{ mg adult dose} = \text{Approximate child dose} \qquad \text{Equation 13}$$

$$\frac{50}{1} \times \frac{1}{1} = 50 \text{ mg child dose}$$

Fried's rule (infant younger than 1 year)

This method is based on the age in months. The adult dose is multiplied by the following fraction (150 months is the age of a 12-year-old child):

$$\frac{\text{Age (in months)}}{150 \text{ mo}} \qquad \text{Equation 14}$$

$$\frac{\text{Age (in months)}}{150 \text{ mo}} \times \text{Adult dose} = \text{Approximate infant dose}$$

$$\frac{9 \text{ mo}}{150 \text{ mo}} \times 200 \text{ mg} = \text{Infant dose}$$

$$\frac{9}{150} \times \frac{200}{1} = \frac{9}{15} \times \frac{20}{1} = \frac{9}{3} \times \frac{4}{1} = \text{Infant dose}$$

$$\frac{9}{3} \times \frac{4}{1} = \frac{36}{3} = 12 \text{ mg infant dose}$$

Young's rule (child of 2 years and older)

This method is based on the age of the child in years. The adult dose is multiplied by the following fraction:

$$\frac{\text{Age of child in years}}{\text{Age in years} + 12} \times \text{Adult dose} = \text{Approximate child dose}$$

Adult dose of penicillin—500 mg   Equation 15

Child age—8 years

Child dose = x mg

$$\frac{8 \text{ yr}}{8 \text{ yr} + 12} \times 500 \text{ mg} = \text{Approximate child dose}$$

$$\frac{8}{8+12} = \frac{8}{20} = \frac{2}{5}$$

$$\frac{2}{5} \times \frac{500}{1} = \frac{2}{1} \times \frac{100}{1}$$

$$\frac{2}{1} \times \frac{100}{1} = \frac{200}{1} = 200 \text{ mg} = \text{Child dose}$$

BSA method

A nomogram is used to correlate the height (centimeters or inches) with the weight (kilograms or pounds) to determine BSA in square meters. The drug dose is ordered in milligrams per square meter.

Height—23 in   Equation 16

Weight—44 lb

$m^2 = 0.50$ (BSA)

Dose—1 mg/m^2

0.50×1 mg = x dose

$\qquad x = 0.50$ mg of drug

Other methods using BSA include the following:

$$\frac{\text{BSA in } m^2}{1.75} \times \text{Adult dose} = \text{Approximate child dose}$$

$$\frac{\text{BSA of child}}{\text{BSA of adult}} \times \text{Adult dose} = \text{Approximate child dose}$$

Rule of Six to Calculate IV Infusion in a Pediatric Crisis Situation*

The rule of six is a simplification of a complicated mathematical equation used to calculate the amount of drug needed to make an infusion. The rule of six is as follows:

6 × Weight (wt) in kilograms (kg) = Milligrams (mg) of drug to add to 100 ml of IV fluid. When the fluid is infused at 1 ml/hr, it will deliver drug at the rate of 1 μg/kg/min.

Desired dose = μg/kg/min   Equation 17

$$= \mu g \times \frac{1 \text{ mg}}{1000 \text{ μg}} \times kg \times min \times \frac{1 \text{ hr}}{60 \text{ min}}$$

$$= 0.06 \text{ mg} \times kg \times hr$$

$$\frac{\text{Desired dose}}{\text{Desired rate}} = \frac{0.06 \text{ mg} \times kg \times hr}{ml/hr} \qquad \text{Equation 18}$$

$$\frac{\text{Desired dose}}{\text{Desired rate}} = \frac{kg \times 0.06 \text{ mg}}{ml} = \frac{\text{mg drug}}{100 \text{ ml}} \qquad \text{Equation 19}$$

$$\text{Amount of drug (mg)} = \frac{kg \times 0.06 \text{ mg} \times 100 \text{ ml}}{ml} \qquad \text{Equation 20}$$

$$\text{Amount of drug (mg/100 ml)} = kg \times 6 \qquad \text{Equation 21}$$

The rule of six can be used with the following drugs: amrinone, dobutamine, dopamine, nitroglycerin, and nitroprusside. Doses of these drugs are given in terms of 1 μg/kg/min or multiples thereof.

When using epinephrine, isoproterenol, norepinephrine, or prostaglandin E_1, multiply by 0.6 instead of 6. Doses of these drugs are given in terms of 0.1 μg/kg/min because of their potency.

For lidocaine, multiply by 60 instead of 6 because doses are usually started at 20 to 50 μg/kg/min.

Example: A 7-kg infant is in heart failure and requires continuous dobutamine infusion to run at 5 ml/hr to deliver 5 μg/kg/min. How many milligrams of dobutamine must be added to a 100-ml IV fluid bag?

Rule of six: 6 × 7 kg = 42 mg

---

*Consult with a pharmacist or physician regarding calculations, drug concentrations, and compatible IV fluids and solutions. From McLeroy PA: *Hosp Pharm* 29(10):939, 1994.

Therefore 42 mg of dobutamine is added to 100 ml of IV fluid and 1 ml/hr = 1 µg/kg/min. Label the bag *dobutamine 42 mg/100 ml DSW 1 ml/hr = 1 µg/kg/min.*

Study Questions

Refer to flow rate and drug dosage calculation examples provided earlier in this chapter.

1. Calculate an infusion rate for 1000 ml every 10 hours using a 10 drop/ml infusion set.

$$\frac{\text{gtt/ml of set}}{60 \text{ min}} = \text{Total hourly volume} = \text{gtt/min}$$

_____ ml over _____ hours = _____ gtt/min

2. Calculate an infusion rate for 500 ml every 12 hours using a 12 drop/ml infusion set.

gtt/ml of set × total hourly volume = gtt/min

_____ ml over _____ hours = _____ /hr

3. If a medication is to be added to 50 ml of normal saline and administered over 30 minutes, what should the flow rate be set at if a 60 gtt/ml calibration is used?

$$\frac{50 \text{ ml} \times 60 \text{ gtt}}{30 \text{ min}} = \text{Flow rate}$$

4. Calculate the flow rate for 250 ml of D_5W given over 2 hours with a 15 gtt/ml infusion set.

$$\frac{250 \text{ ml} \times 15 \text{ gtt}}{120 \text{ min}} = \text{Flow rate}$$

5. You are to administer Ancef 500 mg IV piggyback using a 15 gtt/ml secondary infusion set. If the medication is diluted in 100 ml of D_5W, how fast should the drop per minute rate be set to administer the medication in 30 minutes?

_____ ml × _____ gtt = flow rate of _____ minutes

6. Agency standard solution for heparin is 25,000 units in 500 ml of D_5W. The order is to administer 1000 units/hr. Calculate the infusion rate using a 60 gtt/ml set.

First calculate the volume of D$_5$W that contains 1000 units using the proportion formula.

$$\frac{25,000}{500 \text{ ml}} = \frac{1000 \text{ units}}{x}$$

You must then calculate the flow rate per hour and the drops per minute using the 60 gtt/ml infusion set.

7. The order is to infuse dopamine 200 mg diluted in 250 ml of D$_5$W at 5 µg/kg/min. The patient's weight is 132 lb. The infusion set = 60 gtt/ml.
   a. Convert 132 lb to kilograms.
   b. How many milligrams of dopamine will each milliliter contain?
   c. What dose is the patient to receive per minute?
   d. How many gtt/min? How many ml/hr?

8. Calculate the BSA (m^2) for an adult 66 inches tall and weighing 200 lb. Then calculate the drug dosage mg/m^2 (order: cyclophosphamide 650 mg/m^2; doxorubicin 50 mg/m^2; and 5-fluorouracil 300 mg/m^2).

   Body surface area (BSA) = 2.00 via nomogram

9. Rule of six: A child weighing 10 kg requires a continuous lidocaine infusion to deliver at the rate of 20 µg/kg/min. (Rule of 6 for lidocaine: Multiply by 60 instead of 6 because doses are usually started at 20 to 50 µg/kg/min.)
   a. _____ kg × 60 = _____ mg/100 ml IV fluid
   b. _____ ml/hr = _____ µg/kg/min

10. Rule of six: A 7-kg infant is in heart failure and requires a continuous dobutamine infusion to run at 5 ml/hr to deliver 5 µg/kg/min. How many milligrams of dobutamine must be added to a 100-ml IV fluid bag?
    a. Rule of six: _____ × 7 kg = _____ mg
    b. Therefore, _____ of dobutamine is added to 100 ml of IV fluid and _____ ml/hr = _____ µg/kg/min.

ANSWERS:
1. 1000 ml divided by 10 hr = 100 ml/hr

$$\frac{10 \text{ gtt/ml}}{60 \text{ min}} = \frac{1}{6} \times \frac{100 \text{ ml/hr}}{1} = \frac{1}{6} \times \frac{100}{1} = 16.6 = 17 \text{ gtt/min}$$

2. 500 ml divided by 12 hr = 41.6 = 42 ml/hr

$$\frac{12 \text{ gtt/min}}{60 \text{ min}} = \frac{1}{5} \times \frac{42 \text{ ml/hr}}{1} = \frac{1}{5} \times \frac{42}{1} = 8.3 = 9 \text{ gtt/min}$$

3. $\dfrac{50 \times 60}{30} = \dfrac{3000}{30} = 100$ gtt/min over 30 min

4. $\dfrac{250 \times 15}{120} = \dfrac{3750}{120} = 31.25 = 32$ gtt/min over 120 min

5. $\dfrac{100 \times 15}{30} = \dfrac{1500}{30} = 50$ gtt/min

6. $\dfrac{25,000 \text{ units}}{50 \text{ ml}} = \dfrac{1000 \text{ units}}{x \text{ ml}}$

$\qquad = 500,000 = 25,000 \, x$

$x = 20$ ml/hr

$\dfrac{60 \text{ gtt set}}{60 \text{ min}} = \dfrac{1}{1} \times 20 \text{ ml/hr} = 20 \text{ gtt/min}$

7. a. $132 \div 2.2 = 60$ kg

b. $\dfrac{200 \text{ mg}}{250 \text{ ml}} = 0.8$ mg/ml concentration

$0.8 \text{ mg} = x \text{ μg}$
$0.8 \times 1000 = 800 \text{ μg/ml}$ concentration

c. 5 g × 60 kg/min
$\qquad = 300$ μg/min

d. $\dfrac{800 \text{ μg}}{1 \text{ ml}} = \dfrac{300 \text{ μg}}{x \text{ ml}} = \dfrac{0.375 \text{ ml} \times 60 \text{ gtt/ml set}}{1 \text{ minute}}$
$\qquad = 23$ gtt/min = 23 ml/hr

8. BSA = 2.0
Cyclophosphamide: 650 mg × 2 = 1300 mg
Doxorubicin: 50 mg × 2 = 100 mg
5-Fluorouracil: 300 mg × 2 = 600 mg

9. a. 10 kg × 60 = 600 mg/100 ml of IV fluid
b. 1 ml/hr = 10 μg/kg/min (Therefore 2 ml/hr would deliver 20 μg/kg/min.)

10. a. 6 × 7 = 42 mg
b. Therefore 42 mg of dobutamine is added to 100 ml of IV fluid and 1 ml/hr = 1 μg/kg/min.

Professional Resources

14

Education

The professional resource chapter is designed to provide a variety of information regarding education principles, pharmaceutical and device research and development, and nurse-related risk management information. The initial section on adult learning principles and consideration can readily be adapted for nursing staff, patient, and/or family education. The second section addresses the key objectives essential for any Intravenous Therapy Course for varied skill mix levels of nursing staff (e.g., licensed practical nurse, registered professional nurse), and/or some topics could be provided to para-professional staff in extended care settings.

Pharmaceutical and device research and development, with clinical implementation, continues to challenge nurses in all practice settings. This section describes the research process with clinical testing and implementation for patient care uses. Nursing responsibility and accountability regarding use and/or suspect product or nonfunctional equipment reporting is provided.

Risk management with professional practice issues covers the essential topics to make the nurse more aware of professional duties and responsibilities. Topics such as reporting a "needlestick injury" and legal issues are provided.

The remaining section of this chapter includes the following:

- IV infusion therapy device company listings
- Manufacturers of PICCs and related equipment
- Government and regulatory websites
- Professional organization websites

Adult Learning Principles and Considerations (See Chapter 11 for Pediatric Information)

A. Knowles adult education principles
   1. Adults are independent learners.
   2. Adults' past experiences are resources for learning.
   3. Adults' readiness to learn emerges from life's developmental stages.
   4. Adults' time perspective in learning is related to immediacy of application.
   5. Adults' orientation for learning is problem-centered.
   6. Adults learn well by doing.
   7. Adults resist learning under conditions that are incongruent with their self-concepts.
B. Adult education assessment principles
   1. Physical: age, visual or hearing acuity, mobility, fatigue, illness
   2. Psychologic: anxiety, stress response, time, family responsibilities, adaptation to life/illness
   3. Sociocultural: coping mechanisms, occupation, education, income, recreation
   4. Cultural issues: language, communication, religious beliefs, cultural remedies/healers
   5. Environmental: noise, space, room temperature, travel to/from
C. Application of the learning domains
   1. Cognitive domain: knowledge, comprehension, application, analysis, synthesis, evaluation, information application and retention (how and what we learn and retain)
   2. Psychomotor domain: perception, readiness, guided response, complex response, adaptation, performance skills, involves use of skeletal muscles and dexterity (the ability to learn and/or become competent in a skill or activity)
   3. Affective domain: awareness, responding, valuing organization, value characterization, attitudes, values, beliefs (how and what we believe, value, respond)
D. Special education needs
   1. Language barriers: consider family member, friend, professional to interpret information.
   2. Use concrete examples to clarify information; provide opportunity for learner to demonstrate new skill, or technique.

3. Use simply written materials (e.g., graphics, large print), proceed from simple to complex; allow ample time for learning new skill or information; consider social support.
4. Teach only the essentials.
5. Minimize distractions while learning new information or skill.
6. Identify the patient objectives of teaching with measurable outcomes; start with most important information; minimize anxiety; encourage questions; reinforce; plan periods of review; rest.

E. Educational materials options
   1. Multimedia
      Videotape: illustrate procedures; no opportunity for interaction or return demonstration
      Computer-assisted information (CIA): process controlled by learner; potential to be time-consuming
      CD-ROM compact disc: interactive limitations with video; multiple levels learning needs
      Virtual reality: requires dedicated computer for software
   2. Audio cassette tapes: opportunity to listen to information multiple times
   3. Working models: allow learner to have hands-on experience
   4. Chalkboards, posters, flip-charts: multiple ways to present information to groups and facilitate group process
   5. Written materials: able to individualize to specific agency protocol

Intravenous Therapy Course Objectives

A. Be knowledgeable of the state nurse practice act as it relates to IV therapy.
   1. Maintain active and current license related to your specific scope of practice.
   2. Become aware and active in professional organizations (e.g., Intravenous Nurses Society, Oncology Nursing Society, American Association of Critical-Care Nurses, and National Association for Home Care).
   3. Participate in your agency's continuous performance improvement projects.

B. Understand anatomy and physiology as applied to IV therapy.
   1. Identify protective functions of the skin.
   2. Differentiate between arteries and veins.
   3. Identify venous anatomic structures.

4. Demonstrate appropriate vein selection for prescribed IV treatment.
5. Know measures that reduce the vasovagal response.
6. List IV therapy–related factors that can cause alterations of the cardiopulmonary system.
7. Identify factors that can alter normal blood clotting.
8. Know and practice aseptic technique, universal blood and body secretion precautions, and disposal of supplies in appropriate disposal system.
9. Become informed and select the appropriate product specific to the IV therapy procedure according to the purpose, type, and duration of designated IV therapy.
10. Review and become familiar with all IV therapy products and infusion pumps used in the agency clinical setting.

C. Understand fundamental concepts of fluid and electrolyte balance and relate these to prescribed treatment modalities. Understand the relationship between IV fluids and the body's homeostatic and regulatory functions.

1. Identify the major homeostatic mechanisms that regulate fluid and electrolyte balance.
2. Describe the influence of age and/or specific illness on maintenance of fluid and electrolyte balance.
3. Name the function of the following laboratory parameters: albumin, bilirubin, calcium, chloride, creatinine, glucose, magnesium, potassium, sodium, blood urea nitrogen, complete blood count, prothrombin time, partial thromboplastin time, and urine specimen analysis.
4. Recognize the importance of abnormal parameters for the following laboratory panels: arterial blood gases, complete blood count, electrolyte profile, liver function studies, and renal function profile.
5. Describe the nursing responsibilities for monitoring a patient's fluid and electrolyte status.
6. List types of fluid and electrolyte imbalances.
7. List types of acid-base imbalances.
8. Identify specific IV fluids and indications for use.
9. Recognize major adverse patient outcomes related to fluid and electrolyte IV therapy.

D. Demonstrate competency in venipuncture techniques.

1. Prepare the patient for IV therapy by providing patient education.
2. Select the correct-size IV catheter for the therapy prescribed.

   3. Assemble all equipment.
   4. Select the appropriate vein for the prescribed therapy.
   5. Insert the catheter following agency policy.
   6. Secure the catheter according to policy.
   7. Follow agency guidelines for IV dressing, flushing, heparinization, and/or discontinuing the IV access procedure.
   8. Document the procedure according to policy.
E. Recognize measures that prevent IV therapy–related infections.
   1. List ways in which the system may become contaminated.
   2. Demonstrate aseptic assembly of IV infusion.
   3. Identify Centers for Disease Control and Prevention guidelines for prevention of intravascular infections and transmission of blood-borne infections.
   4. Rotate the IV site every 72 to 96 hours or in the presence of redness or inflammation.
   5. Identify indications for changing the entire IV administration set.
F. Demonstrate knowledge and competency in the administration of IV fluids.
   1. List nursing responsibilities when monitoring fluid administration.
   2. Assemble required products, infusion pump, and/or designated equipment.
   3. Identify principles and equipment used to maintain an accurate flow rate.
   4. Change tubing and bags using aseptic technique.
   5. Maintain and monitor heparin lock patency.
   6. Calculate flow rates correctly.
   7. Discontinue infusion.
G. Demonstrate knowledge and competency in the administration of IV medications.
   1. State objectives of IV drug administration.
   2. Name factors that affect patient response to drugs.
   3. List factors that influence drug compatibility and stability.
   4. State the five rights of medication administration.
   5. Demonstrate IV piggyback, IV push, and/or continuous infusion for drug administration.
   6. Know drug, side effects, and/or potential contraindications.
   7. Set up a medication infusion using a pump.
   8. Calculate the rate required to administer the prescribed dose.
   9. Assess the patient for adverse effects.

     10. Follow agency guidelines for documentation, physician consultation, and/or drug hypersensitivity interventions.

H. Demonstrate knowledge and competency in the administration of blood and blood products.

    1. Report the clinical objective for the patient's blood transfusion.

    2. State the indications for administration of the various blood products.

    3. State the IV solution used for the initiation of blood or component therapy.

    4. Identify signs and symptoms of blood transfusion reactions.

    5. Describe the identification and verification procedure that must be followed before transfusing a blood product.

    6. Demonstrate appropriate blood and/or blood production administration via selection of equipment, patient and product identification, transfusion monitoring guidelines, and documentation requirements.

I. Demonstrate knowledge and competency in the administration of total parenteral nutrition (TPN).

    1. Define TPN.

    2. Recognize terms used to describe TPN.

    3. Identify indications for TPN administration.

    4. List potential complications of TPN.

    5. Identify principles of TPN administration.

    6. Follow agency guidelines for patient monitoring, documentation, and patient teaching for self-care home administration.

J. Demonstrate knowledge and clinical competency for nursing management of venous access devices.

    1. Compare and contrast the varied devices related to the patient issues: device selection, insertion procedure, type, purpose, and duration of therapy.

    2. Become familiar with and competent in the venous access device procedure for blood sampling, heparinization, and dressing changes.

    3. Describe potential complications related to venous access devices.

    4. Summarize sequential steps for declotting catheter/ implantable port and for repair procedure for tunneled catheters.

K. IV therapy courses that have defined didactic course presentation and verification of clinical competency.

1. Peripherally inserted central catheters (see Chapter 4)
2. Chemotherapy administration (see Chapter 8)
3. Critical care drug, infusion therapy, and monitoring catheter insertion (see Chapter 10)
4. Pediatric drug and infusion calculation and administration, venous access device and therapeutic patient monitoring of chemotherapy, blood products, and TPN infusions (see Chapter 11)

Pharmaceutical and Device Research and Development

Objectives

1. Discuss the research process for pharmaceutical products and health care devices and their impact on patient care delivery.

2. Identify international and federal laws that mandate the research and development process for the new health care technologies.

3. Describe the reporting and investigation processes for suspicion of or actual problems encountered during use of pharmaceutical products or devices.

4. List the sequential steps to follow if a needlestick injury occurs.

In today's highly regulated health care industry, interdisciplinary clinical and management practitioners provide specialized care to their patients using increasingly complicated and efficient technologies. All types of technologies used to improve the health of individuals and groups, including pharmaceutical products, health care devices, and health care delivery business systems, are required by international and federal laws to meet certain standards of research and development as well as manufacturing practices. These standards are defined in mandated processes used during their development to protect the public from unsafe, untested, and nonvalidated pharmaceuticals, products, and systems or unscrupulous corporations who market such ineffective goods for use in the health care industry.

All health care products, pharmaceuticals, and business systems through which new technologies are provided to the public are the direct result of rigorous research and development processes.

Specific laws are cited, definitions are provided, and user and consumer rights are articulated to improve practitioners' ability to effectively use health care devices as they are intended. Health care practitioners are required by law to file reports that are designed to protect the public from problems encountered using technologies that have and have not been validated for clinical use.

Professionals who perform research on health care–related topics continuously and meticulously follow these mandated scientific process and research methods to examine and explore the outcomes and impacts of hypotheses and theories of health care and wellness enhancement. The results of these research processes are their discovering, designing, prototyping, manufacturing, testing, and advancing all manner of technologies designed to improve human health care.

Pharmaceutical Industry

This industry had its infancy in ancient times when the scientific or discovery process was informal. Health care practitioners of the day used their own potions, advanced as they were then, and their own experience with them to improve care. There are still large areas of the world today where much of this has not changed significantly.

The increased globalization of commercial efforts for both pharmaceuticals and health care devices seen currently has been advanced by the direct and near instantaneous communication facilitated by use of cellular phones, computers, and the Internet, as well as by extraordinarily mobile transportation technologies. These advances in communication and transportation technology have virtually shrunk the miles connecting effective information and goods to many practitioners who were previously unable to obtain access to these advanced products for application and use.

Five steps of research and development constitute this approved development process for pharmaceuticals. The first step, the *medicine and preclinical discovery or research phase,* requires documentation of the scientific basis or rationale for the product. An extensive computerized search and analysis of available compounds, which can affect a certain condition in the human population, is conducted. The results are then screened for use within human cell lines. From this information, pharmaceutical companies formulate a stable and usable form of the compound and manufacture the large quantities required to conduct toxicology studies for the compound. In these preclinical and animal trials, use of the pharmaceutical compound is studied and its effects are documented. If the compound passes the expected toxicologic, safety, and efficacy tests within the defined animal population to the satisfaction of the U.S. Food and Drug Administration (FDA), the study then is approved for human clinical trials.

The next four steps in the development process are human clinical trials, which are conducted according to FDA clinical trial guidelines through the following phases. In *phase 1 trials,* the compound is tested for safety in normal healthy or ill human subjects and an attempt is made to establish an acceptable pharmacologic dose range. In *phase 2 trials,* the compound is tested for effectiveness and continued safety of treatment in selected and relatively small populations with the disease or condition to be treated, diagnosed, or prevented. *Phase 3 trials* are conducted in larger patient populations for which the medicine is eventually intended after efficacy has been established. These trials produce additional safety and efficacy data for relatively large number of patients and for special groups of patients in both controlled and uncontrolled trials directed specifically by the nature of the medicine or the disease it treats. Results often are compared to data for standard treatments available to the general population. At this phase a *new drug application* (NDA) is filed with the FDA, and if the drug is approved, a marketing dossier is filed.

After the NDA is FDA approved, *phase 4 trials* are conducted to provide additional details about the medicine's safety and/or efficacy profile. Different formulations, dosages, durations of treatment, interactions with other medications, and other comparisons may be evaluated; new age groups, races, and other types of patients can be studied; and postmarketing surveillance, observational, or nonexperimental studies are conducted to further demonstrate the medicine's use in the human population.

Health Care Device Industry

The health care device industry had its roots in ancient times, just as the pharmaceutical industry did. For example, when someone broke a leg, individuals responsible for the care of the injured person created or invented devices to keep the leg stable and enable it to heal properly. Splints, bandages, and crutches evolved, and additional practitioners modified these tools for other newly designated purposes over time.

Today, international and federally mandated device research and development processes known as *design control documents* are used to record such advances from many perspectives and sources in four steps.

Like the first step for the pharmaceutical research and development process, the *health care device concept* or *idea phase* is typically formulated by individuals or groups of individuals who applied a problem-solving approach or formal research method to solve a personal, patient, or health care practice-related dilemma. The device developer or group articulates information about the concept, which forms the development source history for the new device.

If this device is robust and complete enough to lend itself to further research and development and subsequent commercial protection as intellectual property under U.S. Patent, trademark or service mark, trade secret, or copyright law, a comprehensive review and documentation of the device concept, including a comparison of its features with similar or like devices (known as *prior art*) must be completed. This process is described by the United States Patent and Trademark Office (www.uspto.gov) and Department of Commerce law (www.loc.gov).

In addition, device predevelopment templates for evaluating the commercial potential for the product must be used to determine whether the need for the product and market reimbursement funding are adequate to cover the continued cost of development to ensure the future success of the product in the marketplace. One such predevelopment device assessment formula can be found at www.healthcareinvention.com.

The second formal device research and development phase is the *reduction-to-practice phase,* also known as *alpha testing,* during which the new device is actually made or a prototype is made for bench testing to demonstrate the device's intended value, function, and features. The alpha bench test results are articulated and described in a *patent application* filed with the United States Patent and Trademark Office, which enumerates the device's specific claims of use, manufacture, and or application.

The third step in the device research and development process is the *beta test product phase,* in which a single or multiple identical products are developed from the results and input of the alpha testing. Additional product development input is obtained from those who prescribe or use the health care device and have a personal and professional responsibility to enhance and advance the product by ensuring that the special needs and criteria for the product's use are specifically addressed throughout the continuing device development process. In formal research and development of health care devices, engineers, designers, users, and prescribers refine the original design by applying input from their discipline's perspective to the development process. Suggestions and feedback from alpha and beta testing and clinical device testing are integrated into the new applications of the device, known as the *production model*.

Throughout the development process, health care business delivery systems that fund the development of the device are responsible for determining how to most effectively and efficiently deliver the product to those who need it. These companies apply international and federal device research and development methods found at www.fda.gov/device controls to receive approval to market the medical device developed as either class I, II, or III, depending on its application and the potential for risk to the patient on whom it will be used. These classifications have implications for the extent of testing required for the product to be marketed in the health care device industry.

If the devices resulting from such a mandated device development process are to be used effectively and then be commercially distributed, they, just like the products of the pharmaceutical industry, are required by international and federal law to operate within established guidelines specified by regulatory organizations like the FDA. The goal is "to safeguard the consumer by applying its" requirements to articles from the moment of conception all the way through the process of their use, ensuring the safety and efficacy of all pharmaceuticals and medical devices introduced into interstate commerce. The FDA accomplishes this by reviewing and approving applications for new products, tracking product performance after approval, inspecting manufacturing facilities, and providing guidance for manufacturers of health care devices.

In today's sophisticated health care device environment, the top 20 manufacturers of medical devices spend approximately $5.64 billion annually to spawn advancing technologies, which results in many novel and valuable tools and devices designed for health and wellness uses. As the sophistication of business development processes advanced the development of their health care devices, so too the FDA has refined the medical device classification system to include only three classes according to the 1976 and 1992 Medical Device Amendments Acts. Class I devices are products that have been demonstrated by the FDA to meet all of the general controls. Class II devices must meet the general controls plus additional standards or controls by demonstrating that they are 510 K approved. Class III devices must meet all of the class I and II criteria and in addition must meet additional controls to ensure their safety and effectiveness when used for humans.

When these research tasks are completed and a health care technology has been refined to the point at which it is deemed by the FDA to be safe and effective to bring about its positive and expected outcomes, the additional process of commercial development prepares the technology for widespread public use and availability. This is known in the industry as approval for marketing or *launch* and is accomplished through the use of existing or newly developed health care delivery business systems.

Nursing Responsibilities: Clinical Use and Reporting Problems for Pharmaceuticals and Devices

One of the most important responsibilities nurses have is to be the patient advocate in the complicated environment that delivers health care. This requires the nurse to be knowledgeable and resourceful regarding the use, administration, and management of the technologies that patients and agencies use. Included in this responsibility are the following two requirements.

Feedback requirement

Although all of the previously identified processes involved in the development of pharmaceutical and device technologies are the responsibility of the inventors, researchers, and commercial developers of the technologies, a part of a nurse's role in the health care industry today is to be aware of the many varied health care–related research professionals and resources available. These professionals team with the nurse during clinical device evaluations or failures to obtain information regarding the product's function, failure, and ease of use during actual clinical uses of the product. The information provided to the developers of the technology regarding its use, suggestions for improvement, and positive features in the product evaluation of the alpha or beta test phase is the feedback mechanism that ensures enhanced product and device improvement. The nurse's part in this phase of the research process is to assist in the development of effective and creative new ways of meeting the critical and informed needs of individuals and populations.

Suspect product reporting

In addition, after the commercial launch or release of the device for use, the laws set up to protect the public from fraudulent products offer practitioners, product prescribers, and end users of product the opportunity to send feedback in formal ways to the manufacturers, developers, and those responsible for ongoing safe use and availability of such effective products.

For example, if the nurse has an IV therapy pump that does not work according to the steps described in its operation manual, the device should be taken out of service immediately, labeled with the agency's "suspect product failure report" (Figure 14-1) that documents observations according to the agency's risk management protocol, and replaced with a different pump that does function according to the device specifications. Other agency resources should be accessed by having the agency's biomedical division test the "suspect" device according to the device manufacturer testing protocols and, if necessary, by calling the manufacturer to report the model and serial numbers and the documented problem. In addition, a report for "suspect devices" should be filed with the FDA by using the voluntary MedWatch device reporting form (No. 3500 available by demand fax by calling 1-800-FDA-1088). Confidentiality regarding the reporting of problems associated with pharmaceuticals and devices is explained on the actual form. If the device or pharmaceutical problem results in a serious adverse event in an agency outside of a physician's office, the facility may be legally required to file the report with the FDA as well as the manufacturer of the suspect technology.

In addition, *The Physicians Desk Reference* is published and updated annually with all approved and regulated over-the-counter pharmaceutical preparations to give health care providers exhaustive FDA information regarding the published use, indications, and prescribing instructions for each pharmaceutical.

All FDA-approved medical device manufacturers and their device listings are published annually in the *Medical Device Register.* This publication documents manufacturers' telephone numbers and other contact information available to health care providers and the public for use in filing product-related failure or benefit reports.

Suspected Nonfunctional
Equipment Notice

Attach tag, place in dirty utility, call BioMed if stationary.

Date ___/___/___ | Time ____ : ____ am pm

Patient involvement? ☐Yes ☐No

Patient harm? ☐Yes ☐Possibly ☐No

If yes or possibly, complete UOR/incident report and page Risk Management

UOR # _____

Problem
☐Battery ☐Power Cord ☐Alarm ☐Sensor
☐ Preventive Maintenance Needed
☐ Error Code _____

Comments_____

_____

Department/Unit	Room/Bed #
Your Name Phone #	Equipment Type
Bar Code #	Control # Equipment ID

Phone ext: UHS SFC-8505   BioMed SFC-6931
            SJC-5128   SJC-5350
Via Christi Regional Medical Center

Fig. 14-1
Example Suspected Nonfunctional Equipment Notice.

Risk Management
Nursing Responsibilities Regarding Professional Practice Issues

To practice nursing, one must meet the state's or government's minimum educational requirements and demonstrate clinical competency for professional practice as defined by each state's or government's nurse practice act. For a copy of the nurse practice act from the governing body of your state or jurisdiction, write to the state or government licensing body, usually located in the state or governmental capital city and request a personal copy. This information can be accessed at the American Nursing Association's website www.ana.org. IT IS YOUR RESPONSIBILITY to know and practice within the specific guidelines of these laws. Any act of yours, documented to be outside of these practice guidelines, is reportable and can be cause for the loss or suspension of your professional license to practice.

In addition, because of the rapidly changing and expanding nature of scientific knowledge and the health care environment many state and government licensing bodies now require that nurses update their education annually or biannually by earning a specified number of continuing education units (CEUs) to continue to practice the nursing profession. Just as states and governments define nursing practice acts differently, there are different requirements for each practitioner's practice scope within the professional jurisdiction. Accordingly, there are nursing education standards that address the accepted curriculum requirements these accredited continuing educational units must meet to be acceptable as CEUs for licensure renewal. These guidelines can be requested from your licensing agency and are articulated in your state's or government's licensing renewal documents. Furthermore, related formal education from accredited colleges and universities or other accredited professional educational providers are good sources to obtain CEUs for license renewal and are often obtainable while advancing your educational base at the same time.

However, in all circumstances, to get your license renewed, you must meet these practice-specific guidelines for renewal by submitting documentation of the CEUs earned when applying for license renewal. Failure to do so may result in the suspension or revocation of your license and the resulting loss of your ability to continue to practice, at least temporarily, in your practice setting.

Each nurse is responsible for the acts performed during his or her professional duties. Nursing professionals are more frequently named in malpractice lawsuits in potentially different roles in clinical practice (e.g., education and/or research). As identified earlier, the nurse has many responsibilities to patients regarding professional practice standards. Therefore, to minimize personal exposure be informed of your particular practice standards, assume personal responsibility for your actions and provide reasonable and prudent care in all circumstances. Never provide a treatment or perform skills that you are not competent and knowledgeable or skilled in performing. To best avoid and prevent unwanted legal situations related to your profession from arising, the following guidelines should be followed.

- Know and follow the state's or government's practice guidelines and standards of care for your professional level. This includes practicing within the parameters of your nurse practice act, community and agency procedures, and policies and practice guidelines.

- Know and uphold patients' rights: the right to privacy, the right to obtain and refuse treatment, and the right to know the caregiver, and proactively resolve conflicts as they may occur.

- Communicate caring and competence to each patient, patient's family members, or attending caregivers by addressing their concerns as appropriate, remembering that each person has dignity and has a right to respectful care, and by offering appropriate support and encouragement as adjustments in a patient's health status changes are integrated and accepted.

- Maintain positive communication skills with all related interdisciplinary health care providers. This includes professional written, verbal, and nonverbal communication tasks such as documentation of test results and procedures and their outcomes, reports to attending and consulting professionals, reports to professionals and family members in attendance who are about to take responsibility for a patient upon transfer, and demonstration of problematic or highly detailed skills that must be performed for the patient by his or her new caregiver.

- Educate your patients regarding their care in language they can understand, giving them realistic procedural and treatment explanations before the procedures occur and allowing them the opportunity to define, question, or clarify their care expectations.

- Prudently document the facts surrounding all care, procedures, treatments, and education provided to your patients and the circumstances of the professional intervention provided. Include all professional actions to demonstrate and correct problems identified and their resolution to appropriate authorities and interdisciplinary team members involved up and down the chain of professional command.

- Do not provide care or professional opinions that are outside the parameters of your level of responsibilities within the nursing practice act of your state or government. To do so represents practicing without a license.

- Whenever unusual occurrences take place during your tour of duty, document them factually using your agency protocol. These documents inform the agency of potential legal exposures and responsibilities.
- IV therapy situations requiring incident reports include, but are not limited to, events such as medication extravasations, flow rate errors, equipment failures or difficulties, unexpected drug reactions, medication errors, infection control and chemical spill situations, patient care procedure breakdowns, laboratory gathering or processing delays that may affect expected patient outcomes, blood or blood product reactions, reactions to latex and other allergic reactions, and potential legal problems communicated by patients, families, or other health care providers.
- Report all safety threats and potential or actual violence-related issues to the proper authorities in the chain of professional, legal, and agency command according to your agency's policy and procedure.
- When or if you become aware that potential or actual fraudulent or illegal care activities have occurred with your patient, you have a professional responsibility to document the event and report it according to your agency and within legal guidelines to the appropriate authorities. Some of these may include alternative, complementary, integrative, or unproven quackery therapies and unlicensed providers of such services who may have made claims that are untrue, and whose actions or therapies have resulted in documented worsening health condition of the patient. In such events, consult the lists provided in "Resources" section for agencies to report such events and occurrences to and do so according to your agency's risk management reporting guidelines.

Needlestick Injury and Fluid-Borne or Environmental Contamination Reporting Requirements

These events are the most common high-risk occurrences for nursing professionals since the incidence of blood-borne and drug-resistant diseases and the use of toxic chemical therapeutic agents and radiologic technologies have increased.

- If you experience a needlestick or are exposed to bodily fluid or radiation during your course of duty, your agency has a specific infection control reporting protocol that must be followed completely when all such exposures occur. Failure to do so, as soon as the professional needs of the patient are attended to, may result in the loss of your legal rights and any care available to you immediately and in the future related to the incident should you contract a blood-borne or drug-resistant disease or have health problems related to chemical or radiation exposure.

- Cleanse the area according to agency protocol.
- Immediately report the event to your supervisor.
- Document facts of the event as they occurred. Include date; time; procedure being performed; patient name and case number; witnesses to the event; actions taken with the patient, family, and other staff; and method of addressing the event with each.
- Report as appropriate to your agency's infection control officer or health officer within the accepted time frame.
- Inform the patient and family, if necessary, of required follow-up steps to document staff exposure potential, indicating that it will be done at agency expense.
- Continue to follow-up with all ongoing personal care requirements according to your agency's protocol until all health-related requirements are met, your safety and health status have been demonstrated, and you have been released from further care requirements by your agency.

Resources

In the previous sections, professional resources were referred to during the related discussions. Included here are the many available governmental, state, legal, professional, pharmaceutical, device and health care industry contacts that exist to assist you, the health care provider, to provide the most informed and responsible care available. Included are not only names and addresses, but also Internet websites, which will facilitate your immediate contact and required information search needs. In addition, Table 14-1 lists a variety of IV catheters/stylets and blood collection equipment and their safety features. These products demonstrate some of the advances in technology that help protect the health of the patient and the health care professional.   *Text continued on p. 479*

Table 14-1   Product table

Product Name	Manufacturer	Safety Feature Activation	Size	Comments
IV Catheters/Stylets				
BD Insyte* Autoguard* Shielded IV Catheter	BD Medical Systems Sandy, UT (888) 237-2762 www.bd.com/infusion	With the push of a button the needle instantly retracts into a transparent safety barrel.	14, 16, 18, 20, 22, 24 gauge	One-handed technique. Available in winged and non-winged designs. BD Vialon* biomaterial.
Introcan† Safety* IV Catheter	B. Braun Medical Bethlehem, PA (800) BBRAUN2 www.bbraunusa.com	A safety clip, preassembled inside the catheter hub, automatically engages and covers needle tip as user withdraws needle from the hub.	14, 16, 18, 20, 22, 24 gauge	Passive safety feature; requires no user activation. Catheter hub is also available with wings.

Continued

From RN, Market Choices, Oct. 99, vol. 62, no. 10, p. 63, Medical Economics, 2000, Montvale, N.J.
*Trademark.
†Registered trademark.

Table 14-1   Product table—cont'd

IV Catheters/Stylets—cont'd

Product Name	Manufacturer	Safety Feature Activation	Size	Comments
Protectiv* Acuvance* IV Safety Catheter	Johnson & Johnson Medical Arlington, TX (800) 255-2500 www.jnjmedical.com	A D-shaped, solid, blunt rod is built within the sharp, outer needle. The rod automatically extends beyond the sharp needle tip as user threads catheter into the vein.	14, 16, 18, 20, 22, 24 gauge	Passive safety feature; requires no user activation. Accommodates all insertion techniques. Catheter hub is also available with wings.
Protectiv IV* Catheter Safety System	Johnson & Johnson Medical Arlington, TX (800) 255-2500 www.jnjmedical.com	User withdraws needle into protective shield by retracting the needle housing until needle is locked in place.	14, 16, 18, 20, 22, 24 gauge	One-handed or two-handed technique, depending on user preference. Catheter hub is also available with wings.

Product	Company	Description	Gauge	Features
BD Saf-T-Intima* Integrated IV Catheter Safety System	BD Medical Systems Sandy, UT (888) 237-2762 www.bd.com/infusion	Combines needlestick safety with a virtually bloodless catheter system. Needle shield telescopes out over stylet as it is withdrawn.	18, 20, 22, 24 gauge	Passive safety feature. Catheter has flexible wings, pre-attached extension tubing and PRN adapter. Available in straight and "Y" designs. BD Vialon* biomaterial.

Blood Collection Equipment

Product	Company	Description	Gauge	Features
Angel Wing Safety Needle System	Kendall Mansfield, MA (800) 962-9888 www.kendallhq.com	User advances safety shield over needle tip as the needle is withdrawn from patient.	19, 21, 23, 25 gauge	One-handed technique. Available with multi-sample luer adapter and tube holders.

Continued

From RN, Market Choices, Oct. 99, vol. 62, no. 10, p. 63, Medical Economics, 2000, Montvale, N.J.

Table 14-1 Product table—cont'd

Product Name	Manufacturer	Safety Feature Activation	Size	Comments
Blood Collection Equipment—cont'd				
Eclipse* Blood Collection Needle	Becton Dickinson Franklin Lakes, NJ (888) 237-2762 www.bd.com	After the blood draw, user presses down on the plastic shield, which snaps over needle.	21, 22 gauge	One-handed technique. For use with Becton Dickinson's Vacutainer brand blood collection tubes.
ProGuard II	Kendall Mansfield, MA (800) 962-9888 www.kendallq.com	Single-use needle/tube holder. After use, user retracts needle completely into the tube by moving a latch.	Fits 1" or 1½" blood draw needles	One-handed technique. For use with any standard blood draw needle. Disposaable holder reduces risk of cross-contamination.

| Punctur-Guard† Blood Collection Needle | Bio-Plexus Vernon, CT (800) 223-0010 www.bio-plexus.com | Needle has internal blunting mechanism that is activated prior to removal from the patient. A hollow blunt cannula, within an otherwise standard needle, is retracted before insertion. Upon completion of the blood draw, but before removal from the patient, the inner blunt is advanced and locked beyond the sharp tip of the outer needle. When the needle is removed from the patient, the contaminated sharp is in the safe mode. | 21, 22 gauge | One-handed technique. For use with Bio-Plexus needle holders. |

Sharp entry

Blunt exit

Punctur-guard

Continued

From RN, Market Choices, Oct. 99, vol. 62, no. 10, p. 63, Medical Economics, 2000, Montvale, N.J.

Table 14-1   Product table—cont'd

Product Name	Manufacturer	Safety Feature Activation	Size	Comments
Blood Collection Equipment—cont'd				
Safe-Point* M-D Blood Collection Needle with Sheath	North American Medical Products Albany, NY (800) 488-6267 www.nampinc.com	User pushes protective sheath up with finger to cover needle tip as needle is withdrawn from vein.	21, 22 gauge	One-handed technique. Attaches to any standard tube holder. Safe-Point is also available as a blood collection needle/sheath with tube holder pre-attached.
Safety-Lok* Blood Collection Set	Becton Dickinson Franklin Lakes, NJ (888) 237-2762 www.bd.com	User pushes protective shield forward to cover needle after it is removed from patient.	21, 23, 25 gauge	Two-handed technique. Winged catheter hub. Tubing comes with or without a multiple sample luer adapter.

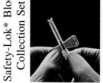

Product	Manufacturer	Description	Gauge	Technique
Saf-T Clik Shielded Blood Needle Adapter	Maxxim Medical Clearwater, FL (800) 456-7701 maxximmedical.com	Single-use needle/tube holder. After removal of the needle from patient, user slides protective sheath up to completely cover needle.	One size fits standard blood collection needles and tubes.	One-handed technique. Disposable holder reduces risk of cross-contamination.
Shamrock Safety Winged Set	Maxxim Medical Clearwater, FL (800) 456-7701 maxximmedical.com	After needle is withdrawn, user pulls it backward into its protective shield.	21, 23, 25 gauge	Two-handed technique. The luer hub can be connected to a syringe or a multiple sample luer adapter with pre-attached tube holder.

Continued

Table 14-1 Product table—cont'd

Product Name	Manufacturer	Safety Feature Activation	Size	Comments
Blood Collection Equipment—cont'd				
Vanish Point[†] Blood Collection Tube Holder	Retractable Technologies Lewisville, TX (888) 703-1010 www.vanishpoint.com	After drawing blood but before removing needle from patient's vein, user closes cap at the back of the tube holder, causing needle to retract and encapsulating both ends of the needle within the holder.	Compatible with standard multiple sample blood collection needles up to 1½" long and standard vacuum collection tubes.	One-handed technique. Activated in patient. Not for use with winged needle sets or luer adapters. Latex-free. Disposable holder reduces risk of cross-contamination.
Venipuncture Needle-Pro[†]	SIMS/Portex Keene, NH (800) 258-5361 www.portexusa.com	Single use sheath and needle/tube holder. Sheath locks over the contaminated needle when user presses sheath against a hard surface.	One size fits all needles and vacuum tube blood sampling systems.	One-handed technique. Swiveling sheath allows for repositioning of the needle as desired during venipuncture. Disposable holder reduces risk of cross-contamination.

From RN, Market Choices, Oct. 99, vol. 62, no. 10, p. 63, Medical Economics, 2000, Montvale, N.J.

The information in Table 14-1—alphabetical by product name—is not a complete listing of the many devices on the market; it does include products from all the major manufacturers, however. The omission of a product from this review does not indicate a negative assessment of that product, nor does the appearance of a product on this list indicate an endorsement. The source *(RN Journal)* did not individually evaluate devices.

IV Therapy Device Companies

Abbott Laboratories, Hospital Products Division, Abbott Park, IL, 847-937-6100, www.abbott.com

ALARIS Medical Systems (formerly IMED/IVAC), San Diego, CA, 800-854-7128, www.alarismed.com

Arrow International Inc., Reading PA, 800-523-8446, www.arrowintl.com

Baxa Corporation, Englewood, CO, 800-567-2292, www.baxa.com

Pall Corporation, www.pall.com/industry/health.asp

Gish Biomedical, Inc., Irvine, CA, 800-938-0531, www.gishbiomedical.com

I-Flow Corporation, Irvine, CA, 800-448-3569, www.i-flowcorp.com

Medtronic, Inc., Columbia Heights, MN, 800-328-0810, www.medtronic.com

MicroJect, Salt Lake City, UT, 888-642-7646, www.microject.com

Sabratek, Niles, IL, 800-556-7722, www.sabratek.com

SIMS Deltec, Inc., St. Paul, MN, 800-426-2448, www.deltec.com

Manufacturers of PICCs and Related Equipment

Arrow International Inc., 800-523-8446, www.arrowintl.com

Bard Access Systems, 800-545-0890, www.bardaccess.com

Becton Dickinson, 800-453-4538, www.bd.com

B. Braun Medical Inc., 800-523-9695, www.bbraunusa.com

CONMED, 800-527-2462, www.conmed.com

Cook Critical Care, 800-457-4500, www.cookcriticalcare.com

HDC Corporation, 800-227-2918, www.hdccorp.com

Luther Medical Products Inc., 800-227-2918, www.luthermedical.com

SIMS Deltec, Inc., 800-426-2448, www.deltec.com

Venetec International, 800-833-3895, www.venetec.com

Vygon Corporation, 800-544-4907, www.vygonusa.com

Professional Organization Websites

American Association of Blood Banks, www.aabb.org

American Association of Critical-Care Nurses, Inc., www.accn.org

American Cancer Society, www.cancer.org

American Medical Association, www.ama-assn.org

American Nursing Association, www.nursingworld.org

American Red Cross, www.redcross.org

American Society of Enteral and Parenteral Nutrition, www.clinnutr.org

Association of Perioperative Registered Nurses, Inc, www.aorn.org

Association of Pediatric Oncology Nursing, www.apon.org

Hospice and Palliative Nurses Association, www.hpna.org

Hypertension, Dialysis & Clinical Nephrology, www.hdcn.com

Intravenous Nurses Society, www.ins1.org

Joint Commission on Accreditation of Healthcare Organizations, www.jcaho.org

National Association for Home Care, www.nahc.org

Oncology Education Services, Inc., www.oesweb.com

Oncology Nursing Society, www.ons.org

Government and Regulatory Websites

Agency for Health Care Policy and Research (AHCPR), www.ahcpr.gov

Centers for Disease Control and Prevention(CDC), www.cdc.gov

CDC Hospital Infections Program, (HIP), www.cdc.gov/ncidod/hip

Food and Drug Administration, www.fda.gov

FDA MedWatch Program, www.fda.gov/medwatch

International Organization for Standardization, www.iso.ch

National Institutes of Health (NIH), www.nih.gov

Occupational Safety and Health Administration, (OSHA), www.osha.gov

United States Post Office, www.uspo.gov

World Health Organization (WHO), www.who.int

Bibliography

Infusion Guidelines

Arrants J: Reliability of IV intermittent access port (saline lock) for obtaining blood samples for coagulation studies, *Am J Crit Care* 8(5):344, 1999.

Carroll P: Latex allergy: what you need to know, *RN* 62(9):40, 1999.

Centers for Disease Control and Prevention: Recommendations for prevention and control of hepatitis C virus (HCV) infection and HCV-related chronic disease, *MMWR Morb Mortal Wkly Rep* 47(RR-19):1, 1998.

Chaly PS, Loriz L: Ethics in the trenches: decision making in practice, *Am J Nurs* 98(1):17, 1998.

Gritter M: Latex allergy: prevention is the key, *J Intraven Nurs* 22(5):281, 1999.

Hanchett M, Kung LY: Do needleless intravenous systems increase the risk of infection? *J Intraven Nurs* 22(3):117, 1999.

Horner KA: Technology assessment of two needleless systems, *J Intraven Nurs* 21(4):203, 1998.

Intravenous Nursing Society: Revised intravenous standards of practice, *J Intraven Nurs* 21(1 suppl):S1, 1998.

Jagger J, Perry J: Shield staff from occupational exposure, *Nurs Manag* 30(6):53, 1999.

Lipson JE, Dibble SL, Minarik PA, editors: *Culture and nursing care: a pocket guide,* San Francisco, 1996, USCF Nursing Press.

Marsee V: Ethical perspectives. In Chernecky C, Berger B, editors: *Advanced and critical care oncology nursing,* Philadelphia, 1998, WB Saunders.

Perry AG, Potter PA: *Clinical nursing skills and techniques,* ed 4, St Louis, 1998, Mosby.

Terry J and others, editors: *Intravenous therapy, clinical principles and practice,* Philadelphia, 1995, WB Saunders.

Thomas CS: Management of infectious waste in the home care setting, *J Intraven Nurs* 20(4):188, 1997.

Venipuncture

Beecroft PC and others: Intravenous lock patency in children: dilute heparin versus saline, *J Pediatr Pharm Pract* 2(4):211, 1997.

Corrigan AM, Pelletier G, Alexander M: *Core curriculum for intravenous nursing,* ed 2, Cambridge, Mass, 1999, Intravenous Nurses Society.

Garner JS: Guideline for isolation precautions in hospitals, *Infect Control Rounds* 18(2):1, 1996.

Heilskoy J and others: A randomized trial of heparin and saline for maintaining intravenous locks in neonates, *J Soc Pediatr Nurs* 3(3):111, 1998.

Homer LD, Holmes KR: Risks associated with 72- and 96-hour peripheral intravenous catheter dwell times, *J Intraven Nurs* 21(5):301, 1998.

Hospital Infection Control Practices Advisory Committee: Guideline for prevention of intravascular device-related infections. Part I. Intravascular device-related infections: an overview, *Am J Infect Control* 24:262, 1996.

Hudson T: AQ sharper point on using safer needles, *Hosp Health News* 73(9):46, 1999.

Infusion Management Update: Needlestick safety legislation steadily moving forward, *Infusion Manag* 9(1):4, 1999.

Jagger J, Perry J: Shield staff from occupational exposure, *Nurs Manag* 30(6):53, 1999.

Little black book of home care cues, Springhouse, Pa, 1997, Springhouse Corporation.

McConnell EA: Infection control: more than a matter of economics, *Nurs Manag* 30(6):64, 1999.

Orenstein R: The benefits and limitations of needle protectors and needless intravenous systems, *J Intraven Nurs* 22(3):122, 1999.

Pearson ML and others: CDC guideline for prevention of intravascular device-related infections, *Am J Infect Control* 24:262, 1996.

Perry AG, Potter PA: *Clinical nursing skills and techniques,* ed 4, St Louis, 1998, Mosby.

Central Venous Catheters

Abbokinase (urokinase for catheter clearance) prescribing information. North Chicago, Ill, 1999, Abbott Laboratories.

Angeles T: Removing a nontunneled central catheter, *Nursing 98* 28(5):52, 1998.

Bagnall-Reeb H: Diagnosis of central venous access device occlusions: implications for nursing practice, *J Intraven Nurs* 21(5 suppl): S115, 1998.

Calia KA, Herbst SL, Sidawy EN: *Management of central venous catheter venous catheter occlusions: the emerging role of Alteplase,* 1999, Gardiner-Caldwell SynerMed.

Hadaway LC: Major thrombotic and nonthrombotic complications, *J Intraven Nurs* 21(5S):S143, 1998.

Hadaway LC: Vascular access devices: meeting patients' needs, *MedSurg Nurs* 8(5):296, 1999.

Holmes KR: Comparison of push-pull versus discard method from central venous catheters for blood testing, *J Intraven Nurs* 21(5):282, 1998.

Jones GR: A practical guide to evaluation and treatment of infections in patients with central venous catheters, *J Intraven Nurs* 21(5 suppl): S134, 1998.

Krzywda KA: Predisposing factors, prevention, and management of central venous catheter occlusions, *J Intraven Nurs* 22(6 suppl):S11, 1999.

Maki DG and others: Prevention of central venous catheter-related bloodstream infection by use of an antiseptic-impregnated catheter, *Ann Intern Med* 127(4):257, 1997.

Mohler M, Sato Y, Bobick K, Wise LC: The reliability of blood sampling from peripheral intravenous infusion lines: complete blood counts, electrolyte panels, and survey panels, *J Intraven Nurs* 21(4):209, 1999.

Oncology Nursing Society: *Access device guidelines,* Pittsburgh, 1996, Oncology Nursing Press.

Oncology Nursing Society: *Cancer chemotherapy guidelines and recommendations for practice,* Pittsburgh, 1999, Oncology Nursing Press.

Orr ME: Vascular access device selection for parenteral nutrition, *Nutr Clin Pract* 14(8):172, 1999.

Ray CE Jr: Infection control principles and practices in the care and management of central venous access devices, *J Intraven Nurs* 22(6 suppl):S18, 1999.

Steele CA: Access devices, administration of chemotherapy. In Yasko JM, editor: *Nursing management of symptoms associated with chemotherapy,* Bala Cynwyd, Pa, 1998, Meniscus Health Care Communications.

Viale PH, Yamamoto DS, Geyton JE: Extravasation of infusate via implanted ports: two case studies, *Clin J Oncol Nurs* 3(4):145, 1999.

Peripherally Inserted Central Catheters

Bean CA and others: High-tech homecare infusion therapies, *Crit Care Nurs Clin North Am* 10(3):287, 1998.

Cole D: Selection and management of central venous access devices in the home setting, *J Intraven Nurs* 22(6):315, 1999.

Gabriel J: PICCs—how Doppler ultrasound can extend their use, *Nurs Times* 95(6):10, 1999.

Intravenous Nurses Society: Position paper: peripherally inserted central catheters, *J Intraven Nurs* 20(4):172, 1997.

Macklin D: How to manage PICCs, *Am J Nurs* 97(9):26, 1997.

Masoorli S: Removing a PICC? Proceed with caution, *Nursing 98* 28(3): 56, 1998.

Mazzola JR, Schott-Baer D, Addy L: Clinical factors associated with the development of phlebitis after insertion of a peripherally inserted central catheter, *J Intraven Nurs* 22(1):36, 1999.

Poole SM: Quality issues in access device management, *J Intraven Nurs* 22(6 suppl):S26, 1999.

Renner C: Polyurethane vs. silicone PICC catheters, *J Vasc Access Devices* 2:16, 1998.

Sansivero GE: Venous anatomy and physiology: considerations for vascular access device placement and function, *J Intraven Nurs* 21(5 suppl):S107, 1998.

Smith JR: Peripherally inserted central catheters revisited, *Am J Surg* 176(2):208, 1998.

IV Fluids

Brown SL and others: Infusion pump adverse events: experience from medical device reports, *J Intraven Nurs* 20(1):41, 1997.

Chung M, Akahoshi M: Reducing home nursing visit costs using a remote access infusion pump system, *J Intraven Nurs* 22(6):309, 1999.

Hadaway LC: I.V. infiltration: not just a peripheral problem, *Nursing* 29(9):41, 1999.

Lefevee J: Infusion pumps, *Prof Nurse* 13(9):621, 1998.

Mohler M and others: The reliability of blood sampling from peripheral intravenous infusion lines, *J Intraven Nurs* 21(4):209, 1998.

Mulligan MA: The innovative use of a PCA pump for the management of cardiac angina, *J Palliat Care* 14(4):47, 1998.

Pagana KD, Pagana TJ: *Mosby's diagnostic and laboratory test reference,* St Louis, 1998, Mosby.

Phipps WJ, Cassmeyer VL, Sands JK, Lehman MK: *Medical-surgical nursing: concepts and clinical practice,* ed 6, St Louis, 1999, Mosby.

Powers FA: Your elderly patient needs I.V. therapy: can you keep her safe? *Nursing* 29(7):54, 1999.

Saladow J: Infusion devices, the newest products and features, *Infusion* 2(6):15, 1996.

Sheff B: VRE and MRSA: putting bad bugs out of business, *Nurs Manag* 30(6):42, 1999.

Weinstein SM: *Plumer's principles and practice of intravenous therapy,* ed 6, Philadelphia, 1997, Lippincott.

IV Medication Administration

Alcoser PW, Burchett S: Bone marrow transplantation: immune system suppression and reconstitution, *Am J Nurs* 99(6):26, 1999.

American Geriatric Society Panel on Chronic Pain in Older Persons: Clinical practice guidelines: the management of chronic pain in older patients, *J Am Geriatr Soc* 46:635, 1998.

American Pain Society: *Principles of analgesic use in the treatment of acute pain and cancer pain,* ed 4, Glenview, Ill, 1999, American Pain Society.

Berger A, Portenoy R, Weissman D: *Principles and practices of supportive oncology,* Philadelphia, 1998. Lippincott-Raven.

Berenson J and others: Long-term pamidronate treatment of advanced multiple myeloma patients reduces skeletal events, *J Clin Oncol* 16(2):593, 1998.

Born, Lepore & Associates, Inc: *Current clinical perspectives on Aredia,* Fair Lawn, NJ, 1997, Novartis Pharmaceuticals.

Dahl JL: New JCAHO standards focus on pain management, *Oncol Issues* 9:27, 1999.

Dalakas MC: *Autoimmune peripheral neuropathies, pathogenesis and treatment,* Omaha, 1998, University of Nebraska Medical Center, Clinical Communications Inc.

Derby SA: Opioid conversion guidelines for managing adult cancer pain, *Am J Nurs* 99(10):62, 1999.

Downs C: The pain relief promotion act of 1999, *Oncol Iss* 9:7, 1999.

Engstrom C, Hernandez I, Haywood J, Lielenbaum R: The efficacy and cost effectiveness of new antiemetic guidelines, *Oncol Nurs Forum* 26(9): 1453, 1999.

Fiesta J: Legal aspects of medication administration, *Nurs Manag* 29(1): 22, 1998.

Gahart BL, Nazareno AR: *Intravenous medications,* ed 16, St Louis, 2000, Mosby.

Hineman L, editor: *Clinical management of chemotherapy-induced nausea and vomiting,* Springfield, NJ, 1999, Scientific Therapeutics Information, Inc.

Hodgson BB, Kizior RJ: *Saunders nursing drug handbook,* 2000, Philadelphia, WB Saunders.

Hoffman-Terry ML and others: Adverse effects of outpatient parenteral antibiotic therapy, *Am J Med* 106(1):44, 1999.

Lechner DL: Sizing up your patients for heparin therapy, *Nursing 98* 28(8):36, 1998.

McCaffery M, Pasero C: *Pain: clinical manual,* ed 2, St Louis, 1999, Mosby.

Paice JA, Citari AA: Cancer pain management: new therapies, *Oncol Nurs Updates* 4(2):1, 1997.

Paice JA, DuPen A, Schwertz D: Catheter port cleansing techniques and the entry of povidone-iodine into the epidural space, *Oncol Nurs Forum* 26(3):603, 1999.

Pasero C, McCaffery M: Providing epidural analgesia, how to maintain a delicate balance, *Nursing* 29(8):34, 1999.

Poole SM, Nowobilski-Vasilios A, Free F: Intravenous push medication in the home, *J Intraven Nurs* 22(4):209, 1999.

Smith KH: A multidose IV additive program using the Abbott Plum Pump, *Infusion Manag Update* 8(1):14, 1999.

Tam VH and others: Vancomycin peak serum concentration monitoring: implications for homecare, *J Intraven Nurs* 22(6):336, 1999.

Weitz JL: Low-molecular weight heparins, *N Engl J Med* 337(10): 688, 1997.

West VL: Alternate routes of administration, *J Intraven Nurs* 21(4): 221, 1998.

Blood and Blood Component Administration

American Association of Blood Banks: *Technical manual,* ed 13, Bethesda, Md, 1999, The Association.

American Association of Blood Banks: *Blood transfusion therapy: a physician's handbook,* ed 7, Bethesda, Md, 1998, The Association.

American Association of Blood Banks: *Standards of blood banks and transfusion services,* ed 18, Bethesda, Md, 1998, The Association.

Buchsel PC, Leum E, Rudolph SR: Nursing care of the blood cell transplant patient, *Semin Oncol Nurs* 13(3):172, 1997.

Dalakas MC, Filipi M, Cihunka C: *Current concepts in autoimmune peripheral neuropathies, pathogens and treatment,* Omaha, 1998, University of Nebraska Medical Center, College of Nursing, Clinical Communications Inc.

Foelber R: Autologous stem cell transplant plus interleuken-2 for breast cancer: review and nursing management, *Oncol Nurs Forum* 25(3): 563, 1998.

Gorski LA, editor: *Best practices in home infusion therapy,* Gaithersburg, Md, 1999, Aspen.

Harmening DM, editor: *Modern blood banking and transfusion practices,* ed 4, Philadelphia, 1999, FA Davis.

Herrmann RP and others: Clinical care for patients receiving autologous hematopoietic stem cell transplantation in the home setting, *Oncol Nurs Forum* 25(8):1427, 1998.

Kapustay PM: Blood cell transplantation: concepts and concern, *Semin Oncol Nurs* 13(3):151, 1997.

Kennedy MS: Undertransfusion or the prudent, cautious, and wise use of blood? *J Intraven Nurs* 22(3):131, 1999.

Pall Medical: *IV filtration: choice or necessity?* Technical Report, Ann Arbor, Mich, 1999, Pall Medical.

Poliquin CM: Overview of bone marrow and peripheral blood stem cell transplantation, *Clin J Oncol Nurs* 1(1):11, 1997.

Rieger PT: Emerging strategies in the management of cancer, *Oncol Nurs Forum* 24(4):728, 1997.

Wagner ND, Quinones VW: Allogeneic peripheral blood stem cell transplantation: clinical overview and nursing implications, *Oncol Nurs Forum* 25(6):1049, 1998.

Weiskopf RB: Do we know when to transfuse red cells to treat acute anemia? *Transfusion* 38:517, 1998.

Whedon MB, Wujcik D: *Blood and marrow stem cell transplantation,* ed 2, Boston, 1997, Jones and Bartlett.

Yoder LH: Diseases treated with blood cell transplants, *Semin Oncol Nurs* 13(3):164, 1997.

Chemotherapy Administration

Berg D: Irinotecan hydrochloride: drug profile and nursing implications of a topoisomerase I inhibitor in patients with advanced colorectal cancer, *Oncol Nurs Forum* 25(3):535, 1998.

Berg D and others: Overcoming multidrug resistance: Valspodar as a paradigm for nursing care, *Oncol Nurs Forum* 26(4):711, 1999.

Camp-Sorrell D: Developing extravasation protocols and monitoring outcomes, *J Intraven Nurs* 21(4):232, 1998.

Camp-Sorrell D: Surviving the cancer, surviving the treatment: acute cardiac and pulmonary toxicity, *Oncol Nurs Forum* 26(6):983, 1999.

Comley AL and others: Effect of subcutaneous granulocyte colony-stimulating factor injectate volume on drug efficacy, site complications, and client comfort, *Oncol Nurs Forum* 26(1):87, 1999.

Davis L, Drogasch M: Triple check procedure prevents chemotherapy errors, *Oncol Nurs Forum* 24(4):641, 1997.

DeVita VT Jr, Hellman S, Roseman SA, editors: *Cancer: principles and practice of oncology,* ed 5, Philadelphia, 1997, JB Lippincott.

Dorr VJ: A practitioner's guide to cancer-related alopecia, *Semin Oncol* 25(5):562, 1998.

Engstrom C, Hernandez I, Haywood J, Lilenbaum R: The efficacy and cost effectiveness of new antiemetic guidelines, *Oncol Nurs Forum* 26(9): 1453, 1999.

Fall-Dickson JM, Rose L: Caring for patients who experience chemotherapy-induced side effects: the meaning for oncology nurses, *Oncol Nurs Forum* 26(5):901, 1999.

Gotaskie G, Robinson KD: Routes of administration and error precautions, administration of chemotherapy. In Yasko JM, editor: *Nursing management of symptoms associated with chemotherapy,* Bala Cynwyd, Pa, 1998, Meniscus Health Care Communications.

Hineman L, editor: *Clinical management of chemotherapy-induced nausea and vomiting: focus on oral 5-HT3-receptor antagonists,* Springfield, NJ, 1999, Scientific Therapeutics Information, Inc.

Hogan CM: The nurse's role in diarrhea management, *Oncol Nurs Forum* 25(5):879, 1998.

Itano JK, Taoka KN, editors: *Core curriculum for oncology nursing,* ed 3, Philadelphia, 1998, WB Saunders.

Johnson BL, Gross J: *Handbook of oncology nursing,* ed 3, Boston, 1998, Jones and Bartlett.

McCorkle R and others: *Cancer nursing: a comprehensive textbook,* ed 2, Philadelphia, 1997, WB Saunders.

Myers JS: Supportive care in preventing and reducing cancer therapy-induced toxicities, In *New therapies symposia highlights,* p. 10, Bala Cynwyd, Pa, 1999, Meniscus Health Care Communications.

National Cancer Institute. *Common toxicity criteria,* Bethesda, Md, 1998, The Institute.

Oncology Nursing Society: *Cancer chemotherapy guidelines and recommendations for practice,* Pittsburgh, 1999, Oncology Nursing Press.

Otto SE: Radiopharmaceuticals (strontium 89) and radiosensitizers (IudR)—innovative therapies for pain management and cancer care, *J Intraven Nurs* 21(6):335, 1998.

Reiger PT: *Clinical handbook of biotherapy,* Boston, 1999, Jones and Bartlett.

Robert H. Lurie Comprehensive Cancer Center of Northwestern University: *Evaluation and management guidelines for the treatment of chemotherapy-induced diarrhea: a primer,* Evanston, Ill, 1999, The Center.

Rutledge DN, Engelking C: Cancer-related diarrhea: selected findings of a national survey on oncology nurse experiences, *Oncol Nurs Forum* 25(5):861, 1998.

Singleton LC, Connor TH: An evaluation of the permeability of chemotherapy gloves to three cancer chemotherapy drugs, *Oncol Nurs Forum* 26(9):1491, 1999.

Thomas CS: Management of infectious waste in the home care setting, *J Intraven Nurs* 20(4):188, 1997

US Department of Labor, Office of Occupational Medicine, OSHA: *Controlling occupational exposure to hazardous drugs,* CPL 2-2.20B CH-4, Washington, DC, 1995, US Government Printing Office.

Viele CS, Holmes BC: Amifostine: drug profile and nursing implications of the first pancytoprotectant, *Oncol Nurs Forum* 25(3):515, 1998.

Williams J, Wood C, Cunningham-Warburton P: A narrative study of chemotherapy-induced alopecia, *Oncol Nurs Forum* 26(9):1463, 1999.

Parenteral Nutrition

Andris DA: Total parenteral nutrition in surgical patients, *MedSurg Nurs* 7(2):76, 1998.

Archer SB and others: Current uses and abuses of total parental nutrition, *Adv Surg* 29:165, 1996.

American Society for Parenteral and Enteral Nutrition: *Nutrition support practice manual,* Silver Spring, Md, 1998, The Society.

Galica L: Parenteral nutrition, *Nurs Clin North Am* 32(4):705, 1997.

Kudski KA, Teasley-Straysburg K: Parenteral nutrition: guidelines for formula selection, administration and potential complications. Enteral and parenteral nutrition. In Irwin RS, Cerra FB, Rippe JM, editors: *Intensive care medicine,* vol II, ed 4, Philadelphia, 1999, Lippincott-Raven.

Kimbrell JD: Acquired coagulopathies, *Crit Care Nurs Clin North Am* 5(3):453, 1993.

Ryder J, Viall C: Total parenteral nutrition. In Boggs RL, Wooldridge-King M, editors: *AACN procedure manual for critical care,* ed 3, Philadelphia, 1998, WB Saunders.

Trujillo EB, Jacobs DO: Parenteral nutrition in adults. In Rakel RE, editor: *Conn's current therapy,* Philadelphia, 1999, WB Saunders.

Trujillo EB, Robinson MK, Jacobs DO: Nutritional assessment in the critically ill, *Crit Care Nurse* 19(1):67, 1999.

Williams SR: Nutrition and diet therapy, St Louis, 1997, Mosby.

Vascular Access in Adult Critical Care

Ahrens TS: Hemodynamic monitoring, *Crit Care Nurse Clin North Am* 11(1):19, 1999.

Ahrens TS, Taylor RW: The PA catheter goes under the microscope, *Crit Care Nurse* 18(1):88, 1998.

Brandstetter RD and others: Swan-Ganz catheter: misconceptions, pitfalls, and incomplete user knowledge—identified trilogy of need of correction, *Heart Lung* 27(4):218, 1998.

Connors AF and others: The effectiveness of right heart catheterization in the initial care of critically ill patients. *JAMA* 18:889, 1996.

Darovic GO: *Hemodynamic monitoring: invasive and noninvasive clinical application,* Philadelphia, 1995, WB Saunders.

Gahart BL, Nazareno AR: *Intravenous medications,* ed 16, St Louis, 2000, Mosby.

Gawlinski A: Cardiac output monitoring, protocols for practice. In Chulay M, Gawlinski A, editors: *Hemodynamic monitoring,* Aliso Viejo, Calif, 1998, American Association of Critical-Care Nurses.

Grap MJ and others: Hemodynamic monitoring: a comparison of research and practice. *Am J Crit Care* 6(6):452, 1997.

Imperial-Perez F, McRae M: Arterial pressure monitoring. Protocols for practice. In Chulay M, Gawlinski A, editors: *Hemodynamic monitoring,* Aliso Viejo, Calif, 1998, American Association of Critical-Care Nurses.

Keckeisen M: Pulmonary artery pressure monitoring, Protocols for practice. In Chulay M, Gawlinski A, editors: *Hemodynamic monitoring,* Aliso Viejo, Calif, 1998, American Association of Critical-Care Nurses.

Kinney MR and others: *AACN clinical reference for critical care nursing,* ed 4, St Louis, 1998, Mosby.

Lichtenthal PR, editor: *Quick guide to cardiopulmonary care,* Irvine, Calif, 1998, Edwards Critical Care, Baxter Healthcare Corp.

Pearson ML: Hospital infection control practices advisory committee. Guideline for prevention of intravascular device-related infections, *Infect Control Hosp Epidemiol* 17:438, 1996.

Pulmonary artery catheter consensus conference: consensus statement, *New Horizons* 5(3):175, 1998.

Pediatrics Intravenous Therapy

Ball J, Bindler R: *Pediatric nursing: caring for children,* ed 2, Stamford, Conn, 1999, Appleton & Lange.

Dugger B: Intravenous nursing competency: why is it important? *J Intraven Nurs* 20(6):287, 1997.

Fann BD: Fluid and electrolyte balance in the pediatric patient, *J Intraven Nurs* 21(3):153, 1998.

Frey AM: When a child needs peripheral I.V. therapy, *Nursing* 28(4): 18, 1998.

Harris JL, Maguire D: Developing a protocol to prevent and treat pediatric central venous catheter occlusions, *J Intraven Nurs* 22(4):194, 1999.

Hazinski MF: *Manual of pediatric critical care,* St Louis, 1999, Mosby.

Intravenous Nurses Society: Position paper: peripherally inserted central catheters, *J Intraven Nurs* 20(4):172, 1997.

Intravenous Nurses Society: Position paper: the registered nurses' role in vascular access device selection, *J Intraven Nurs* 20(2):71, 1997.

Intravenous Nurses Society: Revised intravenous nursing standards of practice, *J Intraven Nurs* 21(1 suppl), 1998.

Pillitteri A: *Child health nursing: care of the child and family,* Philadelphia, 1999, Lippincott.

Rogers JS, Soud TE: *Manual of pediatric emergency nursing,* St Louis, 1998, Mosby.

Whaley LF, Wong DL: *Nursing care of infants and children,* ed 6, St Louis, 1999, Mosby.

Wheeler C, Frey AM: Intravenous therapy in children. In Terry J and others, editors: *Intravenous therapy: clinical principles and practice,* Philadelphia, 1995, WB Saunders.

Wiener ES, Albanese CT: Venous access in pediatric patients, *J Intraven Nurs* 21(5 suppl):S122, 1998.

Wood D: A comparative study of two securement techniques for short peripheral intravenous catheters, *J Intraven Nurs* 20(6):280, 1997.

Home Care Infusion Therapy

Barrio D: Antibiotic and anti-infective agent use and administration in homecare, *J Intraven Nurs* 21(1):50, 1998.

Gahart BL, Nazareno AR: *Intravenous medications,* ed 16, St Louis, 2000, Mosby.

Gorski L, Grothman L: Home infusion therapy, *Semin Oncol Nurs* 12(3):193, 1996.

Gorski LA, editor: *Best practices in home infusion therapy,* Gaithersburg, Md, 1999, Aspen Publishers.

Johndrow P: Phlebotomy techniques in the home, *Home Healthcare Nurse* 17(4):246, 1999.

Kaye L, Davitt J: *Current practices in high-tech home care,* New York, 1999, Springer.

Little black book of home care cues, Springhouse, Pa, 1997, Springhouse Corporation.

Oncology Nursing Society: *Access device guidelines,* Pittsburgh, 1996, Oncology Nursing Press.

Oncology Nursing Society: *Cancer chemotherapy guidelines and recommendations for practice,* Pittsburgh, 1999, Oncology Nursing Press.

Pagana KD, Pagana TJ: *Mosby's diagnostic and laboratory test reference,* St Louis, 1998, Mosby.

Phipps WJ, Cassmeyer VL, Sands JK, Lehman MK: *Medical-surgical nursing: concepts and clinical practice,* ed 6, St Louis, 1999, Mosby.

Stoker J: Defining homebound status, *Home Healthcare Nurse* 17(2): 119, 1999.

Terry J and others, editors: *Intravenous therapy, clinical principles and practice,* Philadelphia, 1995, WB Saunders.

Weinstein SM: *Plumer's principles and practice of intravenous therapy,* ed 6, Philadelphia, 1997, Lippincott.

Calculations for IV Therapy

Bates DW and others: Effect of computerized physician order entry and a team intervention on prevention of serious medication errors, *JAMA* 280:1311, 1998.

Cohen MR: *IV drug safety,* Huntingdon Valley, Pa, 1999, Institute for Safe Medication Practice.

Cohen MR, editor: *Medication errors,* Washington, DC, 1999, American Pharmaceutical Association.

Curren AM, Mundy LD: *Math for meds: dosages and solutions,* ed 7, San Diego, 1995, WI Publications Inc.

Institute for Safe Medication Practices: ISMP medication safety alert, *ISMP* 4(20):1, 1999.

Katzung BG, editor: *Basic and clinical pharmacology,* Stamford, Conn, 1998, Appleton & Lange.

Marrelli TM: *Nursing documentation handbook,* St Louis, 1999, Mosby.

McLeroy PA: The rule of six: calculating intravenous infusion in a pediatric crisis situation, *Hosp Pharm* 29(10):939, 1994.

Opfer KB, Wirtz DM, Farley K: A chemotherapy standard order form: preventing errors, *Oncol Nurs Forum* 26(1):123, 1999.

Schulmeister L: Chemotherapy medication errors: descriptions, severity, and contributing factors, *Oncol Nurs Forum* 26(6):1033, 1999.

Professional Resources

Czaplewski LM: Marketing your expertise, *J Intraven Nurs* 22(2):75, 1999.

DeFife SW: The Internet, now is the time to go on-line, *Surg Serv Manag* 2(10):37, 1996.

Ehrenberger H, Murray PJ: Issues in the use of communications technologies in nursing research, *Oncol Nurs Forum* 25(10):11, 1998.

Garity J: Creating a professional presentation: a template for success, *J Intraven Nurs* 22(2):81, 1999.

Gomez EG, DuBois K, King CR: Improving oncology nursing practice through understanding and exploring the Internet, *Oncol Nurs Forum* 25(10):4, 1998.

Hadaway LC: Developing an interactive intravenous education and training program, *J Intraven Nurs* 22(2):87, 1999.

Henderson L: *Medical device grants markets soar,* CenterWatch Publication, 6, 1999

Kanaskie ML, Arnold E: New ways to evaluate chemotherapy competencies, *Nurs Manag* 30(11):41, 1999.

Kansas Nurse: OSHA directive emphasizes safety product use, *Legislative News* 74(10):16, 1999.

Kawabata K: Online for continuing education and more, *Infusion Manag Update* 8(1):9, 1998,

Knowles MS: *Modern practice of adult education from pedagogy to andragogy,* ed 2, New York, 1980, Cambridge Books.

Knowles MS: *Andragogy in action,* San Francisco, 1984, Jossey-Bass.

Lamb KV and others: Help the health care team release its hold on restraint, *Nurs Manag* 30(12):19, 1999.

McConnell EA: Technology update: vascular access devices: lines to live by, *Nurs Manag* 30(12):49, 1999.

Medical Device Register®, Montvale, NJ, 1999, Medical Economics Press. URL: www.medec.com.

National Institutes of Health Clinical Center. URL: www.cc.nih.gov.

Nicholas J. Webb Consulting Group: Resources. URL: www.healthcareinvention.com.

Phillips LD: Patient education: understanding the process to maximize time and outcomes, *J Intraven Nurs* 22(1):19, 1999.

Physicians' Desk Reference®: Montvale, NJ, 1999, Medical Economics Company. URL: www.pdr.net.

Pozgar GE, editor: *Legal aspects of health care administration,* ed 7, Gaithersburg, Md, 1999, Aspen.

Rudzik J: Establishing and maintaining competency, *J Intraven Nurs* 22(2):69, 1999.

Spilker B: *Guide to clinical trials,* New York, 1991, Raven.

United States Food and Drug Administration: Code of Federal regulations, title 21, 211, 800, 1999.

United States Food and Drug Administration Center for Devices and Radiological Health: Design control guidance for medical device manufacturers. URL: www.fda.gov/cdrh/comp/designgd.html.

United States Food and Drug Administration:MedWatch, the FDA medical products reporting program, FDA form 3500. Phone: 1-800-FDA-1088. URL:www.fda.gov/medwatch.

United States Library of Congress Copyright Office: General information. URL: www.loc.gov/copyright.

United States Patent and Trademark Office: General information concerning patents, trade and service marks, and trade secrets. URL: www.uspto.gov.

Webb N: Does your invention pass the "laugh test"? *Rev Ophthalmol* 9, 1994.

Index

Page numbers followed by f indicate illustrations; t indicates material in tables; *n* indicates material in footnotes.